In-Vitro Fertilization
The Pioneers' History

In-Vitro Fertilization
The Pioneers' History

Edited by

Gabor Kovacs
Monash University, Melbourne

Peter Brinsden
Bourn Hall Clinic, Cambridge

Alan DeCherney
National Institutes of Health, Bethesda, MD

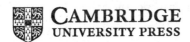
CAMBRIDGE
UNIVERSITY PRESS

CAMBRIDGE
UNIVERSITY PRESS

University Printing House, Cambridge CB2 8BS, United Kingdom

One Liberty Plaza, 20th Floor, New York, NY 10006, USA

477 Williamstown Road, Port Melbourne, VIC 3207, Australia

314-321, 3rd Floor, Plot 3, Splendor Forum, Jasola District Centre, New Delhi - 110025, India

79 Anson Road, #06-04/06, Singapore 079906

Cambridge University Press is part of the University of Cambridge.

It furthers the University's mission by disseminating knowledge in the pursuit of education, learning and research at the highest international levels of excellence.

www.cambridge.org
Information on this title: www.cambridge.org/9781108427852
DOI: 10.1017/9781108551946

© Cambridge University Press 2018

First published 2018

A catalogue record for this publication is available from the British Library

Library of Congress Cataloging in Publication data
Names: Kovacs, Gabor, 1947 April 6- editor. | Brinsden, Peter R., editor. |
    DeCherney, Alan H., editor.
Title: In-vitro fertilization and assisted reproduction : a history / edited
    by Gabor Kovacs, Peter Brinsden, Alan Decherney.
Description: Cambridge, United Kingdom ; New York, NY : Cambridge University
    Press, [2018]
Identifiers: LCCN 2018011569 | ISBN 9781108427852 (hardback)
Subjects: | MESH: Fertilization in Vitro—history | Reproductive Techniques,
    Assisted—history | History, 20th Century
Classification: LCC RG135 | NLM WQ 11.1 | DDC 618.1/780599—dc23 LC record
    available at https://lccn.loc.gov/2018011569

ISBN 978-1-108-42785-2 Hardback

....

Contents

List of Contributors vii
Preface xi

1 **A Brief Outline of the History of Human In-Vitro Fertilization** 1
John D. Biggers and Catherine Racowsky

2 **The Track to Assisted Reproduction: From Animal to Human In-Vitro Fertilization** 8
Jacques Cohen

3 **The American Roots of In-Vitro Fertilization** 21
Frederick Naftolin, Jennifer Blakemore, and David L. Keefe

4 **The Story of Patrick Steptoe, Robert Edwards, Jean Purdy, and Bourn Hall Clinic** 28
Peter R. Brinsden

5 **Professional Hostility Confronting Edwards, Steptoe, and Purdy in their Pioneering Work on In-Vitro Fertilization** 37
Martin H. Johnson

6 **The Development of In-Vitro Fertilization in Australia** 46
Alex Lopata and Gabor Kovacs

7 **The Joneses and the Jones Institute** 66
Charles C. Coddington III and Sergio C. Oehninger

8 **The Development of In-Vitro Fertilization in North America After the Joneses** 75
Matthew Connell and Alan H. DeCherney

9 **The Brussels Story and the Eureka Moment of Intracytoplasmic Sperm Injection** 84
André Van Steirteghem

10 **The Development of In-Vitro Fertilization in Austria** 87
Wilfried Feichtinger

11 **The Development of In-Vitro Fertilization in France** 102
René F. Frydman

12 **The Development of In-Vitro Fertilization in Italy** 104
Luca Gianaroli, Serena Sgargi, Maria Cristina Magli, and Anna Pia Ferraretti

13 **The Development of In-Vitro Fertilization in Scandinavia** 111
Lars Hamberger, Torbjörn Hillensjö, and Matts Wikland

14 **The Development of In-Vitro Fertilization in Spain** 120
Antonio Pellicer

15 **The Development of In-Vitro Fertilization in Greece, Germany, and The Netherlands** 125
Basil C. Tarlatzis, Klaus Diedrich, and Bart Fauser

16 **The Development of In-Vitro Fertilization in Israel** 132
Zion Ben-Rafael

17 **The Development of In-Vitro Fertilization in Latin America** 141
Fernando Zegers-Hochschild

18 **The Development of In-Vitro Fertilization in India** 148
Rina Agrawal and Elizabeth Burt

19 **The Development of In-Vitro Fertilization in China** 152
Daimin Wei, Jianfeng Wang, Yingying Qin, and Zi-Jiang Chen

20 **The Development of In-Vitro Fertilization in Africa** 158
Willem Ombelet

21 **The Development of In-Vitro Fertilization in Russia** 172
Vladislav Korsak and Anatoly Nikitin

v

22 **The Application of In-Vitro Fertilization in the Management of the Infertile Male** 177
David M. de Kretser

23 **The Development of Preimplantation Genetic Diagnosis for Monogenic Disease and Chromosome Imbalance** 180
Leeanda Wilton

24 **The Development of Embryo, Oocyte, and Ovarian Tissue Cryopreservation** 192
Debra A. Gook and David H. Edgar

25 **The Development of Ovarian Stimulation for In-Vitro Fertilization** 202
Colin M. Howles

26 **The Development of Microsurgery for Male and Female Infertility** 208
Sherman J. Silber

27 **Embryonic Stem Cells, Medicine's New Frontier** 214
Ariff Bongso

28 **The Regulation and Legislation of In-Vitro Fertilization** 224
Louis Waller and Sandra Dill

29 **Research on Assisted Reproduction Families: A Historical Perspective** 232
Susan Golombok

30 **The Commercialization of In-Vitro Fertilization** 240
G. David Adamson and Anthony J. Rutherford

Index 249

Contributors

G. David Adamson MD FRCSC FACOG FACS
ARC Fertility, Cupertino, CA, USA

Rina Agrawal MD FRCOG PhD FICOG
Centre for Reproductive Medicine and
Fertility one2one, London, UK

Zion Ben-Rafael MD
Department of Obstetrics & Gynecology, Rabin
Medical Center and Golda Medical Center and
Tel Aviv University, Petah-Tikva, Israel

John D. Biggers DSc PhD
Department of Cell Biology, Harvard
Medical School, Boston, MA, USA

Jennifer Blakemore MD
Department of Obstetrics & Gynecology, New York
University School of Medicine, New York, NY, USA

Ariff Bongso PhD MSc FRCOG DSc DVM FSLCOG
Department of Obstetrics & Gynaecology, NUS
Yong Loo Lin School of Medicine, Singapore

Peter R. Brinsden FRCOG
Bourn Hall Clinic, Cambridge, UK

Elizabeth Burt MRCOG
Department of Obstetrics & Gynaecology,
University College London, London, UK

Zi-Jiang Chen MD PhD
Department of Obstetrics & Gynecology,
Shandong Provincial Hospital; Director, Center for
Reproductive Medicine; Dean, Cheeloo College of
Medicine; Vice President, Shandong University;
Vice President, Ren Ji Hospital, School of Medicine,
Shanghai Jiao Tong University, Jinan, China

Charles C. Coddington III MD FACOG CPEFACPE
Department of Obstetrics & Gynecology,
Mayo Medical School; Division of
Reproductive Endocrinology & Infertility,
Mayo Clinic, Rochester, MN, USA

Jacques Cohen PhD HCLD
ART Institute of Washington, Bethesda, MD;
Althea Science, Livingston, NJ, USA

Matthew Connell DO
Reproductive Endocrinology & Gynecology
Branch, Combined Federal Fellowship in
Reproductive Endocrinology & Infertility,
NICHD/NIH, Bethesda, MD, USA

Alan H. DeCherney, MD
Reproductive Endocrinology and Gynecology
Branch, Combined Federal Fellowship in
Reproductive Endocrinology & Infertility,
NICHD/NIH, Bethesda, MD, USA

David M. de Kretser AC MD FRCCP LLD FRACOG FRCOG FRAGP
Hudson Centre for Reproductive Health,
Monash University, Melbourne, Australia

Klaus Diedrich MD PhD
Department of Obstetrics & Gynecology,
University of Lübeck, Lübeck, Germany

Sandra K. Dill AM BComm MLS GAICD
Access Australia, Silverwater, NSW, Australia

David H. Edgar PhD
Reproductive Services, Royal Women's Hospital,
Melbourne IVF, Melbourne, Australia

Bart C. J. M. Fauser MD PhD
Department of Reproductive Medicine,
University Medical Center Utrecht and University
of Utrecht, Utrecht, The Netherlands

Wilfried Feichtinger MD
Department of Obstetrics & Gynecology,
Medical University of Vienna and Wunschbaby-
Institut Feichtinger, Vienna, Austria

Anna Pia Ferraretti MD PhD
SISMeR Reproductive Medicine Unit, Bologna, Italy

René F. Frydman MD
Dep;artent of Obstetrics & Gynecology,
Hôpital Foch, Paris, France

Luca Gianaroli MD
SISMeR Reproductive Medicine Unit, Bologna, Italy

Susan Golombok PhD
Centre for Family Research, University
of Cambridge, Cambridge, UK

Debra A. Gook PhD
Reproductive Services, Royal Women's Hospital,
Melbourne IVF, Melbourne, Australia

Lars Hamberger MD PhD
Department of Obstetrics & Gynecology,
University of Gothenburg, Gothenburg, Sweden

Torbjörn Hillensjö MD PhD
Department of Obstetrics & Gynecology,
University of Gothenburg, Gothenburg, Sweden

Colin M. Howles PhD
ARIES Consulting sarl, Geneva, Switzerland

Martin H. Johnson MA PhD FRCOG FRSB FMedSci FRS
Department of Physiology, Development
& Neuroscience, University of
Cambridge, Cambridge, UK

David L. Keefe MD
Department of Obstetrics & Gynecology, New York
University School of Medicine, New York, NY, USA

Vladislav Korsak MD
International Center for Reproductive
Medicine, St. Petersburg, Russia

Gabor T. Kovacs AM MD FRCOG FRANZCOG CREI FAICD Grad Dip Mgt (Macq)
Department of Obstetrics & Gynaecology,
Monash University and Obstetrics & Gynaecology
Institute, Epworth Healthcare, Australia

Alex Lopata PhD
CancerProbe, Melbourne; formerly Department of
Obstetrics & Gynaecology, University of Melbourne
Royal Women's Hospital, Carlton, Australia

Maria Cristina Magli MSc
SISMeR Reproductive Medicine Unit, Bologna, Italy

Frederick Naftolin MD DPhil
Department of Obstetrics & Gynecology, New York
University School of Medicine, New York, NY, USA

Anatoly Nikitin MD
Baltic Institute of Human Reproduction,
St. Petersburg, Russia

Sergio C. Oehninger MD PhD
Jones Institute for Reproductive Medicine,
Department of Obstetrics & Gynecology, Eastern
Virginia Medical School, Norfolk, VA, USA

Willem Ombelet MD PhD
Genk Institute for Fertility Technology, Department
of Obstetrics & Gynecology, Genk, Belgium

Antonio Pellicer MD
Department of Obstetrics & Gynecology,
Valencia University School of Medicine,
Valencia, and IVIRMA Global, Spain

Yingying Qin MD PhD
Center for Reproductive Medicine, Shandong
Provincial Hospital, Jinan, China

Catherine Racowsky PhD HCLD
Department of Obstetrics & Gynecology,
Brigham & Women's Hospital, Harvard
Medical School, Boston, MA, USA

Anthony J. Rutherford FRCOG
Leeds Centre for Reproductive Medicine,
Seacroft Hospital, Leeds, UK

Serena Sgargi BA
SISMeR Reproductive Medicine Unit, Bologna, Italy

Sherman J. Silber MD
Infertility Center of St. Louis, St. Luke's
Hospital, St Louis, MO, USA

Basil C. Tarlatzis MD PhD
First Department of Obstetrics &
Gynecology, Aristotle University of
Thessaloniki, Thessaloniki, Greece

André Van Steirteghem PhD
Emeritus Professor, Centre for Reproductive
Medicine, Vrije Universiteit Brussel, Brussels, Belgium

Louis Waller AO LLB(Hons) BCL Hon LLD FASSA FAAL
School of Law, Monash University, Melbourne, Australia

Jianfeng Wang
Center for Reproductive Medicine, Shandong Provincial Hospital, Jinan, China

Daimin Wei MD PhD
Center for Reproductive Medicine, Shandong Provincial Hospital, Jinan, China

Matts Wikland MD PhD
Department of Obstetrics & Gynecology, University of Gothenburg, Gothenburg, Sweden

Leeanda Wilton PhD
Formerly Melbourne IVF, East Melbourne, Australia

Fernando Zegers-Hochschild MD
Unit of Reproductive Medicine, Clinica las Condes, Santiago and Progam of Ethics & Public Policies in Human Reproduction, Universidad Diego Portales, Santiago, Chile

Preface

The 40th anniversary of the birth of Louise Brown, the first baby in the world to be born after conception in vitro, seemed to us and to Nick Dunton at Cambridge University Press, to be the ideal time to produce a book on the history of in-vitro fertilization (IVF) worldwide. Our aim has been to invite friends and colleagues from many different countries to write their own personal views on how IVF developed in their own countries or regions. Other authors were asked to review the stories behind other topics, like the early history leading up to human IVF, scientific and pharmaceutical developments, ethical and legal challenges, and how parents and children have fared after treatment by IVF.

This is a collection of personal anecdotes from many colleagues who were there at or near to the beginnings of human IVF, which we intend should inform and entertain future generations of clinicians and embryologists on the origins of our specialty; it is not intended as an academic historical work. We have been very fortunate in attracting some of the very best known names in our specialty to contribute to this book, which, we

hope, will particularly attract the readership of the younger generation of physicians, scientists, nurses, counselors, and other members of IVF teams worldwide. Without a volume such as this, much of the early history of IVF will be lost, as many of the first or early generation of IVF specialists who have contributed chapters are nearing the end of their careers.

We regret that we have been able to have contributions from only a small number of specialists in our field. There are many more of our international friends and colleagues from whom we would also like to have received their personal recollections, but space precludes us including everyone – we hope that omission from our list of eminent authors will not cause offence!

If any of we Editors of this volume are still around on the 50th anniversary of Louise Brown's birth, perhaps we should then produce an updated and enlarged edition. We are certain that there will be many, some as yet undreamed of, advances during the next ten years in IVF and the assisted reproductive technologies that will bear recording.

A Brief Outline of the History of Human In-Vitro Fertilization

John D. Biggers and Catherine Racowsky

Introduction

Any account of the history of in-vitro fertilization and embryo transfer (IVF-ET) is not complete unless descriptions of the hostility from members of the public and the media are included. Nearly all studies on mammalian fertilization and preimplantation development encountered significant opposition from the time they began in the 1930s. Immediately following the announcement in 1978 of the birth of the first IVF baby, Louise Brown, praise for a new treatment for human infertility was accompanied by loud opposition from the press and members of the public. This chapter, therefore, not only discusses the scientific underpinning of clinical IVF-ET, but also includes a brief historical perspective of the public backlash encountered along the way.

The need for an effective treatment for infertility due to blocked Fallopian tubes had been recognized for a long time, originally to help with inter-generational problems relating to the distribution of family wealth. An early attempt to unblock the tube involved passing through it a whalebone bougie (Smith, 1849). This barbarous procedure was never adopted. The discovery that an ovary can function in an ectopic site led Morris in 1895 to graft an ovary below the obstruction; however, this also was unsuccessful. Then, in 1909, Estes proposed inserting the ovary into the uterus while retaining its pedicle, leaving the blood vessels and nerves intact. This operation became known as the Estes operation, which was used occasionally until the introduction of IVF-ET, despite it being frequently unsuccessful.

The Scientific Underpinning of Clinical IVF-ET

One of the first significant discoveries in the history of IVF-ET was the embryo transfer work of Walter Heape who, in 1891, reported the successful transfer of an embryo from one rabbit to another (Heape, 1891). In this experiment, he was testing the hypothesis that phenotypic characteristics of the surrogate mother could be transmitted to the transferred embryo. Although there is no evidence that Heape thought of using this route to overcome infertility due to blocked Fallopian tubes, his work is, nevertheless, important since he demonstrated the feasibility of embryo transfer in mammals (reviewed by Biggers and Kountz, 2016).

Heape was a gentleman scientist who worked in the newly created Laboratory of Animal Morphology, University of Cambridge, under Professor Francis Balfour. He never registered as a student nor did he earn a degree. Nevertheless, he went on to become an Instructor in the Laboratory teaching embryology, which included a practical class that taught students to recover living preimplantation embryos from rabbits for observation under the microscope. The manual for this class can be found as an appendix to the second edition of *The Elements of Embryology* by Foster and Balfour (1883) [Edited by Sedgewick and Heape]. It required little for Heape to apply these techniques for the transfer of one rabbit embryo to a foster mother and obtain newborn rabbits. There is strong circumstantial evidence that this landmark work was done in Heape's private laboratory on his father's estate near Manchester in England (Biggers, 1991). Whether or not a coincidence, Manchester was where Steptoe and Edwards (1978) succeeded in producing the first IVF baby.

Perhaps Heape's more important contribution, however, concerned systematizing the description of reproductive cycles. His first studies in this area, done during his tenure of the prestigious Balfour Studentship in Cambridge, UK, involved describing the menstrual cycle in two species of monkey based on histological changes in the uterus (Heape, 1894, 1896). This work soon attracted the interest of gynecologists and resulted in invitations to speak at the Obstetric Society of London (Heape, 1898). Moreover, Johnstone in the USA, reproduced some of his drawings in the American Journal of Obstetrics and Diseases of Women and Children (Johnstone, 1895). Heape then turned his attention to the description of mammalian reproductive cycles in general, in which he introduced such terms as oestrus, proestrous, diestrous, etc. (Heape, 1900). This work provided the basis for Marshall to demonstrate that reproductive cycles in dogs, sheep and ferrets are all under endocrine control which, in turn, paved the way for the discovery of the reproductive hormones (review: Marshall, 1910).

Heape's work on reproductive cycles had an immediate and lasting influence on our understanding of the endocrinology of reproductive cycles. By contrast, his work on the transfer of embryos between rabbits received little attention during the next 30 years, except in the field of science fiction.

Between 1930 and 1937, Gregory Pincus, an Assistant Professor in the Department of Biology at Harvard University, published several important papers, some with E. V. Enzmann, on the physiology of fertilization and preimplantation development in the rabbit. One of these papers reported successful IVF-ET in rabbits (Pincus and Enzmann, 1934) and another described meiotic maturation of rabbit oocytes in vitro (Pincus and Enzmann, 1935). The following year, results on the activation of rabbit ova were reported, and some of these parthenotes were documented to have undergone cleavage divisions (Pincus and Enzmann, 1936). Pincus (1936) summarized his work in a monograph entitled *The Eggs of Mammals* containing three chapters: "Methods employed in the experimental manipulation of mammalian ova," "Fertilization and cleavage," and "The activation of unfertilized eggs."

Pincus's work immediately encountered controversy in the press and the general public. W. L. Lawrence wrote a conjectural op-ed in the *New York Times* on March 27, 1936:

As rabbits and men belong to the mammalian group, the work is viewed as pointing towards the possibility of human children being brought into the world by a 'host-mother' not related by blood to the child.

It is reasoned that eventually women capable of having children whose health does not permit them to do so may 'hire' other women to bear their children for them, children actually their own flesh and blood.

To one who desires to speculate at this point the Harvard experiment offers another possibility. Theoretically, at least, it may become possible for a woman so inclined, particularly in a country influenced by eugenic considerations, to bring into the world twelve children a year by 'hiring' twelve 'host-mothers' to bear their test-tube-conceived children for them.

Advocates of 'race-betterment' might urge such procedures for men and women of special aptitudes, physical, mental or spiritual.

The following day the *New York Times* published an emotional negative editorial under the title Brave New World. The next year, J. D. Radcliff, writing in the widely circulated *Collier's Magazine*, March 20, 1937, in an article "No father to guide them," commented:

In the resulting world man's value would shrink. It is conceivable that the process would not even produce males. The mythical land of the Amazons would then come to life. A world where woman would be self-sufficient; man's value precisely zero.

In 1937, Pincus took a sabbatical leave at the University of Cambridge, UK, with the knowledge that his academic appointment at Harvard would not be renewed. Despite the scientific recognition of Pincus's work some believe that one of the reasons he went to Cambridge was that the Harvard administration felt its reputation was being tainted by the press (Speroff, 2009). Pincus and Enzmann's claim that they had successfully achieved IVF-ET in rabbits was accepted by the scientific community for several years until the work was challenged by later work on fertilization done in the 1950s, particularly with regard to capacitation.

While Pincus was in Cambridge, UK, Professor John Rock and his colleagues at the Boston Lying-In Hospital, an affiliate of Harvard Medical School, published a paper in the *New England Journal of Medicine* where they claimed to be able to detect an electrical sign that determined the time ovulation occurred in women (Rock et al., 1937). In the same issue, John Rock also wrote anonymously the following remarkable editorial:

Contemplating this new discovery, one's mind travels much further. Lewis and Hartman have fertilized a monkey ovum and photographed its early cleavage *in vitro*. Pincus and Enzmann have started one step earlier with the rabbit isolating an ovum, fertilizing it in a watch glass, and reimplanting it in a doe other than the one that furnished the egg, and have thus successfully inaugurated pregnancy in an unmated animal. If such an accomplishment with rabbits were to be duplicated in human beings, we should, in the words of 'flaming youth', be 'going places'. The difficulty with human ova has been that those recovered from tubes have regressed beyond the possibility of fertilization *in vitro*. But by using the electric sign we may be able to obtain them from the follicle at the peak of their maturity. If the new peritoneoscope can be developed along the lines of the operating cystoscope, laparotomy may even be dispensed with. What a boon for the barren woman with closed tubes.

He wrote the above editorial anonymously, perhaps to avoid the problems that Pincus had encountered with the Harvard Administration.

Rock, with the assistance of Miriam Menkin and the advice of Pincus, went on to establish a research program to develop a method for fertilizing human ova in vitro (*Science News Letter*, 1944). They claimed to have succeeded in a paper published in *Science* in 1944 (Rock and Menkin, 1944; see also Menkin and Rock, 1948). Although the United States was fighting World War II, the potential public health importance of this work was recognized by the *Boston Globe*, which published a front page article in which belief was expressed that the work would contribute to treating serious problems of infertility.

Several of Rock's medical colleagues at Harvard hailed his work for opening up a way to treat intractable forms of human infertility (Marsh and Ronner, 2008). However, the work was not free of criticism: The President of Harvard received a letter from a Missouri woman telling him "when you interfere with the laws of Nature, you interfere with the laws of God, and when you interfere with the laws of God, you insult the intelligence of Christian people" (preserved in the Harvard Medical School Archives, quoted by Marsh and Ronner, 2008).

Despite the acclaims given to Rock's work, the independent discovery of capacitation by Austin (1951) and Chang (1951) raised questions about the criteria required for unequivocal proof that fertilization in vitro had been achieved. In 1962, Austin, after reviewing about 30 claims of IVF in various mammals (including the rabbit, guinea-pig, sheep and human), listed the following four required criteria: (1) use of capacitated spermatozoa, (2) avoidance of aged ova, (3) confirmation that a spermatozoon had entered the ovum, and (4) conditions that exclude parthenogenesis. None of the claims fulfilled Austin's criteria. The ultimate convincing proof of successful IVF-ET is the birth of young whose origin can be identified by phenotypic by or genotypic characteristics, preferably the latter. Eight years elapsed before Chang (1959) reported that he had achieved fertilization in vitro in rabbits, having met Austin's four criteria. However, it was Whittingham who unequivocally demonstrated the in-vitro fertilization of mouse ova using a genetic marker (eye color) to identify native and in-vitro produced offspring (Whittingham, 1968).

The independent discovery of capacitation by Austin and Chang raised doubts that fertilization in vitro had been attained by Pincus in the rabbit and Menkin in the human. A letter, preserved in the Harvard Medical School Archives, was written on June 6, 1954, to John Rock by Carl Hartman, one of the doyens of mammalian reproduction. It reads:

I don't believe you ever got *in vitro* fertilization. . . Have a dozen reasons to question your conclusions, chief of which is the simultaneous and independent discovery by Chang, Austin and Blandau [Braden?] that 'raw' sperms won't fertilize any egg even *in vivo*! Sperms must be 'capacitated'(Austin) in the female tract, either in the uterus or the tube.

Now, I want you to go back to the problem and clean it up and really immortalize yourself, inject 50,000,000 sperm into a woman's uterus, in 2 h take out the sperms and add to the ovarian egg (but only from a 16-18 mm follicle, eggs in lesser ones are N.G.). I'm betting heavy odds on the outcome of the experiment.

Neither Rock nor Menkin took up Hartman's suggestion. They discontinued their studies after 1948. Rock may have been discouraged by the low success rate of Menkin's experiments and by the objections of antagonists at Harvard (McLaughlin, 1982). He and Pincus left this area of research to begin their major contributions to the development of the oral contraceptive pill. Menkin moved to another institution where she had no possibility of carrying the work further.

John Rock's ideas were not completely abandoned, for others tried to repeat his experiments. The best known clinician was Landrum Shettles, at Columbia University in New York City, who, in 1954, claimed to have successfully fertilized human ova in vitro. Further results were reported in 1958 at a meeting of the New York Obstetrical Society, which was attended by John Rock who was excited by the work. Rock commented:

> The time may be rapidly approaching when the poor woman whose tubes had been excised, yet who still wants a baby, will rejoice that Dr Shettles will be able to extract an ovum from her ovary, probably not by laparotomy, but through an operating telescope (which can be done – we have done it); then fertilize the egg *in vitro* by the husband's spermatozoa; and finally put it back in the uterus. Thus will he impregnate the woman in spite of the fact she has no tubes.

In the years that followed, Shettles' work was sharply criticized and caused controversy.

The 1950s and 1960s saw major advances in the field of developmental reproductive biology as investigations focused on identifying the conditions needed to achieve in-vitro fertilization. In addition to discovery of capacitation (Austin, 1961; Chang, 1951), and identification of the evidence needed to prove fertilization in vitro (Austin, 1962) as discussed above, the following key milestones were achieved: (1) the demonstration that mouse preimplantation embryos could develop in chemically defined media (Whitten, 1956, 1957); (2) the demonstration that cultured mouse preimplantation embryos would develop in surrogate mothers, using differences in coat color to distinguish in the young native and cultured offspring (McLaren and Biggers, 1958); and (3) the demonstration that the maturation of mouse oocytes and the early cleavage of mouse preimplantation embryos in vitro required pyruvate in the medium (Biggers et al., 1967).

Between 1964 and 1971, Sir Robert Edwards and his colleagues published the following four key papers, two in *Nature* and two in *The Lancet*, that paved the way to successful in-vitro fertilization in women.

Key Paper (1) Maturation In Vitro of Human Ovarian Oocytes. *The Lancet* (Edwards, 1965)

Edwards' initial work on the meiotic maturation of human oocytes in vitro used the technique for maturing human oocytes, originally described by Pincus who estimated the time for maturation as 12 h.

Edwards' work proceeded slowly because human oocytes were hard to obtain in the UK. Fortunately, he received an invitation from Howard Jones who worked at the Woman's Clinic, Johns Hopkins Hospital, to conduct the tests in Baltimore, where human oocytes were easier to obtain. Edwards' main result showed that Pincus and Saunders had underestimated the time for meiotic maturation to occur in vitro in human oocytes and that the required time was 36–43 h. The results were described in the first of the four key papers, which was published from Johns Hopkins Hospital. Unfortunately, attempts to fertilize these matured ova in vitro failed (Edwards, 1966).

Key Paper (2) Fertilization and Cleavage In Vitro of Preovular Human Oocytes. *Nature* (Edwards et al., 1970)

This advance, made by Edwards and his colleagues, was the production of human blastocysts by exposing human ova to human spermatozoa in vitro. At least five media were tested: two modified physiological salines developed for the study of animal fertilization and three that were used in general cell culture. All allowed modest development only if they contained pyruvate. Two of the media were modifications of physiological salines. The first medium to be tested was a modified Tyrodes solution used by Barry Bavister to study capacitation in the hamster (Bavister, 1969). Later, a modified Krebs–Ringer bicarbonate solution was tested by David Whittingham to study in-vitro fertilization in the mouse. The medium used by Whittingham was a medium developed by Whitten and Biggers (1968) for the culture of mouse preimplantation embryos. Both Bavister and Whittingham were working in the same department, the Physiological Laboratory in Cambridge, as was Edwards.

Key Paper (3) Laparoscopic Recovery of Preovulatory Human Oocytes after Priming of Ovaries with Gonadotropins. *The Lancet* (Steptoe and Edwards, 1970)

The notion of an "operating telescope" envisioned by John Rock was shown to be possible in France by Klein and Palmer (1961) who used a cystoscope to recover an oocyte from a single human follicle. Steptoe and Edwards adapted the laparoscope to recover human oocytes from patients hyper-stimulated with gonadotropins. However, finding optimal doses of the gonadotropins that did not interfere with implantation was difficult, so Edwards and Steptoe reverted to collecting oocytes from a natural cycle without ovarian stimulation; this was the approach they used to achieve the first successful IVF-ET birth.

Key Paper (4) Birth after the Reimplantation of a Human Embryo. *The Lancet* (Steptoe and Edwards, 1978)

The birth of the first in-vitro human baby was achieved after innumerable failures. Indeed, through December 1980, the live birth rate per embryo transfer was only 5.4% (three babies born from 56 embryo transfers; Lopata, 1980). However, this rate was likely considerably lower if cycle start is used as the denominator.

Without doubt, Steptoe and Edwards' achievement of the first IVF-ET success was remarkable and marked the beginning of what was to become a major advance that has resulted in the successful treatment of millions of cases of human infertility. The persistent work done by Edwards and Steptoe over many years is a superb example of translational research.

The Public Backlash to Louise Brown's Birth

The day after the announcement of the birth of the first in-vitro baby, there was worldwide and often frenzied coverage by the media, with commentaries ranging from those heralding a major scientific achievement to those that maintained it was a dangerous or amoral procedure which should be outlawed. This is not surprising since similar comments had been made when artificial insemination was introduced at the end of the twentieth century (Schellen, 1957), and similar reactions were evoked by the experiments of Gregory Pincus and John Rock and Miriam Menkin.

Edwards and Steptoe met praise and resistance to their work in the United Kingdom before and after the birth of Louise Brown. This history has been summarized in a book by Edwards and Steptoe in 1980 entitled *A Matter of Life*, and an article by Edwards written a decade later entitled "A bumpy road to human in vitro fertilization," in which he states that "popes were critical and rigid Protestants were sometimes vicious" (Edwards, 2001). Edwards acknowledges being influenced by a particular friend, Gordon Dunstan, a leading senior ethicist of the Church of England, who wrote

a book entitled *The Artifice of Ethics* with four chapters on IVF-ET and a "penetrating and ethical analysis" (Dunstan, 1974). Edwards and Steptoe had other setbacks. For example, the Medical Research Council did not approve an application to support setting up an IVF-ET clinic in Cambridge and they had to seek private funds to set up the famous clinic at Bourn Hall, near Cambridge. Importantly, Edwards and Steptoe made a major contribution to the many public policy debates surrounding IVF-ET in the years that followed that, collectively, resulted in the gradual adoption of IVF-ET as an acceptable medical procedure.

The British Government established a committee in 1982, under the chairmanship of Dame Mary Warnock called The Committee of Inquiry into Human Fertilisation and Embryology. The general conclusion of their Report, published in 1984, recommended that the human embryo should be protected, but that research on human embryos and IVF-ET would be permissible given appropriate safeguards. A regulatory committee was established and eventually the British Parliament passed the Human and Fertilisation Embryology Act (1990), which has led to countless worthwhile studies on human preimplantation development.

The birth of the first test-tube baby had immediate individual reactions in the United States, which can only be illustrated by individual experiences. At the time, one of us (JDB) was Program Director of a grant at Harvard Medical School from the National Institutes of Health (NIH), which had a specific aim to study human oocyte maturation, under the direction of Melvin Taymor at the Peter Bent Brigham Hospital. A day after Louise Brown's birth, JDB received a call from the NIH informing him that the NIH was immediately freezing the funds allotted to the human oocyte maturation work. Shortly thereafter, a conference was held at the NIH in Bethesda, MD under the co-chairmanship of JDB and Luigi Mastroianni on Fertilization and Embryonic Development In Vitro and its proceedings were published the following year, in 1981. The book contains no papers on human in-vitro fertilization because officials at the NIH instructed the co-chairmen to disallow discussion of the subject at the meeting and in the published papers.

President Carter activated on September 15, 1978, a dormant Ethics Advisory Board of the Department of Health, Education and Welfare, to consider whether or not research using human ova and preimplantation embryos should be controlled or forbidden. The members of the Committee represented comprehensive scientific, medical, legal and philosophical interests and an infertile couple gave testimony of their struggles with infertility. JDB was scientific advisor to this committee and CR also attended these hearings. Among the many topics discussed, in addition to the incidence of infertility in the US population and the likely efficiency of the procedure, was the safety of the procedure particularly regarding the production of abnormal fetuses, and the conflicting views on the morality of IVF-ET. A report was finally produced and it recommended that human embryos used for research could be kept in culture no longer than 14 days and not replaced in a human patient. Further, the ova could only be obtained from married couples. No grants for research on human preimplantation embryos or oocytes, either exposed to sperm or induced to undergo activation, has since been funded by the NIH.

The formation of the first IVF clinic in the USA at the Eastern Virginian Medical School, Norfolk, Virginia, was a particularly turbulent process, as is well documented by the late Dr. Howard W. Jones in his book *In Vitro Comes to America* (2014). Starting a clinic involved getting a Certificate of Need that necessitated a public hearing as required by the State of Virginia. JDB testified at the public hearing, which lasted approximately six hours, where right-to-lifers on one side of the hall shouted insults at infertile couples who shouted back "you want to prevent me having a baby." Some testifiers opposing the Certificate of Need were particularly objectionable and rude to Dr. Jones and his wife, Dr. Georgiana Jones, who were trying to set up the IVF Clinic. A few weeks later JDB was a speaker at a symposium on IVF held by the Virginia Bar Association. The meeting was held at Virginia Beach, home of the Christian Broadcasting Network and Regent University founded by the southern Baptist televangelist Pat Robertson, who at one time ran for the republican nominee for President of the United States. On the day of the symposium, a hostile crowd formed at the entrance to the hotel causing the speakers to be taken into the hotel through the kitchens! Fortunately the Certificate of Need was granted, which allowed the Joneses to begin forming what became the renowned Norfolk Clinic.

Concluding Remarks

As is usually the case when a remarkable medical treatment is established, much precedes the first success.

The establishment of clinical IVF-ET is no exception. Mammalian reproduction entails a remarkably complex system of processes involving not only the production of fully developmentally competent gametes, but also a uterus that is receptive to implantation and to maintenance of pregnancy. However, reproduction in the human is unique in that it is remarkably inefficient. Therefore, it is of no surprise that rigorous and exhaustive scientific investigations in a multitude of species were required to fill the necessary knowledge gaps for the first clinical IVF-ET success. Indeed, it took more than eighty years of painstaking research before Louise Brown's birth. However, the remarkable team of Edwards and Steptoe must be given all the credit in the world for their accomplishment and for the joy that they have brought to millions of couples worldwide. This is all the more noteworthy in light of the ethical and religious hurdles that not only needed to be overcome during the decade leading up to their success, but also during subsequent years as research on human reproduction continues to advance.

References

Austin CR (1951) Observations on the penetration of the sperm into the mammalian egg. *Aust J Sci Res* 4, 581–596.

(1961) *The Mammalian Egg*. Blackwell, Oxford.

Bavister BD (1969) Environmental factors important for in vitro fertilization in the hamster. *J Reprod Fertil* 18 (Suppl. 3), 544–545.

Biggers JD (1991) Walter Heape, FRS: a pioneer in reproductive biology. Centenary of his embryo transfer experiments. *J Reprod Fert* 93, 173–186.

Biggers JD, Kountz C (2016) *Walter Heape, FRS. A Pioneer of Reproductive Biology*. JamesTowne Bookworks, Williamsburg, Virginia.

Biggers JD, Whittingham DG, Donahue RP (1967) The pattern of energy metabolism in the mouse oocyte and zygote. *Proc Natl Acad Sci USA* 58, 560–567.

Chang MC (1951) Fertilizing capacity of spermatozoa deposited in the fallopian tube. *Nature* 168, 697–698.

(1959) Fertilization of rabbit ova in vitro. *Nature* 184, 466–467.

Dunstan G (1974) *The Artifice of Ethics*. SCM Press, Lancaster.

Edwards RG (1965) Maturation in vitro of human ovarian oocytes. *Lancet* 286, 926–929.

(1966) Preliminary attempts to fertilize human oocytes matured in vitro. *Am J Obstet Gynecol* 96, 192–200.

Edwards RG (2001) The bumpy road to human in vitro fertilization. *Nat Med* 7, 1091–1094.

Edwards RG, Steptoe PC (1980) *A Matter of Life*. Hutchinsons, London.

Edwards RG, Bavister BD, Steptoe PC (1969) Early stages of fertilization in vitro of human oocytes matured in vitro. *Nature* 221, 632–635.

Edwards RG, Steptoe PC, Purdy JM (1970) Fertilization and cleavage in vitro of preovular human oocytes. *Nature* 227, 1303–1307.

Estes WL (1909) A method of implanting ovarian tissue in order to maintain organ function. *Pa Med J* 13, 610–613.

Foster M, Balfour FM (1883) In: Sedgewick A and Heape W (Eds.) *The Elements of Embryology*, 2nd edn. MacMillan, London.

Heape W (1891) Preliminary note on the transplantation and growth of mammalian ova within a uterine foster mother. *Proc Roy Soc Lond* 48, 457–459.

(1894) The menstruation of *Semnopithecus entellus*. *Phil Trans Roy Soc B* 185, 411.

(1896) The menstruation and ovulation of *Macacus rhesus*. *Proc Roy Soc B* 60, 202.

(1898) The menstruation of *Semnopithecus entellus*. *Trans Obstet Soc* 40, 161–174.

(1900) The "sexual season" of mammals and the relation of the "pro-oestrum" to menstruation. *Quart J Micr Sci* 44, 1.

Johnstone AW (1895) The relation of menstruation to the other reproductive functions. *Amer J Obstet & Diseases Women Children* 32, 33–48.

Jones HW (2014) *In Vitro Fertilization Comes to America*. Jamestowne Bookworks, Williamsburg, Virginia.

Klein R, Palmer R (1961) technique de prélèvement des ovules humains par ponction folliculaire sous coelioscope. *C R Biol* 155, 1919–1921.

Laurence WL (1936) Life is generated in scientist's tube. *New York Times*, 27 March.

Lopata A (1980) Successes and failures in human in vitro fertilization. *Nature* 288, 642–643.

Marsh M, Ronner W (2008) *The Fertility Doctor*. Johns Hopkins Press, Baltimore.

Marshall FHA (1910) *The Physiology of Reproduction*. Longmans, Green and Co., London.

Mastroianni L, Biggers JD (1981) *Fertilization and Embryonic Development In Vitro*. Plenum Press, New York.

McLaren A, Biggers JD (1958) Successful demonstration and birth of mice cultivated in vitro as early embryos. *Nature* 182, 877–878.

McLaughlin L (1982) *The Pill, John Rock, and the Church*. Little Brown and Co., Boston.

Menkin MF, Rock J (1948) In vitro fertilization and cleavage of human ovarian eggs. *Amer J Obstet Gynecol* 55, 440–452.

Morris RT (1895) The ovarian graft. *NY Med J* 59, 83–87.

Pincus G (1936) *The Eggs of Mammals*. MacMillan Co., New York.

Pincus G, Enzmann EV (1934) Can mammalian eggs undergo normal development in vitro. *Proc Natl Acad Sci USA* 20, 121–122.

Pincus GG, Enzmann EV (1935) The comparative behavior of mammalian eggs in vivo and in vitro: 1. The activation of ovarian eggs. *J Exp Med* 62, 665–675.

(1936) The comparative behavior of mammalian egg in vivo and in vitro: 2. The activation of tubal eggs. *J Exp Zool* 73, 195–208.

Radcliff JD (1937) No father to guide them. *Colliers Magazine*, March 20, 19–20.

Rock J, Menkin MF (1944) In vitro fertilization and cleavage in human ovarian eggs. *Science* 100, 105–107.

Rock J, Reboul J, Wiggers HC (1937) The detection and measurement of the electrical concomitant of human ovulation by the use of the vacuum-tube potentiometer. *N Engl J Med* 217, 654–658.

Schellen AMCM (1957) *Artificial Insemination in the Human*. Elsevier, Atlanta.

Science News Letter (1944) Artificial fertilization, August 12.

Shettles LB (1954) Studies on living ova. *Trans N Y Acad Sci* 17, 99–102.

(1958) The living human ovum. *Amer J Obstet Gynec* 69, 365–371.

Smith WT (1849) On a new method of treating fertility, by the removal of obstructions of the fallopian tube. *Lancet* 1, 529–531.

Speroff L (2009) *A Good Man: Gregory Goodwin Pincus*. Amica Publishing Inc., Portland Oregon.

Steptoe PC, Edwards RG (1970) Laparoscopic recovery of preovulatory human oocytes after priming of ovaries with gonadotropins. *Lancet* 1, 683–689.

(1978) Birth after the preimplantation of a human embryo. *Lancet* 2, 366.

Whitten WK (1956) Culture of tubal mouse ova. *Nature* 177, 96.

(1957) Culture of tubal mouse ova. *Nature* 179, 1081.

Whitten WK, Biggers JD (1968) Complete development in vitro of the preimplantation stages of the mouse in a simple chemically defined medium. *J Reprod Fertil* 17, 399–401.

Whittingham DG (1968) Fertilization of mouse eggs in vitro. *Nature* 220, 592–593.

The Track to Assisted Reproduction: From Animal to Human In-Vitro Fertilization

Jacques Cohen

Introduction

In-vitro fertilization (IVF) has become a routine medical intervention over the past four decades, resulting in the birth of nearly 7 million children. Experimental embryology, which is the foundation for assisted reproduction, has yielded three recent Nobel Prizes in the fields of stem-cell research, nuclear transplantation, and IVF: Martin Evans in 2007, Bob Edwards in 2010, and Shinya Yamanaka and Jon Gurdon in 2012. The 2010 Nobel Prize in physiology or medicine was awarded to Robert G. Edwards for his central role in establishing clinical IVF, a goal he had broadly outlined in a ground-breaking paper in *The Lancet* in 1965 (Edwards, 1965). Mr. Patrick Steptoe, the consultant gynecologist who was instrumental in counseling and treating the patients, collected the eggs by laparoscopy and transferred the embryos trans-vaginally, but he had unfortunately passed away 22 years before the awarding of the Nobel Prize to Edwards. The third member of Edwards' team was his loyal clinical laboratory assistant Jean Purdy, who also passed away at a very young age in 1985 and who is regarded as a pioneer in IVF laboratory quality management. The Nobel Prize is not awarded posthumously. After the births of the first two IVF children, the three pioneers established the world's first IVF clinic near Cambridge, UK, in 1980. This move represented extraordinary courage, as it had taken hundreds of attempts to arrive at the two births. At Bourn Hall Clinic, Jean Purdy hired two laboratory assistants who worked as QC officers, handled the Petri dishes and all sterile specimens and paperwork, and witnessed all procedures. The clinical embryologists were treated and respected like classically trained surgeons. As an embryologist, one showed up on time, scrubbed, checked the schedule, made decisions, did the pipetting, prepared the sperm samples, talked to patients, and performed a small set of embryology procedures that was available at the time: No cryopreservation, no micromanipulation, no sophisticated microscopy, no contemporary embryo selection methods. Bob Edwards performed all procedures for a while, seven days per week, until Simon Fishel was hired, and became the second embryologist at Bourn Hall Clinic in 1981. Carole Fehilly-Willadsen and I joined the team some months later. It was the experience of a lifetime to collaborate with this group in the ensuing three years. I left Bourn Hall Clinic in the spring of 1985. This was probably a mistake on my part.

As astounding as the relatively quick rise of IVF may have been, 50 years ago it was often considered dystopian science fiction drawing on a Brave New World of dark forces in society, to control reproduction, and change its norms. Rarely was the technology viewed as an obvious means for treatment of subfertility. Despite numerous obstacles such as lack of public funding for clinical embryology research in many countries (including the USA), assisted reproduction is now well established as an industry encompassing medicine, genetics, cryobiology, engineering, business, and law. Its path to success in the USA seems to follow Moore's Law with linear improvement of success rates measured as a function of implantation, by about 1% annually, corrected for maternal age, which is considered the most important confounder (Cohen et al., 2012). This linear progression has been constant since the early days and may predict a time in the near future when there is no need for multiple attempts. IVF is certain to see major new changes with further integration of genetics, molecular biology, engineering, and physics. And it seems more and more likely that it will become an obvious form of safe reproduction, controlling unwanted pathogenic mutations, inheritable or *de novo*, and allowing prospective parents to build their families with forethought and deliberation. But to anticipate and help shape such a future, the past must be understood. Where did it begin and how did we arrive here? First there were the experimental embryologists, micromanipulation engineers, and cryobiologists on whose shoulders we stand today. They were studying the basic science of mammalian reproduction and their story begins about 150 years ago in Europe. Before that there was no knowledge of spermatogenesis, oogenesis, steroidogenesis, gamete maturation, fertilization, meiosis, chromosomes, genes and their expression, DNA, cold storage, and cell tissue culture, although cell theory – that living organisms consist of specialized building blocks called cells, which originate from other cells through a process called mitosis – had been formulated in 1839 by a group of scientists, following decades of studies in plants and animals.

My own modest role in this long process has concerned three main areas: developing new techniques and tools, adapting (and improving on) laboratory protocols from animal to human embryology, and bringing attention to quality control in the clinical laboratory. In the mid-1970s, I was fortunate to work in the laboratory of Professor Gerard Zeilmaker and his PhD student Gerard van Marle from Erasmus University in Rotterdam (The Netherlands), first as a Master's student (1976–1978) and later as a PhD student (1978–1981). They were the only team at that time specializing in preclinical preimplantation mammalian embryology in The Netherlands. That experience was concurrent with the years leading up to the birth of Louise Brown across the North Sea in England. We considered the work by Edwards, Steptoe, and Purdy, and its many breakthroughs, and wondered about the first steps towards establishing the new discipline of embryology as part of a road map to clinical treatment. At the same time, others were forging ahead with studies in reproduction in rodents and large domestic species in order to improve farm animal breeding. David Whittingham – a living legend – was responsible for the development of several key technologies including IVF in defined culture media and, together with Stanley Leibo and Peter Mazur, freezing of cleavage stage mammalian embryos (Whittingham, 1968; Whittingham et al., 1972). Their work was contemporaneous with Ian Wilmut's work in sheep. In Rotterdam, we followed this work closely, but we were also interested in other areas of reproductive research. As a developer of products and techniques for clinical embryology, I have enjoyed collaborations with numerous scientists, clinicians, geneticists, experimental embryologists, and engineers who have helped to shape the field of human assisted reproduction. The reader is reminded that this text is not written by a science historian. Though intended to be unbiased, the narrative draws not only on written history gathered from historical documents, but on personal recollection and experience, as well as numerous conversations with scientists and physicians in the field. Also, as I have been asked to describe the events that led to the birth of Louise Brown 40 years ago, and my own experience thereafter, I have used and altered passages from a few textbook chapters that I have written before (Cohen et al., 2012; Cohen, 2013).

The history of IVF can be told in many different ways as is obvious when reading through this book. Here the story is told from the perspective of applied mammalian clinical science, with emphasis on the final steps that led to the birth of the first IVF baby in 1978. Tribute is made to those responsible for paradigm shifts in philosophy that allowed the new reproductive technologies to take form. What is also covered is some of my personal experiences during the first decades following Louise's birth. Moreover, because no medical intervention is possible without the laboratory instruments and tools that have been made available in surgery and laboratory practice, I will discuss this aspect in some detail, in the hope that future reflections on the history of IVF and related technologies will include appropriate reference to this neglected area of science history. Just as the formulation of cell theory was intricately linked to the development of the microscope, IVF, micromanipulation, cryopreservation, and associated technologies have relied on engineering efforts by individuals whose names are often forgotten or not even known.

The first IVF laboratories relied completely on instruments and devices produced for cell tissue culture and microscopy. Egg retrieval and embryo transfer kits were assembled from existing surgical and laboratory tools. Numerous scientific and engineering explorations preceded IVF. For instance, in 1850, only a few years before the Austrian Schenk looked at the fertilization process for the first time, John Lawrence Smith, a faculty member at what is now Tulane University (New Orleans, USA), engineered the inverted microscope. Robert Chambers from New York University (USA) invented the first micromanipulator for cell surgery in 1912 and connected the device and microscope with a motion picture camera to observe the dissection of chromosomes. The first incubators were used for hatching chicken eggs and date back to ancient Egypt. Initially it was just a space with a regulated temperature control system heated by fire. In the nineteenth century this changed to heated bell jars. Carbon dioxide (CO_2) incubators date from the early 1960s and warm jacketed incubators were developed in the 1970s.

Experimental embryologists used such devices for their experiments and later re-engineered these tools to suit the needs of embryology. It is only in the past 35 years that clinical embryologists and surgeons have been modifying cell tissue culture instrumentation and disposables for clinical IVF, the first unique embryology laboratory instrument being the MINC incubator invented by David Mortimer in Australia in the 1990s. The adaptation of small surgical tools and disposables goes back to the early days of IVF.

How One Hundred Years of Experimental Embryology Influenced Genetics and Clinical Medicine

Historians are not always in agreement about who was the first to witness mammalian fertilization and sperm–egg interaction outside the reproductive tract. Was it Schenk in Vienna, Austria, in 1878, or the Swiss physician and zoologist Hermann Fol in 1879? What is evident is that Schenk was the first to describe the dissolution of cumulus cells in rabbit eggs held in follicular and uterine fluids after exposure to epididymal spermatozoa, thereby clearly establishing the field of experimental embryology. This was reported exactly 100 years before the birth of Louise Brown (Steptoe and Edwards, 1978).

Oskar Hertwig, a student of the renowned German biologist and artist Ernst Haeckel, described fertilization in the sea urchin two years before Schenk (in 1876) and it seems that these observations led him to emphasize the important role of sperm and egg nuclei during inheritance and the reduction of chromosomes (meiosis) during the generation of gametes. Another distinguished German biologist and artist, Theodor Boveri, published some of the most significant principles of preimplantation embryology in the late 1880s and early 1890s. Before this, Oscar Hertwig had already proposed that sperm and egg nuclei fuse during fertilization. Fusion of gamete nuclei is typical in invertebrates studied by Hertwig, but does not occur in mammals. The single large pronucleus seen in human zygotes may occasionally be the product of fusion, but this is an unusual and possibly abnormal event associated with artificial conditions.

Boveri studied the maturation of egg cells of *Ascaris megalocephala*, the horse nematode. He observed that, as eggs matured, there came a point when chromosome numbers were reduced in half. Boveri was one of the first to see evidence for the process of meiosis. Boveri and Sutton independently advanced the chromosome model of inheritance in 1902. Boveri performed his studies with sea urchins, in which he found that all the chromosomes had to be present for proper embryonic development to occur. Sutton's work with grasshoppers demonstrated that chromosomes are organized in matched pairs of maternal and paternal chromosomes, which detach during meiosis. The Boveri–Sutton chromosome theory (the chromosome theory of inheritance) is a fundamental theory in genetics. This model identifies chromosomes as the carriers of genetic material. It explains the mechanism essential to the laws of Mendelian inheritance by identifying chromosomes with paired factors as would be required by Mendel's laws. Boveri and Sutton also argue that chromosomes must essentially be linear structures with genes located at specific sites along them. The chromosome as an organelle was discovered at least 60 years earlier by Wilhelm Hofmeister in Germany. Just a few years after Boveri–Sutton, E. B. Wilson and Nettie Stevens (1905) independently discovered the chromosomal XY sex-determination system – that males have XY and females XX sex chromosomes.

Boveri and his partner Marcella Boveri were among the first true experimental embryologists. He was nominated for, but never received, the Nobel Prize before his sudden death in 1912. He not only chronicled the development of normally fertilized sea urchin eggs, he also described development following polyspermic fertilization. Boveri deduced that male sperm and female egg nuclei were similar in the amount of transmissible information. They each had a half set (haploid number) of chromosomes. As long as a set of each was present, defined as the diploid number of chromosomes, there was usually normal sea urchin development. Any more or any less and development would be abnormal. Mendel's laws were rediscovered in 1900. Boveri recognized the correlation between Mendel's findings and his own cytological evidence of how chromosomes behaved.

The centriole, which is integral to cell division and flanks the spindle, was also discovered by Boveri earlier in 1888. A pair of centrioles, one aligned perpendicular to the other, are found in the centrosome, which is the microtubule organizing center of animal cells (although some centrosomes, like that of the mouse are acentriolar). Boveri subsequently hypothesized that cancer was caused by errors during cell division. Although belittled at the time, Boveri was later proved to be right. In addition to playing a critical role in mitosis, the centriole apparently also provides structural support. Boveri correctly argued that only one of the centrioles from the two gametes could survive the fertilization process, the other one being inactivated. In mammals, the male centriole is usually the one that survives; an exception is the mouse, in which acentriolar maternal centrosomes are drivers of cell division. Research in my laboratory in the 1990s demonstrated that human centrioles are derived from the sperm head. We used a similar logic as Boveri to analyze the differences in mitotic behavior, chromosome segregation, and mosaicism, observing differences in chromosome counts in diandric, digynic, and normal zygotes.

Walter Heape (1890) in the UK was the first to successfully transfer "segmented ova" (cleaved embryos) from one animal to another. It was 80 years later that in-vivo fertilized embryos were flushed from the human uterus by Croxatto's team in Chile. Heape used the characteristics of the Angora rabbit from which the embryos were obtained to describe the offspring after transfer into a Belgian hare. The cohort of siblings was of a mixed nature, since the recipient rabbit was mated normally. The embryos were not exposed to laboratory conditions and transfer was done very quickly after washing the embryos from the oviducts. Heape's idea, to use embryo transfer between two animals, apparently did not translate into the concept of artificial fertilization, at least not explicitly stated as such; however, if his experiments did not lead him to the idea directly, they may have inspired others.

The Concept of Ectogenesis

The idea of achieving extracorporeal fertilization was probably first introduced by the great British population geneticist, J. B. S. Haldane, who in a book written for a lay audience and published in 1924 (*Daedalus; or, Science and the Future*) suggested how a process he called "ectogenesis" would soon create individuals outside of the human body (Haldane, 1924). Haldane predicted that the first human birth would occur in 1951, only slightly optimistic since the concept would become validated not long after, and World War II delayed many scientific investigations. Haldane's friend Aldous Huxley, an English author, popularized artificial reproductive technology mixed with liberal sexuality some 600 years into the future in his famous novel, *Brave New World* (1932). As has unfortunately become commonplace when the future of science is portrayed,

Brave New World is a dystopic prophecy. Huxley only admitted to having copied the concept from Haldane's in-vitro conception theory many years after the publication of his book. Now the Heape–Haldane–Huxley concept of alternative forms of procreation was out of the box and the tantalizing possibility that such technologies could soon be available to everyone was on the horizon.

The second modest shift in thought occurred with the idea of applying the ectogenesis model to women with tubal disease. This concept was introduced rather plainly in a short editorial in *The New England Journal of Medicine* in 1937, presumably by Dr. John Rock (suggested by Howard Jones), who was a highly regarded ObGyn at Harvard University. At the time, the idea was perceived to be so outrageous that even the author avoided claiming it, and the editorial was unsigned. The concept had now matured from being proposed as a futuristic way of general procreation to a specific treatment for women with tubal disease. Dr. Rock did not suggest that artificial procreation should include laboratory-supported pregnancy.

Infertility diagnosis and treatment before Louise Brown was more sophisticated than is sometimes believed. Infertility was an established clinical subspecialty well before World War II. By contrast, andrology is a new discipline. The success of treatment was sometimes expressed as a function of the duration of infertility. Treatment rarely produced better results than no treatment. There were notable exceptions; for instance, tubal disease treatment using surgical intervention was well established and relatively successful. Similarly, certain endocrine and immunologic disorders could be treated occasionally. The advent of sperm transfer, artificial insemination using the semen of a donor, may have occurred as early as 1790 in London by Dr. John Hunter. In the early part of the twentieth century, donor insemination was practiced sporadically until the 1950s when the procedure was first described in medical journals. Chris Polge was the first to deep-freeze mammalian spermatozoa in 1949. Human spermatozoa were first successfully frozen in Iowa (USA) a few years later, by Raymond Bunge and Jerome Sherman, who also established the world's first sperm bank at the University of Arkansas around 1960.

Meanwhile, scientists would complete the first steps of "ectogenesis" in the laboratory, planning fertilization experiments in vitro in animal models. Although M. C. Chang's work in 1959 is widely regarded as the first proof of IVF in a mammalian model, there were dozens of scientific publications spanning 80 years of research that paved the way (Austin, 1961). Of note are the remarkable early experiments by Onanoff in 1893 using eggs flushed from the uterus. Most experimental embryologists later used tubal eggs. Gregory Pincus, the father of the contraception pill, claimed to have fertilized rabbit eggs before World War II with his colleague Enzmann; however, the does were inseminated first by a buck and the eggs were flushed quickly from the Fallopian tubes after which they were washed vigorously to remove spermatozoa. In the 1950s when in-vitro inseminations were more commonplace, it became obvious that spermatozoa could interact with the zona pellucida shortly after insemination and that excess spermatozoa could not be easily removed by washing. Other observations published by Pincus such as the presence of two polar bodies after activation (disputed by Chang) and a very short interval of only 12 h between observing the germinal vesicle and the first polar body appearing in the human (disputed by Edwards) were also reasons to perhaps consider the pre-War work in a different light.

John Rock and Miriam Menkin at Harvard would collect hundreds of immature ovarian eggs from patients and attempt to fertilize them with modest results. In the 1950s, Thibault in France and M. C. Chang in the United States carried the field forward by confirming fertilization in vitro and obtaining offspring in the rabbit following transfer of the embryos. However, many of the intricate details of the IVF process were still basically unknown. For instance, it was believed that spermatozoa had to mature in the uterus first. By the time Bob Edwards became interested in treating tubal infertility by IVF in the early 1960s, a few others had also attempted to fertilize human eggs in vitro, although fertilization was not positively proven in any of those cases. A number of important questions needed to be answered first: (1) What was a suitable culture fluid or medium for human embryo culture? (2) What was the best way of culturing the specimens? (3) How could immature eggs be matured in vitro? (4) How could mature rather than immature eggs be obtained routinely? (5) How should spermatozoa be prepared for insemination? (6) How could more than one follicle be recruited in the ovary? (7) How could ovulation be timed accurately? (8) At what stage should embryos be returned to the uterus? (9) How and where should embryos be transferred?

Although some of these questions were being addressed by experimental embryologists working with animal models, it was understood that each species has its own specific requirements. This was certainly the case in the human, partly because women who were candidates for treatment were older and suffered from infertility. Human IVF was also different because oocytes were obtained from and embryos were returned to the same individual rather than the egg donor and embryo recipient being two different individuals as is routine in animal work. The concepts of clinical IVF and PGD were accurately described in 11 key points published in Edwards' remarkable 1965 paper in *The Lancet* (Edwards, 1965).

Culture Media and the Culture System

The first tissue culture media were developed nearly 150 years ago by Ludwig and Ringer. These were simple salt solutions, which were initially based on the chemical properties of blood serum. Knowledge was gained during those early years about the biochemistry of metabolism in mammals and humans, particularly osmolarity, pH, and temperature. This knowledge provided the basis for making many changes to the salt solutions that were already in use. The second generation of culture media was developed more than a century later, in the 1970s, aiming to mimic the reproductive environment (the so-called "Back to Nature" principle). The "Back to Nature" principle still has substantial support from influential culture system specialists like David Gardner, Patrick Quinn, and David Mortimer. The third group of media was designed to optimize growth in vitro, to some extent ignoring existing formulations and principles. To formulate these media, the performance of each ingredient was evaluated separately using a process referred to as "simplex optimization" – a system developed first for the mouse in the laboratory of embryo culture pioneer John Biggers at Harvard University nearly 25 years ago. This work was supported by the United States National Institutes of Health (NIH) in part to define culture media for use in the human while circumventing the ongoing moratorium on human embryo research, which has been in place since 1979. The US National Institute of Child Health and Human Development provided a large program grant bearing the name National Cooperative Program on Non-Human In Vitro Fertilization and Preimplantation Development; this was more colloquially known as "The Culture Club."

John Hammond was the first director of the new Animal Reproduction unit of the Animal Research

Station in Cambridge (UK) in 1949. He was the first to observe mouse embryos cleaving in vitro and eight-cell embryos reaching the blastocyst stage (Hammond, 1949). He was presumably also the first to observe the hatching process in vitro. He is considered the father of embryo culture for having set in motion a host of studies undertaken in the 1950s by experimental embryologists interested in obtaining fertilization and extended embryo culture in vitro, allowing continuous observations to be made on developmental stages from just after sperm penetration to immediately preimplantation. The general plan was to model preimplantation development in vitro, although some scientists also suggested continuing to grow the fetus in vitro. Hammond used a salt solution containing sodium chloride, potassium chloride, calcium chloride, magnesium chloride, and some glucose for culture. To this he added about 5% egg white. The embryos were flushed and placed in a serological tube, sealed, and cultured in air for 48 h. Only a few of the eight-cell embryos could develop further under those conditions. Hammond demonstrated that glucose was essential for compaction and development of the blastocyst. He was presumably the first to publish on the use of test tubes for mouse embryo culture.

In 1956, Wesley Whitten from Australia showed that more than 90% of eight-cell mouse embryos would develop to the blastocyst stage when cultured in KRB supplemented with glucose, penicillin, streptomycin, and bovine serum albumin (Whitten, 1956). In 1958, McLaren and Biggers showed that such blastocysts would produce live young when transferred to recipient mothers (McLaren and Biggers, 1958). This was a significant step on the road to in-vitro fertilization (IVF) in animals. Whitten added lactate to his 1956 formulation and was able to culture two-cell mouse embryos from outbred animals to the blastocyst stage. However, he could not achieve the same with zygotes. This observation led to the discovery of the so-called "two-cell block" in mouse embryo culture. Both Hammond and Whitten used serological or test tubes with volumes of media less than 1 ml to culture the embryos. Before them, Pincus and Enzmann in the 1930s used Carrel flasks with volumes of 2–10 ml of fluid. Work on fertilization in vitro also proceeded actively during those years. Charles Thibault and colleagues observed fertilization of rabbit eggs in 1954 and live kits were obtained by M. C. Chang at the Worcester Foundation in 1959, but defined embryo culture media were not used for IVF in those days.

In a series of papers, Ralph Brinster showed that phosphoenolpyruvate, pyruvate, lactate, and oxaloacetate, but not glucose, could support the development of the two-cell mouse embryo to the eight-cell stage, while glucose could support the development of the eight-cell embryo to the blastocyst stage (Brinster, 1963). Based on these findings, Brinster modified Whitten's medium by reducing the calcium concentration and adding pyruvate to produce BMOC2, which would support the development of the mouse two-cell embryo to the blastocyst stage at high rates. In 1971, David Whittingham modified Brinster's medium by decreasing the concentration of lactate and increasing the concentration of pyruvate to produce M16 medium.

Brinster's medium and M16 were significant advances for embryo culture and were widely used by experimental embryologists. Except for outbred or hybrid strains of mice, these media could not overcome the two-cell block. Blocks to development in vitro were similarly found in hamster (two-cell), cattle (eight–sixteen-cell), and pig (four–eight-cell). All these arresting stages appear to coincide approximately with the onset of major embryonic genome expression.

Although continued culture in vitro of zygotes and particularly two-cell embryos could be achieved readily from the early 1960s onwards and many labs were able to follow the guidelines set by the experimental embryology pioneers, two aspects still needed attention before fertilization outside the Fallopian tube could become reality. First, capacitation is an important step in the maturation of mammalian spermatozoa and is a prerequisite to fertilization. This process occurs in vitro spontaneously when seminal-plasma-free spermatozoa, either ejaculated or isolated from the epididymis, are incubated in culture medium for a few hours. Sperm capacitation in vitro was first described in the hamster by Yanagimachi and Chang in 1963 and this set the stage for a number of sperm preparation methods, which all had in common the separation of seminal plasma and the isolation of motile spermatozoa. Of equal importance and infinitely more complicated was the problem of obtaining cohorts of mature eggs (Edwards, 1965). Fowler and Edwards in the 1950s were the first to succeed with the process of superovulation and pregnancy in mice using high dosage of gonadotrophins (Fowler and Edwards, 1957). In 1962, Gemzell showed that superovulation could be also achieved in the human using pituitary gonadotrophins.

The final step to overcome before routine implementation of assisted reproduction was design of a practical and effective embryo culture system. By 1963, test tubes (Hammond) and Carrell flasks (Pincus) were used to culture embryos or perform in-vitro insemination. Brinster introduced culture of eggs and embryos in small droplets of culture medium under a layer of paraffin oil. With some modifications, this "microdrop" method using the Petri dish, has become the most widely used and successful system for culture of mammalian embryos in vitro, although open culture and test tubes remained in use in some IVF clinics in North America and Australia well into the early 1990s. The Petri dish is used in more than 95% of ART procedures – perhaps as many as 100 million of them! In spite of that, the dish has changed little since its inception in the latter part of the nineteenth century. There have been few secondary changes to adapt the original plain design of the dish to areas of specialized use such as cell tissue culture and microbiology. The same can be said about the adaptations made to the Petri dish after its introduction to preclinical embryo research in the 1940s and 1950s as well as clinical work in the past decade. There have been some recent alterations, such as place markings for droplets, small wells, or identifications on the bottom.

As mentioned above, one of the most important features of contemporary embryo culture was developed by Ralph Brinster (of sperm stem-cell fame) in 1963, when he successfully cultured mouse eggs to the blastocyst stage (Brinster, 1963). He wanted to do away with the "open" culture and protect the small volumes of culture medium in the dish with a transparent but dense overlay. He used paraffin oil for this purpose. The advantages of this ingenuous system were huge. Oil prevented most microbial infections, allowing fertilization and embryo growth to take place in less fluctuating conditions. For example, gametes and embryos could be observed for longer periods since medium evaporation would be essentially avoided. The method also allowed the study of minute quantities of metabolites released or absorbed by the cells; later, this elegant system facilitated the introduction of micromanipulation methods. Intra-cytoplasmic sperm injection (ICSI) and embryo biopsy would have been nearly impossible without the use of oil. The high heat capacity of oil also helped maintain temperature when the dishes were brought outside the incubator for observation or manipulation. Persisting problems were oil toxicity and batch-to-batch variation. Paraffin oil has now been largely replaced by other oils such as mineral oil. This is a variation on light hydrocarbon oils, a distillate of petroleum. Toxicity has been greatly diminished because certain mineral oils are used for human consumption as a lubricant laxative. Brinster's technical marvel was for a long time unappreciated by human IVF specialists, as nearly all early practitioners (particularly in the USA) used either organ culture dishes or small test tubes (Australia) for culture of human gametes and embryos. From the first day of studying experimental embryology in 1976, I used Brinster's method, thanks to Gerard Zeilmaker's culture system. I persuaded Fishel and Edwards to switch back to the Brinster method, when I joined them in 1982 at which point they were experimenting with test tubes based on the experience of the Australian teams. When I moved to the USA in 1985, I changed the culture system in the Atlanta laboratory (and later the Cornell laboratory) from open organ culture dishes (the "Norfolk system") to Brinster's system. I believe that it is thanks to Simon Fishel and me that this system is now universally adopted. We are probably also to "blame" for painstakingly controlling the embryo transfer process, and pointing out how poor technique adversely impacted results in the early days of IVF, when classically trained surgeons/gynecologists had to manipulate microliter volumes while advancing a sharp catheter through the cervix blindly and without visualization by ultrasonography.

Two Decades that Paved the Way for Human IVF

Human fertilization in vitro was first successfully shown by Edwards and Bavister in 1968. Bavister based the culture medium on work done earlier in the hamster. They added spermatozoa to nine human eggs and demonstrated unequivocally that fertilization had occurred when they photographed a sperm tail within one of the eggs and two pronuclei and polar bodies in another (Edwards et al., 1969).

Whereas clinicians probably celebrate the first birth following IVF, many embryologists and scientists celebrated the first evidence of fertilization. The 40-year anniversary celebration of this event was organized by Martin Johnson at Christ College in Cambridge (UK) in the fall of 2009.

The collaboration between Bob Edwards and Patrick Steptoe, one of the most fruitful collaborations ever undertaken between a scientist and a clinician, started in 1968 because Steptoe had been able to introduce laparoscopy successfully after others like Palmer (1944) and Semm (1964) provided the instruments to visualize and manipulate the ovaries. The first infertile patients were invited to participate in IVF treatment in 1970. Unfortunately for those volunteers, it took hundreds of attempts to finally obtain a sustained pregnancy in November 1977 (Edwards and Steptoe, 1980; Elder and Johnson, 2015). The first pregnancy had been achieved a year earlier in 1976, but it was ectopic and had to be terminated. Wood and Leeton in Australia also reported a biochemical pregnancy in 1973. Other teams in Sweden, Holland, the USA, India, and Australia had joined in, but the three UK pioneers remained the most focused and determined. They also publicly shared most of their observations and progress in lectures and publications and kept meticulous records.

Louise Joy Brown was born on July 25, 1978, and quickly became the most famous baby in the world. Her name is still recognized throughout the world. She represents Edwards, Purdy, and Steptoe's quest to make human IVF a reality for infertile couples. After the birth of Louise, a short – and remarkably understated – letter was published in *The Lancet* (Steptoe and Edwards, 1978). Three things stood out in this publication. The first was that the transferred embryo was an eight-cell and not a later stage embryo as was the case during previous transfer attempts. The transfer of blastocysts was based on the assumption that embryos at earlier stages would face physiological hostility, since it was believed that the uterus normally accommodates only morulae and blastocysts. We now know that this is only true in other mammals and that the human uterus can tolerate any stage of development around the time of ovulation, even prefertilization if sperm and eggs are injected together; however, success rates are not the same for every stage.

The second surprising revelation in the letter in *The Lancet* was that Lesley Brown's (Louise's mother) diseased Fallopian tubes were removed and her ovaries had been relocated into a position of easy accessibility. It escaped no one's attention that this maneuver guaranteed that there would be no doubt about the pregnancy having resulted from the IVF embryo and not perchance from spontaneous fertilization of a wandering egg.

A third extraordinary aspect of the announcement was that the mature egg had been retrieved from a naturally growing follicle rather than from follicles that had been developing under exogenous hormonal stimulation, as it had been the case in previous patients. The question that was then posed was whether the natural cycle was requisite to the success of IVF. It was the team of Alan Trounson that provided the answer a few years later, successfully using gonadotropins and clomiphene citrate for ovarian stimulation. Earlier, another team in Melbourne achieved the first IVF pregnancies in Australia (Lopata et al., 1980).

It should be noted that the initial and subsequent successes of IVF occurred without the support of government agencies and under a barrage of criticism. Many ethicists, religious leaders, politicians, lawyers, fellow scientists, and physicians were appalled by the idea. Edwards confronted them head on and even described scenarios new to them in order to focus the debate. His defense of IVF never wavered as he wrote dozens of scholarly articles about the legal, political, and ethical issues surrounding reproductive technologies. Although these battles were not always prominent in Edwards' immediate academic environment, they came to the foreground occasionally and sometimes would have a tremendous effect on the early clinical work at Bourn Hall. I was hired in 1982 to help develop two clinical aspects that the Bourn Hall team felt needed attention: (1) freezing of spare embryos, and (2) methods for micromanipulation to enhance fertilization in cases of extreme male factor infertility. The first project was rather obvious at the time. Extra embryos were not transferred as this was considered unsafe. They were instead discarded during those early days. The team was reluctant to transfer more than one or two embryos at a time. I was trained in the principles of cryopreservation by my PhD supervisor Gerard Zeilmaker and his assistant Camilla Rijkmans-Verhamme. We had frozen more than 10 cleaved human embryos between 1979 and 1981. This work remains unpublished to date. Gerard Zeilmaker did not believe in observations of embryos without embryo transfer and proof of birth. We used DMSO for freezing based on the original Whittingham mouse protocol. The eggs were retrieved by Bert Alberda, a young gynecologist in training at Erasmus University. Survival rate of the thawed embryos was remarkably high. The second project I was asked to develop further at Bourn Hall Clinic was that of applying IVF to cases of extreme male factor infertility. Up to then, men with reduced sperm counts and abnormal semen analysis were counseled for IVF, but fertilization rates remained significantly lower in this group compared to patients with other etiologies. The plan to use micromanipulation to inject a single spermatozoon into the egg goes back to my days in Gerard Zeilmaker's laboratory and it is likely this was contemplated by others as well. We tried to inject mouse spermatozoa in mouse eggs, but were mostly unsuccessful, not surprisingly, as it would take another 25 years before mouse ICSI was technically feasible using piezo-mediated injection.

Establishing and Expanding the Clinical Alternative: the 1980s and 1990s

At the end of 1980, Edwards and Steptoe opened the world's first IVF clinic near Cambridge in an old Manor House called Bourn Hall, which became Bourn Hall Clinic; it had taken the founders some time to establish the facility due to the general lack of interest among financiers. Government funding, both locally and nationally, was quite out of the question after the UK Medical Research Council (MRC) and National Health boards again refused to support IVF; an earlier refusal goes back to 1971 when the MRC declined to fund the emerging field of assisted reproduction. Academic centers also shied away from the project, at least initially. This was common in many countries including The Netherlands, where I was unable to secure funding for an IVF laboratory despite applying to multiple academic institutions. Later in 1983, the MRC would again refuse to grant a broad research application from Bob Edwards, Simon Fishel, and me. Nevertheless, Bourn Hall Clinic became a legendary place complete with in-patient wards, ethics and visitor committees, endocrinology, embryology, and research laboratories, parlors, and a dining hall. Other clinics were opened as well: at the Royal Women's Hospital in Australia (Alex Lopata and Ian Johnson), and Monash University (Carl Wood and Alan Trounson) also in Melbourne, Australia, with some government support, and in London, UK (Ian Craft), using private funding. At the Eastern Virginia Medical School in Norfolk, Virginia (USA), two famous reproductive gynecologists, Drs. Georgianna and Howard Jones, opened the first US-based facility using funds released by the university. Other countries such as India, Austria, France, Holland, Sweden, and Spain followed swiftly and established their own clinics. By 1985 a new discipline was emerging, a field some people were referring to for the first time as ART or Assisted Reproductive Technology.

The enthusiasm generated by the success of IVF in Norfolk in 1981, however, did not persuade the US government to lift the moratorium it had placed on all human embryo research a year earlier. In fact, later (in 1995) a law was enacted that prohibited all funding of "research in which human embryos are destroyed, discarded, or knowingly subjected to risk of injury or death greater than that allowed for research on fetuses in utero" (Dickey-Wicker Amendment, 1995). The US federal government thus does not support clinics or clinical studies and this unfortunate situation has not changed for over a quarter of a century. Though this moratorium has stymied progress, it has not stopped US clinics and academic institutions from performing IVF investigations and clinical trials using private funding.

Although the IVF technology in its basic form became established in the early 1980s, many of its aspects were poorly understood. A number of important observations had been made by the first IVF pioneers. They recognized that timing of ovulation and follicular recruitment were complicated processes often limiting a team's ability to plan ahead while many patients became frustrated because of cancellations shortly before egg retrieval. Drugs were needed to recruit follicles at will and control and time ovarian stimulation. The first such family of drugs were the GnRH agonists. These drugs down-regulate the secretion of gonadotropins luteinizing hormone (LH) and follicle-stimulating hormone (FSH), resulting in a dramatic decline in estradiol levels. This allowed suppression of endogenous gonadotropin production and the LH surge, and planning for egg retrieval following an injection of human chorionic gonadotropin (hCG).

Another clinical bottleneck during the early days of IVF was the requirement for laparoscopy. Although a magnitude more efficient and less traumatic than laparotomy, laparoscopy still had to be performed under general anesthesia in a full operating theater and required considerable recovery time. Moreover, when visualization was hindered, ovaries remained inaccessible and dominant follicles sometimes unreachable. The search for a faster and more efficient means of oocyte recovery was on. Ultrasonography, though in its infancy, had already been applied to track growing follicles. The question was whether it could be used during egg retrieval to visualize the follicle and to allow insertion of an aspiration needle. After all, the ovaries were positioned near the vaginal wall, in very close proximity to a vaginal ultrasound probe, if it had minimal dimensions. Nevertheless, the first aspiration of a follicle using ultrasound was achieved trans-abdominally by Lenz and Lauritsen in Denmark, a considerably longer route requiring access through the bladder. That same year abdominal ultrasound was combined with vaginal follicle aspiration by Norbert Gleicher. The final and determining step was performed by the Swedish team of Lars Hamberger and Matts Wikland in 1985 using a new narrow vaginal ultrasound probe guiding a needle adjacent to it; this method is still in use more than 30 years later.

In the laboratory meanwhile, experimental embryologists, veterinary researchers, and biology technicians were retrained as clinical embryologists. Their first task was to safely handle and observe gametes and embryos, and to make decisions on issues related to sperm preparation, oocyte maturation, and embryo selection. Laboratory and equipment maintenance, and standardization of methods were other important tasks, as was meticulous record keeping. These first clinical embryologists were surprised to notice that human embryo development and morphology varied considerably not just between patients, but also within cohorts. This variability made evaluation of embryos surprisingly difficult. Even more frustrating was the fact that morphology and rate of development seemed only loosely correlated with outcome. The search for important characteristics that could predict implantation has brought under examination many aspects of gamete and embryo development in culture and complicated algorithms have been developed. However, after 30 years, not a single common morphological marker has been identified that can predict the future success of an embryo with certainty. Even algorithms of multiple morphologic (or morphokinetic) criteria do not reveal implanting ability with accuracy. Although time-lapse microscopy has made permanent record keeping a reality, even this elegant tool has shown that reliable embryo selection remains unsettled. During the past few years, researchers have attempted to correlate clinical outcomes with embryo metrics, but only with mixed success. Certainly, one of the major challenges remains development of efficacious (and affordable) embryo selection methods, a crucial step in eliminating multiple pregnancies and facilitating single embryo transfer. Embryologists in the early days experienced a high level of anxiety. So much was unknown, and there was so little guidance. We were aware of the importance of the environment, since cells were mostly unprotected against micro-organisms and

toxic compounds. It was up to the laboratory to set up rules and keep a close eye on the ever-changing circumstances. During the first 20 years of IVF, culture medium was mostly "home-brewed," which exacerbated paranoia and interpretation of downward fluctuations. I quickly became interested in quality control but had few tools to work with. Although I introduced air purification from the mid 1980s in my laboratories, it would be another decade, before I was funded to test for environmental toxins and develop guidelines for air filtration and lab environment optimization. Perhaps partly because of the costs associated with compliance, this concept was for many years embraced by a minority of practitioners and its entry into the "mainstream" is very recent (Sandro et al., 2016).

IVF is the first and only general treatment for infertility and sub-fertility; couples with male infertility can be treated just as successfully as those with female-related infertility. However, this aspect was not generally accepted in the early 1980s. It was feared that spermatozoa from men with male infertility would not be able to penetrate the zona pellucida or that, if they did, fetal development could be abnormal. These concerns were raised during professional meetings in the 1970s and early 1980s. However, when couples with male factor infertility were selected for IVF, many had fertilized eggs although fertilization rate was lower than that in other groups of infertile couples. However, men with severely reduced sperm counts could not be treated as not enough spermatozoa could be prepared for microdroplet insemination. The notion that micromanipulation could further enhance fertilization in male factor cases compared to what was feasible with standard IVF had already been suggested some years back. The first such experiments in spare human eggs may have been conducted in Rotterdam in 1979 and 1980 (Zeilmaker and Cohen), but the work was unpublished. Most of the mouse eggs lysed after piercing. The first birth in mice following micromanipulation was achieved by opening the zona pellucida artificially, an approach called zona drilling (Gordon and Talansky, 1986), achieved by focal reducing of pH to 2.0–2.5. Opening the zona pellucida and allowing multiple spermatozoa into the perivitelline space seemed a step backward compared to direct injection of a single sperm cell into the egg cytoplasm, but in the mouse, unlike the human, the block to polyspermy is controlled at the level of the oolemma. The block to polyspermy in the mouse is very efficient even when there are hundreds of spermatozoa under the zona pellucida.

This is contrary to the situation in the human where the zona pellucida prevents polyspermy. Placing more than one spermatozoon under the human zona pellucida increases the risk of polyspermy. The location of the block to human polyspermy was unknown up to that point. In early 1988, babies were born to couples with male factor infertility, following application of a mechanical form of zona drilling in my laboratory. These were the first pregnancies in human IVF established with the micromanipulator as a surgical tool. This was indeed a team effort but it was particularly Henry Malter's patience and craft that brought about this change (Cohen et al., 1988). That same year the Ng team in Singapore reported on injection of spermatozoa into the peri-vitelline space. Though both alternatives improved the prospects for treatment of more extreme forms of male factor infertility, normal fertilization rates were low due to the absence of a quick block to polyspermy on the membrane level. These first micromanipulation systems were criticized for their low monospermic rates of fertilization, but implantation was as high or higher than in regular IVF patients. Fertilization improved dramatically with the introduction of intracytoplasmic sperm injection (ICSI) by a team of researchers in Brussels, Belgium (Palermo et al., 1992). The single most important factor that determined success was the design of the injection tool (Devroey, personal communication). It was very thin and sharp, unlike the injection tools we had developed earlier in Rotterdam and Atlanta. Credit goes to the team in Brussels who fortunately ignored tool fabrication guidelines from laboratories such as ours. ICSI has been the preferred method of fertilization for those at risk of reduced or failed fertilization for 25 years.

The most exciting events in science are often marked by the merging of seemingly unrelated disciplines. The field of reproductive science had already experienced this in the nineteenth century, when the beliefs of both spermists and ovists were shattered by the observation that spermatozoa penetrate the egg and that this is followed by the formation of two pronuclei in the zygote. Those lucky clinicians and scientists practicing IVF in the 1980s witnessed not one, but three revolutions. The first paradigm shift occurred with the establishment of methods to use IVF-derived technology to treat severe male factor infertility. The interval between the first discussion of this concept in the early 1980s and routine application of ICSI was only about 12 years. The second groundbreaking shift was the development of embryo cryopreservation methods. Here again, the interval from basic science to clinical application was about 12 years.

Cryopreservation of the embryo (and later the egg) allowed clinicians to reduce the number of embryos for transfer. In the human, all stages between the zygote and blastocyst were frozen; however, different cryoprotectants and freezing protocols were required. At Bourn Hall, the embryologists were prohibited by their legal team during the summer of 1982 from investigating freezing of human embryos, due to a number of pending defamation lawsuits against media outlets. This prohibition was lifted after 15 months by Patrick Steptoe when Mohr and Trounson published the first frozen embryo birth in *Nature* in 1983 (Trounson and Mohr, 1983). Steptoe and Edwards were both upset about having lost the opportunity to compete in the race for a first cryo baby. I had been hired earlier to start this research, but had been held back because of the prohibition. The Bourn Hall team, now having added another cryopreservation expert from the veterinary field, Roger Simons, decided to use glycerol as a cryoprotectant. This had been used successfully in cattle embryos. Patrick Steptoe stepped up to the plate in spite of serious illness. Once Bourn Hall's ethical committee approved the research, he personally approached each patient couple who had an excess of zygotes. The central theme of the consenting process was that the embryo donation would be of no benefit to the patient, but possibly to others who would come later. About 50 couples consented to the research over the course of about 3 months. We found that nearly all early-stage embryos would survive the freezing process in glycerol, but our excitement was short lived, once we noticed that the cryoprotectant would not be easily released by the cells. After a day in culture, cells in post-thaw zygotes, cleaved embryos, and morulae swelled and lysed. No division was observed. To our delight and surprise, however, early expanded blastocysts survived and developed for one or more days. Only a few would hatch, but this was not any different from fresh blastocysts, which under culture conditions of the 1980s, rarely hatched in vitro. This later led us to introduce assisted hatching as a response to 1980s culture conditions. It was decided to perform clinical cryopreservation using the glycerol protocol we developed in spare embryos. The third thaw was successful and the first blastocyst cryo baby was born in early 1985.

The many advantages of cryopreservation are now well established. In the 1980s, it became quickly clear that thawing of embryos allowed later transfer in the natural cycle. Some couples did not have to undergo multiple IVF treatments, since the embryos from one cohort would be enough to establish a multi-sibling family. The effort was well founded in science, since pioneers like David Whittingham, Peter Mazur, Stanley Leibo, and Steen Willadsen working with rodents and farm animals had already mastered the technology years earlier. The past 10 years have seen a dramatic further refining of egg and embryo cryopreservation using vitrification, the aims being speed and simplification of methodology, and increasing egg and embryo survival rates.

The third revolution in the 1980s in the world of assisted reproduction was genetic diagnosis of embryos through blastomere biopsy before transfer (Handyside et al., 1989). Interestingly, the general concept had already been introduced 20 years earlier by Bob Edwards and one of his brilliant PhD students at the time, Richard Gardner (Gardner and Edwards, 1968). They performed trophectoderm biopsy in the rabbit embryo, applied a sexing technique, and transferred sexed embryos to the uterus. More than 20 years later and a few years after development of the polymerase chain reaction (PCR), this elegant experiment would form the basis for a new field called Preimplantation Genetic Diagnosis (PGD). The group at Cornell in New York, USA, where I worked at the time, was the second to report on a pregnancy from PGD and the first to report on the high incidence of chromosomal anomalies in embryonic cells and the suggestion that transfer of euploid embryos may increase the chance of implantation (Munné et al., 1995).

The Evolution of Reproductive Clinical Science

IVF is now considered an industry, a field that can stand on its own. More than 6000 clinics specializing in IVF exist worldwide. The largest, in Tokyo, Japan, treats more than 35,000 couples a year! A few forward-looking governments support the IVF effort financially. Other governments, such as the ones in Sweden and Belgium, support and guide the practice with smart laws based on clinical data. Many professional organizations have been formed to support the effort, and special university-based training programs exist for physicians and embryologists sub-specializing in IVF. Hands-on experience is still very much an apprenticeship system. It is estimated that 10 million babies have been born through ART; however, the road to this success has been long and hard. In 1934,

Dr. Gregory Pincus was a young man in his early thirties when he claimed to have achieved in-vitro fertilization in rabbits, just a few years after Haldane's prophecies and Huxley's book. While the discovery made international headlines, he was vilified in the press. The *New York Times* depicted him as Dr. Frankenstein, just like others would later describe the work on in-vitro fertilization by Patrick Steptoe and Robert G. Edwards as bogus. It must have been disconcerting for scientific mavericks like Pincus and Edwards to be disparaged for their sound scientific enquiry. Yet, maybe they found solace in the history of science, since they found themselves in good company – Copernicus, Galileo, Darwin, and Boveri were also unfairly treated during their lifetimes if only for their courage and revolutionary thinking.

Acknowledgment

Mina Alikani is gratefully acknowledged for reading and commenting on the manuscript.

References

Austin CR. Fertilization of mammalian eggs in vitro. *Int Rev Cytol* 1961;12:337–359.

Brinster RL. A method for in vitro cultivation of mouse ova from two-cell to blastocyst. *Exp Cell Res* 1963;32:205–208.

Cohen J. *From Pythagoras and Aristotle to Boveri and Edwards: A History of Clinical Embryology and Therapeutic IVF.* Cambridge University Press, 2013.

Cohen J, Rieger D. Historical background of gamete and embryo culture. *Methods Mol Biol* 2012;912:1–18.

Cohen J, Malter H, Fehilly C, et al. Implantation of embryos after partial opening of oocyte zona pellucida to facilitate sperm penetration. *Lancet* 1988;16(2):162.

Cohen J, Alikani M, Bisignano A. Past performance of assisted reproduction technologies as a model to predict future progress: a proposed addendum to Moore's law. *Reprod Biomed Online* 2012;25:585–590.

Edwards RG. Maturation in vitro of human ovarian oocytes. *Lancet* 1965;2:926–929.

Edwards RG, Steptoe PC. *A Matter of Life: the Story of a Medical Breakthrough.* Morrow, New York, NY, USA, 1980.

Edwards RG, Bavister BD, Steptoe PC. Early stages of fertilization in vitro of human oocytes matured in vitro. *Nature* 1969;15;221:632–635.

Elder K, Johnson MH. The Oldham Notebooks: an analysis of the development of IVF 1969-1978. II. The treatment cycles and their outcomes. *Reprod Biomed Soc Online* 2015; 1:9–18.

Fowler RE, Edwards RG. Induction of superovulation and pregnancy in mature mice by gonadotrophins. *J Endocrinol* 1957;15:374–384.

Gardner RL, Edwards RG. Control of the sex ratio at full term in the rabbit by transferring sexed blastocysts. *Nature* 1968;218(5139):346–349.

Gordon JW, Talansky BE. Assisted fertilization by zona drilling: a mouse model for correction of oligospermia. *J Exp Zool* 1986;239:347–354.

Haldane JBS. *Daedalus; or, Science and the Future* (1924), EP Dutton and Company, Inc., a paper read to the Heretics, Cambridge, on February 4, 1923. Second edition, London: Kegan Paul, Trench & Co, 1928.

Hammond J Jr. Recovery and culture of tubal mouse ova. *Nature* 1949;163:28.

Handyside AH, Pattinson JK, Penketh RJ, et al. Biopsy of human preimplantation embryos and sexing by DNA amplification. *Lancet* 1989;1:347–349.

Lopata A, Johnston IW, Hoult IJ, Speirs AI. Pregnancy following intrauterine implantation of an embryo obtained by in vitro fertilization of a preovulatory egg. *Fertil Steril* 1980;33:117–120.

McLaren A, Biggers JD. Successful development and birth of mice cultivated in vitro as early as early embryos. *Nature* 1958;182:877–878.

Munné S, Sultan KM, Weier HU, Grifo JA, Cohen J, Rosenwaks Z. Assessment of numeric abnormalities of X, Y, 18, and 16 chromosomes in preimplantation human embryos before transfer. *Am J Obstet Gynecol* 1995;172:1191–1199.

Palermo G, Joris H, Devroey P, Van Steirteghem AC. Pregnancies after intracytoplasmic injection of single spermatozoon into an oocyte. *Lancet* 1992;340:17–18.

Sandro C. Esteves, Alex C. Varghese, Kathryn C. *Worrilow. Clean Room Technology in ART Clinics: A Practical Guide.* CRC Press, Taylor and Francis, Boca Raton, FL, USA, 2016.

Steptoe PC, Edwards RG. Birth after the reimplantation of a human embryo. *Lancet* 1978;2:366.

Trounson A, Mohr L. Human pregnancy following cryopreservation, thawing and transfer of an eight-cell embryo. *Nature* 1983;305(5936):707–709.

Whitten WK. Culture of tubal mouse ova. *Nature* 1956;177:96.

Whittingham DG. Fertilization of mouse eggs in vitro. *Nature* 1968;220:592–593.

Whittingham DG, Leibo SP, Mazur P. Survival of mouse embryos frozen to −196 degrees and −269 degrees C. *Science* 1972;178:411–414.

Chapter 3

The American Roots of In-Vitro Fertilization

Frederick Naftolin, Jennifer Blakemore, and David L. Keefe

Introduction

At a time when relatively little was known of the cellular and molecular basis of reproduction, American scientists struck out on a path that forever changed the world's concepts regarding reproductive fates, values, and possibilities. The result of their early work on the mechanisms of fertilization opened the way to in-vitro fertilization and embryo transfer (IVF). Later, the same studies leveraged the development of hormonal contraception. The effects of these early studies on reproductive medicine, veterinary practices and society were indelible. In short, they moved the pivot of the role of women in modern societies.

Some of these pioneers went on to remarkable careers in reproduction and other fields of science/medicine, others have fallen into obscurity. The telling of their contributions at the beginning of this book is both appropriate and underlines how the American melting pot has contributed to more than just the job at hand, even to something so fantastical as IVF and its products like Louise Brown.

This chapter is an abbreviated story of a few of the most consequential American pioneers, told as overlapping personal relations, efforts, and achievements. Certainly, these few stood on the shoulders of many others on all continents to get their peek at early reproduction. And, they made it possible for others to carry the mission into practical clinical application, the story of which is the subject of much of the following chapters. But, let there be no doubt that, from gametes to birth and back, these pioneers played key roles in what was to become the greatest translational science story ever told. And, with the application of modern biological and social science, the end of the story is not in sight.

The story begins in earnest in the early 1930s, and, despite the intrusion of a world-wide conflagration (1939–1945) in the middle of the story its timespan is remarkably short. Because both animals and humans were of interest, the stigma attached to human reproductive studies, and the lack of the tools and techniques to work with humans, the work simultaneously addressed both human and veterinary testing and applications. While this chapter concentrates on outcomes related to assisted human reproduction, the studies discussed below also contributed to the most popular forms of contemporary livestock breeding and development (Gianola & Rosa, 2015).

Reproduction as a Force of Nature and IVF as One of the Effectors of Change

Reproduction is the forge of evolution. It is the main driving force in the history of the earth's flora and fauna. Our anthropomorphic interest in regulating reproductive behavior and reproduction, itself, is as old as recorded history, and this shows no sign of abating (Morin et al., 2014).

Early in evolution the emphasis was on in-vitro, i.e. extra-corporeal, fertilization. With the branching of the evolutionary tree, reproduction was internalized, largely through the re-use of already present cellular and molecular mechanism and structures (Naftolin et al., 1988).

Prospective efforts to change reproduction awaited the development of the prefrontal cortex during speciation of primates. However, until the industrial revolution ignorance, economic disincentives, the lack of biological and social imperatives, and the lack of the tools and techniques to carry out IVF foreclosed the development and acceptance of the prospective control of reproduction. This all changed during the twentieth century, when both hormonal contraception and the successful application of clinical (human and animal) IVF became realities. To be sure, other outlets for bench and clinical scientists' activities also were underway. The literature and lore of reproduction includes very important chapters on assisted reproduction by artificial insemination, ovarian stimulation, surgical approaches to congenital anomalies, inflammatory/hormonal infertility, and mechanical obstruction of

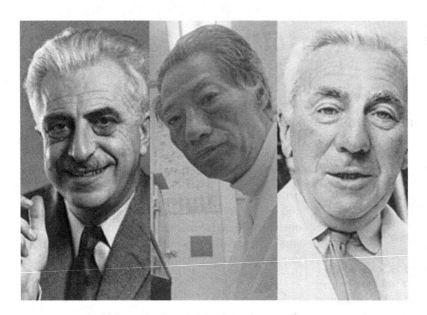

Figure 3.1 Gregory Pincus (left), M. C. Chang (center), and John Rock (right). A 2012 montage by the Planned Parenthood Advocates of Arizona.

fertility in men and women, that cannot be covered in these pages. Their application has in many instances been side-stepped by IVF, but they continue to challenge solution (Rebar & DeCherney, 2004).

America and the Pre-Conception of IVF

Most of the early American contributions were aimed at extra-corporeal formation and maintenance of short gestational species' embryos. They furnished much of the necessary understanding of the very early events necessary for successful clinical IVF. It awaited the optic of "non-purists," often clinician-scientists, to accept that it is permissible to use the half-breed model of IVF and transfer to a maternal hostess to obtain term uterine pregnancies (Edwards & Steptoe, 1980).

The following, then, is the tale of world-class leaders in the field of gametogenesis, fertilization, and animal husbandry, who parted the curtains for clinical events to carry the stage.

Three Horsemen of the Apocalypse...

IVF's early beginnings in America could be analogized to "Pincus to Chang to Rock" as was the case in the storied "Tinker to Evers to Chance" triple-play team of the early 1900s Chicago cubs (Adams, 1910). As in baseball, this team of reproductive scientists literally wiped clean the slate of this inning. They swept from early descriptive studies, to experimental animal testing, to human testing, to successful human in-vitro-fertilized embryo growth. In a subsequent inning, not included in this chapter, they dealt definitively with the discovery, study, and popularization of hormonal contraception. This truly was a tour de force rarely attributable to one small group. This chapter can only skim their combined accomplishments and interject related contributions that were made by contemporaries. Certainly, it is fitting to begin this book with the story of these three individuals (Figure 3.1).

In the Beginning, Gregory Pincus, DSc...

Gregory Goodwin (Goody) Pincus, DSc (1903–1967) (Figure 3.2) wasn't always interested in inhibiting reproduction. A brief recitation of his published work will convince that in addition to being "The Father of the Pill," Pincus was one of the "Fathers of Assisted Reproduction."

Studying at Cambridge after obtaining his DSc at Harvard, Pincus learned of the work of Heape, who reported transfers of rabbit embryos from one pregnant rabbit to another (Heape, 1891). After his return to Harvard in the 1930s, Pincus developed his interest in oocytes and in finding out what started division and development of the fertilized ovum. His pathfinding work resulted in the report of the first ever in-vitro fertilization of rabbit oocytes (Pincus & Enzemann, 1934); however, out of concern over the possibility of parthenogenesis he began a long and deep series of

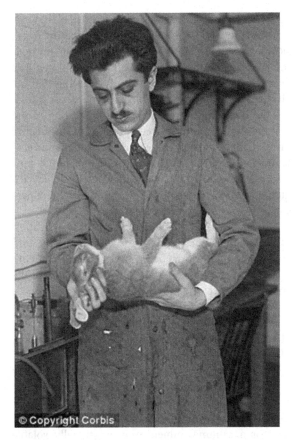

Figure 3.2 Gregory Pincus, circa 1935; source unknown.

experiments on parthenogenesis. He showed that both rabbit and human oocytes at the germinal vesical stage will proceed to the metaphase two stage in tissue culture. During this period, Pincus successfully stimulated division of mammalian eggs into the formation of embryos, even claiming that they grew to delivery. Pincus ultimately claimed that he had successfully delivered a parthenogenic rabbit whose embryonic career had started in vitro (Pincus, 1936). The latter was a disputed claim that may have cost Pincus his reappointment at Harvard (Biggers, 2012). In any case, the controversial nature of this work may be read into Pincus' renunciation of any plans to further apply his knowledge to assisted reproduction in humans (Pincus, 1939).

During his work on rabbit oocyte division, Pincus reported what is likely the first use of pituitary hormones to stimulate the ovary, to obtain increased numbers of oocytes (Pincus, 1940).

Pincus' career at Harvard was a run of imaginative studies that have formed the cornerstone of assisted reproductive technologies. The reasons for James

Conant, the incoming President of Harvard, blocking Pincus' reappointment will never be known. And, work on embryos was to some degree controversial. However, the possible role in the decision of Pincus' being the son of immigrant Jews cannot be overlooked (Urban & Smith 2015). Such thoughts engender the consideration of whether, in the absence of Conant's decision, Pincus would have met and joined forces with Katherine McCormick to change the advent of hormonal contraception (Speroff, 2009).

Before leaving Harvard, Pincus arranged the first Laurentian Hormone Research Conference. These were landmark conferences that captured the cream of endocrine research, and over which Pincus presided for 20 years (Pincus, 1944).

In 1938, after leaving Harvard, Pincus joined Dr. Hudson Hoagland at Clark University. By 1944, they were disillusioned with the academic bickering and started the Worcester Foundation for Experimental Biology, with local businessmens' donations, maintaining their Clark University connections. While its inception indicates that the Foundation was to concentrate on neuropsychiatric issues close to Hoagland's heart (author unknown, 1944) with Pincus as Laboratory Director, the Foundation became most celebrated for its work on reproductive biology. Examples of indelible reports include: 1947 – The effects of serum on spermatozoa (Chang, 1947); 1950 – The effect of seminal plasma on fertilized rabbit ova (Chang, 1950); 1966 – Transport of eggs from the Fallopian tube to the uterus as a function of oestrogen (Chang, 1966); and 1968 – Metabolic clearance rates and interconversions of estrone and 17beta-estradiol in normal males and females (Longcope et al., 1968).

The Foundation has since 1985 been absorbed into the University of Massachusetts. However, during its first four decades, it was the platform for innumerable discoveries in reproductive endocrinology, including the most durable and incisive studies of oocyte fertilization, sperm capacitation, gamete and embryo storage and veterinary in-vitro fertilization, and embryo implantation up to the time of Louise Brown's advent (Chang, 1985).

Although in popular lore the work of the team of Pincus, Rock, and Chang has been most noted for the development of hormonal contraception, their work, and that of Chang's protégé R. Yanagimachi, changed the history of both veterinary and human reproductive endocrinology and assisted reproduction (Chang, 1985). And, while Pincus went on to become known as the "Father of the Pill," Many have put his pioneering work on early events in fertilization at the top of Pincus' scientific contributions.

For a more complete perspective on Pincus, the man and his work, please read *A Good Man : Gregory Goodwin Pincus : the Man, his Story, the Birth Control Pill* (Speroff, 2009), and the paper "IVF and embryo transfer: historical origin and development" (Biggers, 2012).

The Indispensable Role of John Rock, MD. . .

John Rock, MD (1890–1984) (Figure 3.3), was a noted Boston clinician and pelvic surgeon who met and fell-in with Pincus during the latter's Harvard days. They often conversed and shared the excitement of newly-seen visions of the onset of life. Though irrevocably tied to his patients and the clinical side, Rock had the scientist's mind and the wherewithal to carry out experiments in his laboratory at the Free Hospital for Women, in Boston. He hired Miriam Menkin as the laboratory technician, and went to work on the problem of in-vitro fertilization. By the early 1940s, they were making good progress, no doubt with the close consultation of Goody Pincus. The results were truly remarkable. Rock and Menkin became the first researchers to unambiguously fertilize a human egg outside of a human body! Their work was accomplished in February of 1944 and published on

4 August 1944 in a Letter to *Science* entitled "In vitro fertilization and cleavage of human ovarian eggs" (Rock & Menkin, 1944). This experiment marked the first time in history that a human embryo had been produced outside of the body, proving that in-vitro fertilization was possible in humans.

The tenor and thoroughness of the testing of the embryos and the understated approach of Rock come through in this report. These characteristics would also be the hallmarks of his defense of the hormonal contraception (Rock, 1963). In certain ways, Rock played a quiet foil to Pincus' more outgoing and expansive personality. They made a great team.

Rock's breadth in the development and application of clinical reproductive medicine was impressive, and lengthy. In addition to being known as the patient's great friend, he was early in defining the timing of the endometrial cycle by biopsies (Rock & Bartlett, 1937), performed reconstructive surgery on the Fallopian tubes (Rock et al., 1954) and was an early investigator of sperm preservation (Fernandez Cano et al., 1964; Menkin et al., 1964).

In following the events of the times, it becomes clear that Rock represented to Pincus and the others more than a scientific colleague, he represented the needs of women, their situations, and the possibilities for improvement. He was a calming influence on emotionally volatile subjects. This role would become incalculably more

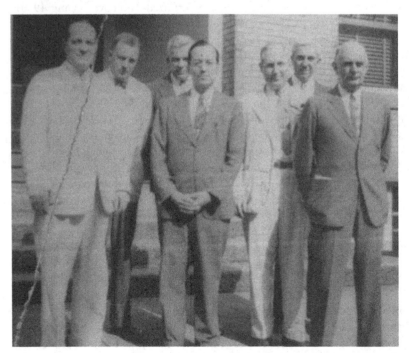

Figure 3.3 John Rock (third from the right) and colleagues.

important when they ventured into the world of hormonal contraception (McLaughlin, 1982).

M.C. Chang Became Central to the Enterprise...

In 1945, M. C. Chang PhD (1908–1991), or "Chang" as he was known by all his colleagues and students, was recruited to the newly developed Worcester Institute by Pincus. Chang and Pincus' lives were inextricably bound from then until Pincus' death in 1967. M. C. Chang was drawn into the IVF story as part of the testing of the validity of rabbit IVF (Chang, 1959; Pincus & Enzemann, 1934). Whether or not Pincus' claim of what would be the first successful mammalian IVF embryo is valid, Chang's involvement had many reverberations, and carried the work forward, especially in terms of understanding the role and mechanisms of sperm function. One of the high points was the first unchallenged mammalian IVF-ET birth. Working with Pincus' oversight, but often on his own, Chang disclosed the synchrony that is necessary for successful implantation of the embryo into the endometrium (Chang, 1950), discovered the need for sperm to prepare for fertilization in 1951 (Chang, 1951), resulting in the first indisputable evidence of successful IVF and delivery in mammals (Chang, 1959). The delay in sperm penetration of the oocyte was termed capacitation by Austin (1952). Perhaps, it was Chang's proof that sperm capacitation followed by in-vitro culture of the embryo until instrumental implantation furnished liveborn heterotopic rabbits that did the most to drive IVF-ET forward (Bavister, 2002).

Chang, always circumspect, credits Pincus and his own students, particularly Drs. Yanagimachi, Pickworth, Iwamatsu, Miyamoto, Toyoda, Hanado, Fukuda, and Maddock, as great factors in his success at the Worcester Foundation (Chang, 1985), but there is no way to hide Chang's contributions to the unraveling of the mysteries of assisted reproduction (Hunter, 2013).

And, Yanagimachi...

Ryuzo Yanagimachi PhD (1928–), was a student of Chang's. He followed the sperm line of research, contributing the details of the acrosome reaction and its role in avoiding polyspermy (Yanagimachi, 2011). In two seminal papers, he and Chang showed in-vitro fertilization of hamster gametes after sperm capacitation (Yanagimachi & Chang, 1963, 1964). However, their work on extra-corporeal in-vitro embryo culture was stymied by the "2-cell block" until long after the human work pulled ahead and resulted in Louise Brown's birth (Bavister, 2002).

Yanagimachi contributed much of what was known of sperm biology at the time of Louise Brown's conception. He remains active today, a living history of the halcyon days of animal IVF research.

And There Was Controversy – Landrum Shettles and What Might Have Been...

Landrum Shettles, MD, PhD (1910–2003) (Figure 3.4) trained as a gynecologist and was an experimentalist in human reproduction. During a turbulent and often controversial life of experimentation, he used the technique reported by Rock and Menkin to attempt in-vitro fertilization of human ova; however, the issue of parthenogenesis versus sperm penetration could not be resolved by the published photographs (Shettles, 1955). He was said to have been an originator of the implantation of fertilized human ova into the Fallopian tube (GIFT), but did not publish documentation.

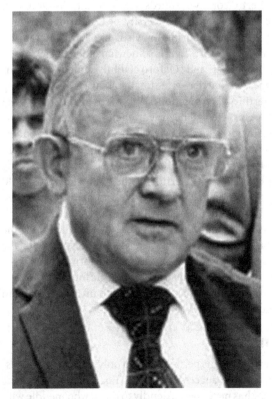

Figure 3.4 Landrum Shettles, MD, PhD, from the *New York Times*, date unknown.

In 1973, Shettles received a surgically harvested oocyte, incubated it using Menkin and Rock's published technique (Rock & Menkin, 1944) and planned to implant the embryo into the donor's uterus. However, since the project had not received institutional review, the supposedly fertilized ovum was discarded by his department head (Lavities & Shettles, 2003). Unfortunately, no evidence to support Shettles' claim of human in-vitro fertilization is recorded.

The Role of Tissue Culture in the Early Experiments on IVF...

Although it was an intercontinental story, the role of the development of tissue culture fluids is an intrinsic part of these early studies. The first experiments used serum or undefined media. Later, the use of defined media and specialized media allowed the development of both veterinary and human IVF. The high points are well-described by Biggers and Bavister (Bavister, 2002; Biggers, 2012).

Bob Edwards and the Joneses...

Robert Geoffrey Edwards was a British developmental biologist at the University of Cambridge whom I (Naftolin) met during my visits to Charles Katangole and Roger Short. To this somewhat older, obstetrician-gynecologist and Oxford DPhil student, Edwards appeared harried and totally focused on attacking infertility. He mentioned his visit to the Joneses at Hopkins. He had been with them for a period of harvesting oocytes from polycystic ovary patients undergoing ovarian wedge resection, a common treatment to lower androgens. The trip was successful in getting oocytes, but not in fertilizing them. But, Edwards could not say enough about his hosts and their openhanded welcome. This relationship went on for decades and was a source of great pleasure to him. Through the years, Edwards maintained his relationship with the Joneses (Figure 3.5), but did not perform formal studies with them. When the Jones Clinic found its success, Edwards rejoiced and continued to interact with them (Edwards, 2003).

Endnote

Reviewing this period, one can only marvel at the prescience and success of Pincus, Rock, and Chang. The USA has never been friendly to those who meddle with reproduction; this continues to this day. Yet, working as biologists, these intrepid pioneers found their way

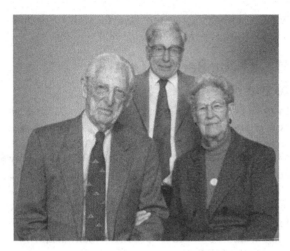

Figure 3.5 Bob Edwards and the Jonses (seated). (Source: Howard Jones.)

to everlasting success in two of the most treacherous and rewarding pursuits – developing in-vitro fertilization and inventing human hormonal contraception. Along the way, they clearly stood on the shoulders of those who had gone before them; and, they gave new perches to those who ran alongside or succeeded them. Their journey is comparable to that of Lewis and Clark, knowing that there was something to reach, making the tough slog and finishing their mission (Ambrose, 1996). Millions of infertile couples are indebted to their contributions to IVF, and hundreds of millions, even billions, to their work on hormonal contraception. While the following chapters will dazzle us with the many accomplishments of those who sought, and continue to seek, to alleviate the agony of infertility and inborn errors of the newborn, we must never forget these pioneers and the gift of both life and the exit from poverty with which they furnished us. May we be worthy of their efforts.

References

Adams, Franklin Pierce, *New York Evening Mail* July 12, 1910.

Ambrose, S. (1996). *Undaunted Courage: Meriwether Lewis, Thomas Jefferson, and the Opening of the American West.* Simon and Schuster, New York.

Austin, CR. (1952). The "capacitation" of the mammalian sperm. *Nature* 170, 326.

Author unknown. (1944). The Worcester Foundation for Experimental Biology. *Science* 99(2570), 259.

Bavister, B. (2002). Early history of in vitro fertilization. *Reproduction* 124, 181–196.

Biggers, JD. (2012). IVF and embryo transfer: historical origin and development. *Reproductive BioMedicine Online* 25, 118–127.

Chang, MC. (1947). The effects of serum on spermatozoa. *Journal of General Physiology* 30(4), 321–335.

(1950). Development and fate of transferred rabbit ova or blastocysts in relation to the ovulation time of recipients. *Journal of Experimental Zoology* 114, 197–226.

(1950). The Effect of Seminal Plasma on Fertilized Rabbit Ova. *Proceedings of the National Academy of Sciences.* 36(3):188–191

(1951). Fertilising capacity of spermatozoa deposited into the Fallopian tubes. *Nature* 168, 697.

(1959). Fertilization of rabbit ova in vitro. *Nature* 179, 466–467.

(1966). Transport of eggs from the fallopian tube to the uterus as a function of oestrogen. *Nature.* 212(5066), 1048–1049.

(1985). Recollections of 40 years at the Worcester Foundation for Experimental Biology. *The Physiologist* 28(5), 400–401.

Edwards, RG. (2003). Tribute to Georgeanna and Howard Jones. *Reproductive BioMedicine Online* 6(3), 352–360.

Edwards, R & Steptoe, P. (1980). *A Matter of Life.* William Morrow, New York.

Fernandez Cano, L, Menkin, MF, Garcia, CR, & Rock, J. (1964). Refrigerant preservation of human spermatozoa. I. Factors influencing recovery in euspermic semen: clinical applications. *Fertility and Sterility* 15, 390–406.

Gianola, D & Rosa, GJ. (2015). One hundred years of statistical developments in animal breeding. *Annual Review of Animal Biosciences* 3,19–56.

Heape, W. (1891). Preliminary note on the transplantation and growth of mammalian ova within a uterine foster mother. *Proceedings of the Royal Society, London.* 48, 447–459.

Hunter, HF. (2013). MC Chang – Reproductive biologist of distinction 1908–1991. *Human Fertility* 16(2), 101–111.

Lavities, S. & Shettles, LB. (2003). *93, Pioneer in Human Fertility.* New York Times Obit. Feb. 16, 2003.

Longcope, C, Layne, DS, & Tait, JF. (1968). Metabolic clearance rates and interconversions of estrone and 17beta-estradiol in normal males and females. *The Journal of Clinical Investigation* 47(1), 93–106.

McLaughlin, L. (1982). *The Pill, John Rock, and the Church: the Biography of a Revolution.* Boston: Little, Brown and Company.

Menkin, MF, Lusis, P, Zaikis JP Jr, & Rock, J. (1964). Refrigerant preservation of human spermatozoa. Ii. Factors influencing recovery in oligo- and euspermic semen. *Fertility and Sterility* 15, 511–527.

Morin, S, Keefe, D, & Naftolin, F. (2014). The separation of sexual activity and reproduction in human social evolution. *Advances in Experimental Medicine and Biology* 814, 159–167.

Naftolin F, Lavy G, Palumbo A, & DeCherney AH. (1988). Poissons, grenouilles, femmes et hommes: The appropriation and retention of archetypical systems for reproduction. *Gynecologic Endocrinology.* 2, 265–273.

Pincus, G. (1936). The parthonogenetic activation of rabbit eggs. *The Anatomical Record.* 67, suppl 1.

Pincus, G. (1939). Ovum culture. *Science.* (2318), 509.

(1940). Superovulation in rabbits.*The Anatomical Record* 77, 1–8.

(1944). The Hormone Conference in Quebec. *Science.* 100(2590), 143.

Pincus, G & Enzemann, EV. (1934). Can mammalian eggs undergo normal development in vitro? *Proceeding of the National Academy of Sciences* 20, 121–122.

Rebar, RW & DeCherney, AH. (2004). Assisted reproductive technology in the United States. *The New England Journal of Medicine* 350(16), 1603–1604.

Rock, J. (1963). *The Time Has Come.* Alfred A Knopf, New York.

Rock, J & Bartlett, MK. (1937). Biopsy studies of human endometrium: criteria of dating and information about amenorrhea, menorrhagia, and time of ovulation. *JAMA* 108(24), 2022–2028.

Rock, J & Menkin, MF. (1944). In vitro fertilization and cleavage of human ovarian eggs. *Science* 100(2588), 105–107.

Rock, J, Mulligan, WJ, & Easterday, CL. (1954). Polyethylene in tuboplasty. *Obstetrics and Gynecology* 3, 21–29.

Shettles, LB. (1955). A Morula stage of Human Ovum Developed in vitro. *Fertility and Sterility* 6(4), 287–289.

Speroff, L. (2009). *A Good Man: Gregory Goodwin Pincus: the Man, his Story, the Birth Control Pill.* Amica Publishing.

Urban, WJ & Smith, M. (2015). Much ado about something? James Bryant Conant, Harvard University, and Nazi Germany in the 1930s. *The International Journal of History and Education* 51, 152–165.

Yanagimachi, R. (2011). Problems of sperm fertility: a reproductive biologist's view. *Syst Biol Reprod Med* 57(1–2), 102–114.

Yanagimachi, R. (2016). M.C. Chang: a pioneer of mammalian in vitro fertilization. *Mol Reprod Dev* 83(10), 846–849.

Yanagimachi, R & Chang, MC. (1963). Fertilization of hamster eggs in vitro. *Nature* 200, 281–282.

(1964). In vitro fertilization of golden hamster ova. *Journal of Experimental Zoology Part A: Ecological Genetics and Physiology* 156(3), 361–375.

Selected Reading

Benagiano, G & Motta, PM. (2001). Robert G. Edwards and Ryuzo Yanagimachi and the Development of Modern Embryology and Human Reproduction. *Italian Journal of Anatomy and Embryology (Archivio italiano di anatomia ed embriologia)* 106(2 Suppl 2), XVII.

Cohen J, Trounson A, Dawson K, et al. (2005). The early days of IVF outside the UK. *Human Reproduction Update* 11(5), 429–459.

Henig, RM. (December 28, 2003). The Lives They Lived; Second Best. *The New York Times.*

Jones, HW. (2008). The use of controlled ovarian hyperstimulation (COH) in clinical in vitro fertilization: the role of Georgeanna Seegar Jones. *Fertility and Sterility* 90(5), e1–e3.

Chapter 4

The Story of Patrick Steptoe, Robert Edwards, Jean Purdy, and Bourn Hall Clinic

Peter R. Brinsden

To understand science it is necessary to know its history.

—*Auguste Compte, 1798–1857*

A thorough comprehension of the history of IVF will improve the depth of appreciation of challenges we are facing today, hopefully resulting in improved outcomes of future treatments.

—*Editorial. Human Reproduction, 2005*

The very close working relationship between physicians, scientists, nurses, counselors, administrators, and ethicists that exists in Assisted Reproductive Technology (ART) programs today is almost unique in the fields of medicine and science. The embodiment of this collaborative effort can be discovered in the close working relationship that existed between the "founding fathers" of ART – Patrick Steptoe and Robert Edwards. The coming together of Steptoe and Edwards in 1968 and their subsequent work, assisted by Jean Purdy, a key member of the team, finally culminated in the birth of Louise Brown, the world's first "Test-tube Baby," in July 1978.

In this chapter, the early history of in-vitro fertilization (IVF) is reviewed from the perspective of Patrick Steptoe, Robert Edwards, and Jean Purdy, who together "created" Louise Brown. An understanding and knowledge of the early history of IVF is important to the practice of IVF today. Although others had been involved in the early development of animal and later human IVF, as described in previous chapters, it was through the determination and dedication of Steptoe, Edwards, and Purdy, often through very difficult times and much opposition from colleagues (see Johnson, Chapter 5 in this volume), that they achieved this first IVF birth. This was some two years before workers in Australia, and later still in the United States, achieved their first births. The story of the Steptoe and Edwards' collaboration, their early years of disappointment and failure, culminating in their eventual success with the birth of Louise Brown

is a fascinating story (Edwards & Steptoe, 1980). Their influence on today's practice of ART, and even on our future practice, is still relevant.

Patrick Christopher Steptoe was born on June 19, 1913, the seventh of ten children. He came from a musical family, studied music as a child and nearly took it up as a career; however, he chose medicine and qualified as a doctor from St. George's Hospital, University of London, in 1939. At the outbreak of the Second World War, he joined the Royal Navy Volunteer Reserve as a surgeon. While serving in the Mediterranean, his ship was sunk and he became a prisoner of war in Italy. It is said that, because of his unique position as a Medical Officer, he was able to help fellow prisoners to escape; however, he was found out and put into solitary confinement. He was released in 1943. On returning to the United Kingdom he specialized in obstetrics and gynecology, with a special interest in infertility, and in 1951 became a Consultant at Oldham General Hospital in the North of England. There he had a large National Health Service (NHS) practice and it was there that he pursued and developed his interest in laparoscopy, which he had studied under both Frangenheim and Palmer in Europe. He developed the technique further, and finally published his seminal textbook *Laparoscopy in Gynaecology* in 1967 (Steptoe, 1967). During the early years of laparoscopy in the United Kingdom, this was the "bible" from which all young gynecologists, including the author of this chapter, learned the technique of laparoscopy. It was because of his ability to visualize the female pelvic organs during laparoscopy that he wrote his first major paper – "Laparoscopy and ovulation," published in *The Lancet* in 1968 (Steptoe, 1968). He also discovered that it was possible to aspirate oocytes from follicles under direct vision using a laparoscope, the experience of which he later published in 1970 (Steptoe & Edwards, 1970). This early pioneering work on laparoscopy caused much criticism and even hostility among Steptoe's peers, who branded it as an unsafe procedure that would "never catch on"!

Robert ("Bob") Geoffrey Edwards was born in 1925 and educated at Manchester Central High School. After doing his National Service in the Army, serving in Palestine, Syria, Jordan, and Iraq, he went to the University of Wales at Bangor in 1948. There, he gained his BSc degree, and then moved on to The Institute of Animal Genetics at Edinburgh University in 1951, where he worked on mouse oocytes and embryos, gaining his PhD in 1955. While he was there he met and later married another young scientist, Ruth Fowler, with whom he published several papers. From Edinburgh he went to California for a year and then, in 1958, moved on to The National Institute of Medical Research, London, where his interests changed from animal to biomedical research. It was during this time that he became interested in human oocyte development and the possibility of achieving in-vitro fertilization of human gametes. At the Institute he did some of the very earliest work on in-vitro maturation of human oocytes derived from small slices of human ovaries provided by a gynecologist in London (Edwards, 1965). He also at this time further pursued his interest in embryonic stem cells derived from mammalian embryos, which he further developed during a year spent at Glasgow University (Cole et al., 1965). However, Edwards then moved to the University of Cambridge in 1963 to join two of the "greats" in animal reproductive physiology - Professors Alan Parkes and "Bunny" Austin. There he continued his work on immunology and oocyte maturation. In 1965 Edwards spent some time in the United States at The Johns Hopkins University, where he collaborated with two other "greats" in the field of human ART - Drs. Howard and Georgeanna Jones (see Coddington and Oehninger, Chapter 7 of this volume). With them he continued his work on human oocytes (Edwards et al., 1966), and forged a lifetime friendship.

On returning to Cambridge, Edwards continued to have difficulty in finding human oocytes, not only for his research, but also in order to pursue his research on the treatment of human infertility. At that time he became aware of the work of Patrick Steptoe, who, by use of the laparoscope as described above, was able to view a woman's ovaries and who had developed a technique to aspirate oocytes from ovarian follicles. Edwards therefore contacted Steptoe in 1968 and expressed his interest in them working together. They subsequently met at the Royal Society of Medicine in London, where Patrick Steptoe was giving a lecture on laparoscopy, during which he showed the first laparoscopic photographs of ovaries in the female pelvis. Edwards approached Steptoe at the end of this meeting, introduced himself and suggested that they should collaborate – a suggestion that was readily accepted by Steptoe.

It was shortly after Steptoe and Edwards started their collaboration that Jean Purdy joined Bob Edwards as a laboratory research assistant in the Physiological Laboratory at the University of Cambridge. Jean was a nurse by training, and had been working at Papworth Hospital near Cambridge when she saw an advertisement for a job with Edwards. She went on to manage the IVF laboratory during the next 10 difficult years, when she and Edwards commuted regularly between Cambridge and Oldham – a distance of more than 200 miles. Without the scientific and managerial talents of Jean, as Edwards later fully acknowledged, they would never have achieved success. It was she who discovered the beautiful old Jacobean manor house near to Cambridge that was to become the famous Bourn Hall Clinic. Jean Purdy died in 1985 at the early age of 39 of a malignancy, having been the mainstay of Steptoe and Edwards in their work and in the development of the IVF program at Bourn Hall.

From 1968 until 1978, Steptoe, Edwards, and Purdy, conducted their early pioneering work on human IVF in Dr. Kershaw's Cottage Hospital at Royton, near Oldham. Very early in their collaboration they started to produce important papers on human IVF, including: "Identification of the mid-piece and tail of the spermatozoon during fertilisation of human eggs *in vitro*" (Bavister, Edwards & Steptoe, 1969), and "Laparoscopic recovery of pre-ovulatory human oocytes after priming of ovaries with gonadotrophins" (Steptoe & Edwards, 1970). They also carried out the first treatment cycles of oocyte recovery with tubal insemination (ORTI) (Edwards, 2009), which was later developed by others, becoming known as gamete intra-Fallopian transfer (GIFT). Other important papers included: "Control of human ovulation, fertilisation and implantation" (Edwards & Steptoe, 1974) and "Induction of follicular growth, ovulation and luteinisation of the human ovary" (Edwards & Steptoe, 1975). All of these papers, and others, were produced during a time of intense activity in Oldham, with Edwards and Purdy travelling hundreds of miles from Cambridge to Oldham and back on a regular basis.

During these early years there was much controversy and criticism of the work of Steptoe and Edwards, especially when they started their first human embryo transfers in 1972 (Edwards & Steptoe, 1980). Difficult

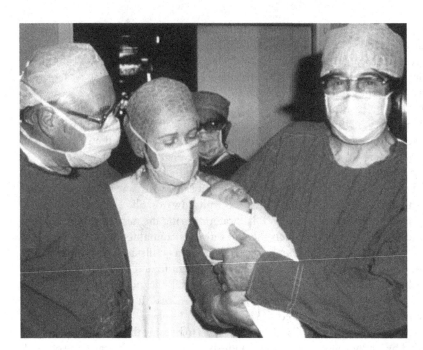

Figure 4.1 Patrick Steptoe, Jean Purdy, and Robert Edwards at the birth of Louise Brown on July 25, 1978.

years followed, in which none of their first 40 patients became pregnant until, in 1976, they did achieve their first IVF pregnancy. There was huge disappointment, however, when it was discovered that this was a tubal ectopic pregnancy (Steptoe and Edwards, 1976; Edwards and Steptoe, 1980). It is of interest to note that this pregnancy was achieved through a single blastocyst transfer! Later in 1976, a Mrs. Lesley Brown was referred to Steptoe for infertility treatment. Having failed to achieve a viable pregnancy after a total of 102 embryo transfers, Lesley Brown became pregnant at her first attempt. This success was achieved in a natural cycle IVF, with one oocyte collected, fertilized and transferred as an eight-cell embryo. Mrs. Brown suffered a difficult pregnancy, but Louise Brown was finally delivered by cesarean section close to midnight on Tuesday, July 25, 1978. Much to the relief of everyone, she was a normal, fit and healthy baby. (Figure 4.1). This momentous achievement was announced with a simple publication in a letter to *The Lancet* (Steptoe and Edwards, 1978), but was reported throughout the world with major headlines (Figure 4.2). The arrival of Louise was heralded as "The Baby of the Century." Indeed, the achievement of this birth has been compared in importance with other major world "firsts'" in medicine, such as the discovery of vaccination and penicillin.

Steptoe and Edwards experienced euphoria at that time, but also suffered intense criticism from a number of quarters. The Vatican stated that this was: "An event which can have very grave consequences for humanity," and Dr. James Watson, of the DNA helix discovery team, was quoted as saying: "This was dabbling with infanticide." The Archbishop of Liverpool, and others, said that it was "morally wrong." In spite of all this criticism, when Steptoe and Edwards presented the results of their work later in 1978 at the Royal College of Obstetricians and Gynaecologists in London, they received a standing ovation, something that had never occurred before in the whole history of the College. At the American Fertility Society meeting in 1978 they also received a standing ovation at the end of their presentation.

On January 14, 1979, they achieved the birth of their second baby, Alastair Macdonald, who was the world's first boy conceived by IVF. During the two years that followed these momentous events, no institution in the United Kingdom would provide any support or funding for Steptoe and Edwards to continue their clinical or research work. The National Health Service, universities, and the Medical Research Council were all unwilling to fund them to set up a clinic, and so they were forced to do so privately (see Johnson, Chapter 5 of this volume). This they did in Bourn, a village near

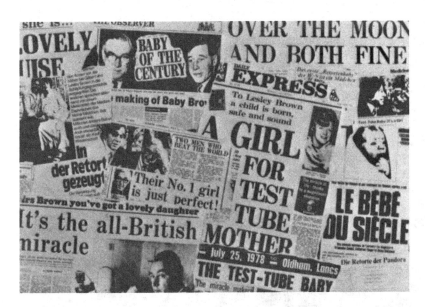

Figure 4.2 International press response to the birth of Louise Brown on July 25, 1978.

to Cambridge, in a beautiful old Jacobean manor house called Bourn Hall, where they founded the world's first IVF treatment and research centre – Bourn Hall Clinic.

On the site of the present building of Bourn Hall there was a moated castle dating from the eleventh century – the only remaining evidence being part of the old moat. The origins of the present house date from the reign of Queen Elizabeth the First, but it has undergone many changes, with the major part being Jacobean, around 1602. The house is surrounded by about 25 acres of parkland. The Hall has been repeatedly upgraded over the past 400 years. After the purchase of the Hall by Steptoe and Edwards in 1980, temporary "Portakabins" were used for the wards, theaters, and laboratories, while the new clinical and laboratory building was being built, which opened in 1987. Later still, a large clinical research unit was added. Meanwhile, elsewhere in the world work on human IVF was progressing and, in Melbourne, Australia, the world's fourth IVF baby, Candice Reed, conceived through the work of the team of Professor Carl Wood and Dr Alex Lopata, was born in June 1980 (Lopata et al., 1980; see also Lopata and Kovacs, Chapter 6 of this volume). The first IVF baby to be born in the United States was conceived in Bourn Hall, but the first baby conceived by IVF through the work of the pioneers Doctors Howard and Georgeanna Jones in America, Elizabeth Carr, was born on 28 December 1981 (Jones et al., 1982; also see Coddington and Oehninger, Chapter 7 of this volume).

Bourn Hall Clinic opened its doors in September 1980. Steptoe, Edwards, Purdy, and their team continued their research, achieving a number of key publications, including: "Current status of in vitro fertilisation and implantation of human embryos" (Edwards & Steptoe, 1983), in which they reported the results of their first 1200 IVF cycles, and noted an increase in clinical pregnancy rates from 16.5% initially, to 30% by 1983. In 1981 the world's first IVF conference was held at Bourn Hall, with many of the early pioneers of human IVF from around the world attending. A total of 30 clinicians and scientists took part in this very relaxed and informal exchange of information on the clinical and scientific aspects human IVF (Figure 4.3). In 1983, Bourn Hall initiated its first embryo cryopreservation program and the first births occurred in 1984.

I (Peter Brinsden) had worked at Bourn Hall for a short period in 1985 under Mr. Steptoe. I well remember being taught the art of laparoscopic oocyte collection under the stern guidance of Steptoe and later with the more gentle guidance of Dr. Jonathan Hewitt! At that time Dr. Rajat Goswamy had just joined the medical staff from King's College Hospital, where he had learnt the art of ultrasound guided oocyte recovery – at that time by the trans-abdominal ultrasound/transvesical needle technique. I well remember being in the operating theater when Mr. Steptoe, while watching Dr. Goswamy do one of these procedures, told him that "ultrasound egg collection will never replace laparoscopic collection." At the time, this view seemed quite reasonable, especially since Steptoe had pioneered

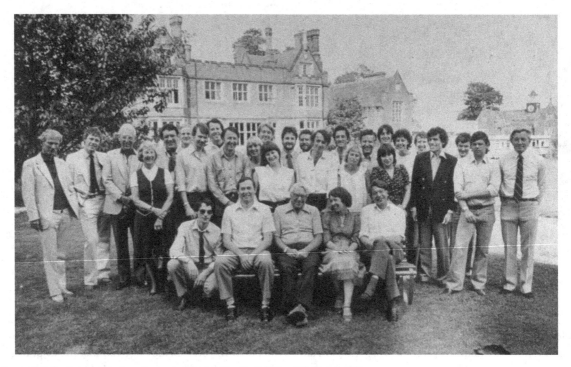

Figure 4.3 First international meeting on In-Vitro Fertilization at Bourn Hall Clinic in 1981.

laparoscopy in the UK in gynecology and later for the collection of oocytes.

After only two months at Bourn Hall, I was invited to join Professor Ian Craft in London as his Deputy Medical Director at The Humana Wellington Hospital, which, over the next four years, became the largest IVF Clinic in the world. Ian Craft should be remembered as another of the pioneers and innovators in IVF in England at that time, along with Dr. John Parsons of King's College Hospital, London, and Dr. Brian Lieberman in Manchester.

By 1986, it was estimated that 2000 babies had been born worldwide, 1000 of these from the Bourn Hall team. The team published their observations on their first 500 births in Human Reproduction in 1986 (Steptoe, Edwards & Walters, 1986). In the same year Drs. Howles and Macnamee published the first paper on tonic levels of luteinizing hormone in the follicular phase, which led to the use of gonadotropin releasing hormone (GnRH) analogs at Bourn Hall, the pioneering work for which had been done by Professor Ian Craft in London (Porter, Smith and Craft, 1984).

Patrick Steptoe was one of the "founding fathers" of the British Fertility Society in 1974. He served as the Society's Chairman from 1974 to 1986, and President from 1986 until his death in 1988. He also served as Chairman of the International Federation of Fertility Societies from 1977 to 1980, and was elected as the first English Vice-President of the American Fertility Society in 1986.

Patrick Steptoe and Robert Edwards were given a number of awards and honors by medical and scientific communities worldwide. They were both awarded the honor Commander of the Order of the British Empire (CBE) by Her Majesty the Queen in the New Years Honours List of 1988. Of particular pride to Patrick Steptoe was his election to Fellowship of the Royal Society (FRS) in 1988, an honor that has been afforded to very few clinicians in the history of the Society. It was unfortunate that, at the height of his achievements and fame, Patrick Steptoe fell ill with prostate cancer and finally died on March 21, 1988. Robert Edwards continued to work as Scientific Director at Bourn Hall and as Editor of the newly formed journal of The European Society for Human Reproduction and Embryology, *Human Reproduction*, which he co-founded. In 1994 he left to start up a new journal – *Reproductive BioMedicine Online*. He was succeeded as Scientific Director at Bourn Hall by Dr. Mike Macnamee.

Most readers of this book will be aware that Edwards, following his retirement from Bourn Hall, continued to write prolifically, lecture worldwide at conferences, and edit *RBM Online*! Two other notable triumphs in his career were for him to receive the Albert Lasker Foundation Award in 2001 and the Nobel Prize in 2010 for "the development of in vitro fertilization." He was knighted by The Queen in 2011 "for services to human reproductive biology," and thus became Professor Sir Robert Edwards, who, notwithstanding, will always be remembered by his friends and colleagues from all over the world as just "Bob." I think Bob would also have been flattered by knowing that in 2007 he was ranked 26th in the *Daily Telegraph* newspaper's list of the world's 100 greatest living geniuses! Bob Edwards died at his home on April 10, 2013, after suffering a long illness.

Following the death of Patrick Steptoe, Dr. Patrick Taylor, who was working with the team at the time as Deputy Medical Director, took over as Medical Director. Towards the end of 1988, however, he decided to return to Canada. He is now retired as Professor Emeritus of the University of British Columbia and has spent his retirement years authoring a series of humorous novels about the life of a country doctor in Northern Ireland, from whence he originally came.

After Patrick Taylor left Bourn Hall, the Clinic was purchased by Ares-Serono SA, a pharmaceutical company that specialized in fertility medications. Bourn Hall then merged with The Hallam Medical Centre, London, which was owned and run by Dr Bridget Mason, to form the Bourn-Hallam Group of IVF Clinics.

In January 1989, I was appointed as Group Medical Director of Bourn-Hallam, based mainly at Bourn Hall, while Dr. John Yovich, from Perth, Western Australia, was appointed Medical Director of The Hallam Centre, where he remained until August 1991, when he returned to Australia.

By the time I had returned to Bourn Hall in 1989, the new clinical and laboratory building was open. To commemorate the life and work of Patrick Steptoe, Bourn Hall invited the 1400 babies who had been born from the work of the Bourn Hall team, and their parents, to a dedication ceremony and a major celebration party. Over 660 children and their parents attended the party in the grounds of Bourn Hall. This was hosted by Professor Edwards and Mr. Steptoe's widow,

Mrs. Sheena Steptoe. They opened the new ward block and dedicated it to the memory of Patrick Steptoe.

In 1989 a program of seminars and workshops was started up under the leadership of Dr. Kay Elder, the Director of Training, with her strong medical and scientific expertise in IVF. Professor Edwards actively participated in these meetings, sharing with delegates his huge knowledge and enthusiasm for the subject. Kay Elder organized a wide range of programs for physicians, scientists, nurses, and others working in the field of IVF. In addition to writing and editing several textbooks on clinical embryology, Kay Elder was a founder member of Alpha – the international society for scientists in reproductive medicine, and, together with Professor Roger Gosden, founded the distance-learning MSc course on Clinical Embryology at the University of Leeds. Dr. Elder remains at Bourn Hall in the role of Senior Research Scientist.

Dr. Mike Macnamee has been at Bourn Hall as a scientist and endocrinologist almost since it first opened. He became deputy to Bob Edwards in 1989 and took over from him as Scientific Director in 1992, but in 1993 he became Director of Operations and then General Manager in 2001, and in 2002 was appointed Vice President Pre-Clinical Development in the Serono research laboratories in Italy. Dr. Sue Avery assumed the duties of Scientific Director in 1993, later moving to Birmingham as Director of the Birmingham Women's Fertility Centre. In 2005 there was a management buyout by the principal managers at Bourn Hall and Mike Macnamee became the Chief Executive, in which role he remains today.

In 1991 Bourn Hall published its first edition of *A Textbook of In Vitro Fertilization and Assisted Reproduction: The Bourn Hall Guide to Clinical and Laboratory Practice*, edited by Paul Rainsbury and Peter Brinsden, with second and third editions edited by Peter Brinsden in 1999 and 2005. Much of the content of these editions was based upon the teaching courses at Bourn Hall as well as our day-to-day clinical and scientific procedures and protocols.

In 2005, I retired from my role as Medical Director at the age of 65, but have remained a Consultant to the Clinic since them. I was succeeded by Dr. Thomas Mathews, who joined Bourn Hall in 1984, spent 10 years working elsewhere in IVF, and then re-joined the Bourn Hall team in 2000, becoming UK Medical Director in 2006, in which role he remains today.

In the past 10 years, Bourn Hall, under the direction of Mike Macnamee, has founded an international group of clinics, with branches in India and Dubai. It has also expanded in the United Kingdom, presently with clinics in six cities in the East Anglia region.

Patrick Steptoe and Robert Edwards, with the strong support of their colleague Jean Purdy, were very much aware of the personal and social consequences of infertility and were passionately committed to helping infertile couples by developing the science of IVF to circumvent the problem of infertility in the knowledge that, in most cases, the infertility itself was not curable.

This passion to help the infertile can be found in many of Patrick Steptoe's pre-Edwards papers. It is exemplified by his sheer dogged determination to pursue his ambitions for infertile couples, in spite of the hostility of the "establishment" and having to perform his pioneering laparoscopic work within the context of a very busy National Health Service gynecological and obstetric practice. Following the birth of Louise Brown in 1978, Steptoe was quoted as saying: "I am not a wizard or a Frankenstein. All I want to do is to help women whose child-producing mechanisms are slightly faulty" (*Time Magazine*, 1978).

Similarly, when one reviews some of the early papers of Bob Edwards, one can fully appreciate the real passion he felt then, to help infertile couples to have children. It is perhaps even more interesting, however,

to see how he displayed such an amazing, almost uncanny, ability to forecast the future clinical and scientific directions along which the field of human assisted reproduction would progress. Many of the advances that we take as recent developments in the field of ART, Edwards himself researched and/or predicted. In 1958 he developed the first embryonic stem cells from rabbit embryos (Cole et al., 1965), and forecast the potential therapeutic use of stem cells developed from human embryos. Many other of his forecasts are now in everyday use; for example, in 1965 he was able to mature human oocytes in vitro that could be developed for stem cell research. He also predicted preimplantation genetic diagnosis of embryos, sex selection, nuclear transfer, human cloning, blastocyst culture and transfer, IVF surrogacy, gamete intra-Fallopian transfer, the importance of avoiding multiple pregnancies, and the cryopreservation of human oocytes and embryos (Edwards, 2009). Looking to the future, it is likely that improved implantation rates will be achieved and single embryo transfer, probably at the blastocyst stage, will become the norm for the majority of patients. Embryo selection using techniques such as preimplantation genetic diagnosis and aneuploidy screening will increasingly be used, and factors affecting implantation, determined by genomic and proteomic

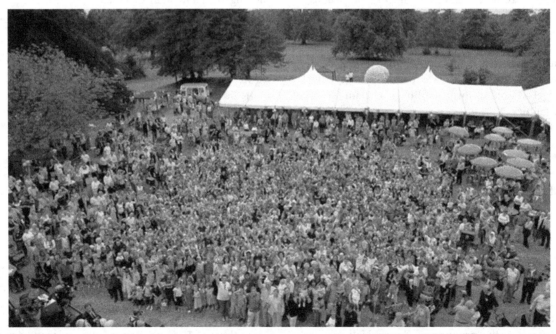

Figure 4.4 Bourn Hall's first "Baby Party" in the grounds of Bourn Hall in 1989. Louise Brown, Alastair Macdonald, and Robert Edwards are in the foreground.

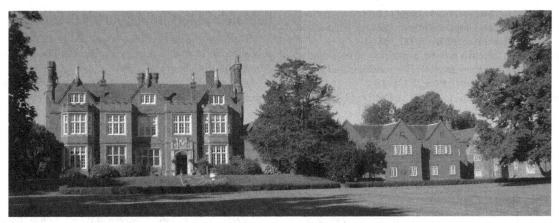

Figure 4.5 Bourn Hall Clinic as it is today.

techniques, increasingly will be employed to improve results of treatment. Cryopreservation of oocytes and ovarian tissue will become common, alongside in-vitro maturation of primordial and immature oocytes; all of which were forecast by Edwards.

It only seems like yesterday that we celebrated Louise's 25th birthday with another big party (Figure 4.4), and in 2018 we will celebrate the 40th anniversary of Louise's birth – now Louise Mullinder, with her own two (naturally conceived!) children. We should pay tribute to all the early pioneers of IVF worldwide, but, in particular to Patrick Steptoe, Robert Edwards, and Jean Purdy, who founded Bourn Hall Clinic, the world's first IVF clinic (see Figure 4.5). Their remarkable achievements are highlighted in this chapter, albeit only briefly. Their story can be followed in more depth by referring to some of the key references and publications given below. We, their scientific and clinical colleagues and friends, who had the privilege of working with them, acknowledge the truly remarkable contribution they made in their chosen field of IVF/ART, for which we all salute them. What greater testament could there be to a lifetime of dedicated work than to have been responsible, in very large measure, for the births of an estimated six million children worldwide!

Pygmaeos gigantum homeris impositos, pleusquam ipsos gigantes videri

(Dwarves on the shoulders of giants see further than the giants themselves).

Quote: Stella Didacus (1524–1578)

There cannot be the slightest doubt that it was he who had the notion that *in vitro* fertilization in the human was possible in spite of previous failures. Perhaps the greatest lesson was the demonstration of the power of intimate collaboration of basic and clinical science for the betterment of the human condition.

Quote from: "In the beginning there was Bob," Howard W. Jones Jr., Human Reproduction 1991

What does it mean to live a good and worthwhile life? One of the simplest ways of thinking about a good life is whether a person leaves the world a better place than they found it. I think in this respect, Patrick led a very good life, helping in his own way to make the world a better place.

Quote from a speech by Professor Andrew Steptoe, son of Patrick, at Bourn Hall Founders Day, July 2008.

References

Bavister, B.D., Edwards, R.G. & Steptoe, P.C. Identification of the midpiece and tail of the spermatozoon during fertilization of human eggs in vitro. *Journal of Reproduction and Fertility*, 1969; 2:159–160.

Cole, R.J., Edwards, R.G. & Paul, J. Cytodifferentiation and embryogenesis in cell colonies and tissue cultures derived from ova and blastocysts of the rabbit. *Developmental Biology*, 1965;13:385–407.

Edwards, R.G. Maturation in vitro of human oocytes. *Lancet*, ii, 1965; 926–929.

Edwards, R.G. 2009. Introduction: the beginnings of human in-vitro fertilization. In: Gradner, D.K. et al. (eds.) *Textbook of Assisted Reproductive Techniques.* Informa UK Ltd;17–30.

Edwards, R.G. & Sharpe, D.J. Social values and research in human embryology. *Nature*, 1971;231:87–91.

Edwards, R.G. & Steptoe, P.C. Control of human ovulation, fertilization and implantation. *Proceedings of the Royal Society of Medicine*, 1974; 67:932–936.

Induction of follicular growth, ovulation and luteinisation in the human ovary. *Journal of Reproduction and Fertility (Supplement)*, 1975;22:121–163.

Edwards, R.G. & Steptoe, P.C. 1980. *A Matter of Life*. Hutchinson, London.

Current status of in vitro fertilization and implantation of human embryos. *Lancet*, ii, 1983;1265–1270.

Edwards, R.G., Donahue, R., Bramki, T. & Jones, H. Jr. Preliminary attempts to fertilise human oocytes matured in vitro. *American Journal of Obstetrics and Gynecology*, 1966;192–200.

Jones, H.W., Jr., Jones, G.S., Andrews, M.C., Acosta, A.A. et al. The program for in vitro fertilization at Norfolk. *Fertility & Sterility*, 1982;38:14–21.

Lopata, A., Johnson, W.I.H., Hoult, I.J. & Spears, A.L. Pregnancy after intrauterine implantation of an embryo obtained by in vitro fertilization of a pre-ovulatory egg. *Fertility & Sterility*, 1980;33:117–120.

Porter, R.N., Smith, W., Craft, I.L., Abdulwahid, N.A. & Jacobs, H.S. Induction of ovulation for in vitro fertilisation using buserelin and gonadotropins. *Lancet*, ii, 1984;1284–1285.

Steptoe, P.C. 1967. *Laparoscopy in Gynaecology*. E. & S. Livingstone, Edinburgh.

Laparoscopy and ovulation. *Lancet*, ii, 1968;913.

Steptoe, P.C. & Edwards, R.G. Laparoscopic recovery of preovulatory human oocytes after priming of ovaries with gonadotrophins. *Lancet*, i, 1970; 683–689.

Reimplantation of a human embryo with subsequent tubal pregnancy. *Lancet*, i, 1976; 880–882.

Steptoe, P.C. & Edwards, R.G. Birth after reimplantation of a human embryo. *Lancet*, ii, 1978;366.

Steptoe, P.C., Edwards, R.G. & Walters, D.E. Observations on 767 clinical pregnancies and 500 births after human in-vitro fertilization. *Human Reproduction* 1986; 1:89–94.

Time Magazine The Test Tube Baby, July 31, 1978.

Research Papers from Bourn Hall Clinic

A full and up-to-date list of the books and research papers published by the staff at Bourn Hall Clinic can be found on our website: www.bournhall.co.uk

Look to the bottom of the "Home Page"; click "Our Family" and then "Research and Publications."

Other Recommended Reading

A Matter of Life, Robert Edwards and Patrick Steptoe. Hutchinson, London, 1980. (Revised 2nd edition published in paperback, 2012.)

Human Conception In Vitro, Robert Edwards and Jean Purdy. Academic Press, London, 1982.

Implantation of the Human Embryo, Robert Edwards, Jean Purdy, and Patrick Steptoe. Academic Press, London, 1984.

Life Before Birth, Robert Edwards. Hutchinson, London, 1989.

Textbook of In Vitro Fertilization and Assisted Reproduction: The Bourn Hall Guide to Clinical and Laboratory Practice, Ed. Peter Brinsden. Taylor and Francis, 2005.

Manual of Intrauterine Insemination and Ovulation Induction, Eds. Richard P. Dickey, Peter R. Brinsden, and Roman Pyrzak. Cambridge University Press, 2010.

In-Vitro Fertilization, Kay Elder and Brian Dale. Cambridge University Press, 2011.

Troubleshooting and Problem-Solving in the IVF Laboratory, Kay Elder, Marc Van den Bergh, and Bryan Woodward. Cambridge University Press, 2015.

My Life as the World's First Test-Tube Baby, Louise Brown. Bristol Books CIC, 2015.

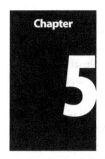

Professional Hostility Confronting Edwards, Steptoe, and Purdy in their Pioneering Work on In-Vitro Fertilization

Martin H. Johnson

Early Inklings of the Hostility

When, in 1965–66, I was in my third undergraduate year at Cambridge University, I experienced the first inklings of the professional hostility to which Bob was exposed. I was reading Physiology Part 2 of the Natural Sciences Tripos, and had started the year with no interest at all in the subject of reproduction. Indeed, I had been put off the subject by some rather dull and incoherent lectures given in the second year by Alan Parkes which featured ground squirrels rather heavily, with little of human interest for the budding doctor that I then intended to become, through my clinical placement the following year at Charing Cross Hospital in London. It was thus with some reluctance that I found myself with my 16 fellow students sitting in a lecture theater one autumn afternoon awaiting the first of eight lectures from a Dr. R. G. Edwards on the subject of Advanced Topics in Reproduction.

Then, three to four minutes late, there was a clatter of feet in the corridor, the doors burst open, and in Bob rushed dropping all his lecture notes as he apologized for being late, gathering them all up – apparently in random order – as his shirt tail flew out of the back of his trousers to flap around characteristically as he bounced about the room waving his arms and scribbling random and largely illegible words on the black board! After eight weeks of being challenged (often to the point of irritation!) by his comprehensive and futuristic vision of reproduction that encompassed endocrinology, immunology, cell biology, ethics, developmental biology, politics, population studies, his beloved genetics, and PEOPLE, I was hooked and inspired! Indeed, both myself and Richard Gardner, a fellow student on the course, were so hooked that we undertook a voluntary project with Bob attempting to visualize cortical granule release by staining them with acridine orange. Although this project was unsuccessful, I decided to postpone my clinical course at Charing Cross Hospital and commenced a PhD with him the following autumn, along with Richard – the happiest, if most daring, career move I could have made (Franklin, 2008).

However, when it became known around the department that two of the students who had got first class degrees had decided to do PhDs with Bob, the other staff members, including the most eminent amongst them, took us to one side and asked why were we going to waste our time on research with that charlatan, who spoke to the press and worked on stuff "down there." Why didn't we transfer to a more respectable and intellectually challenging problem on the brain, eye, ear, or nerve with one of them? This reaction provided us with the first hints, and some of the arguments used to support them, that Bob was not regarded highly by his peers.

And the full extent of the hostility soon became clear to us after we joined his slowly expanding group in October 1966 (Johnson et al., 2010). Thus, we worked at the top of the Physiological Department in a small group of rooms called the Marshall Laboratory, named after the founder of reproduction as a distinct subject: Tibby Marshall (Parkes, 1950). We used to go down mid-morning and afternoon to the first floor departmental tea-room for refreshments, and we soon learnt that if we sat at a table with some staff members they would get up and move tables rather than share with us. However, this ostracism was even worse for Bob, with very few members of the established scientific and medical community prepared to support him in his quest to fertilize human eggs in vitro (Edwards, 1965).

I include Jean Purdy with Edwards and Steptoe in deference to the wishes of both of these men that she should be given joint credit for their work (see Johnson and Elder, 2015b, for more evidence on this point).

However, he rarely showed how it must have been hurting him, usually laughing it off.

The 1969 *Nature* Paper and its Aftermath

Matters got even worse when the *Nature* paper describing evidence of successful IVF in humans came out in 1969 (Edwards et al., 1969). The press went to town on this publication, *Nature* editor John Maddox authoring a piece in the *Times of London* on St. Valentine's Day (the day before the *Nature* paper was published) announcing the "Move towards test-tube babies," which was syndicated round the world. Headlines such as "This human time bomb" and "'Next: chance to choose baby's sex" (*Daily Mail*), "Life outside the body" (*Daily Express*), and "Test tube baby factory" (*Sunday Mirror*) controversially put Edwards, Steptoe, and Purdy in the public eye. This press interest had been fed by the fact that, by 1969, although IVF had only been reported successfully in the rabbit, hamster, and mouse (Chang, 1959, 1968; Yanagimachi and Chang, 1963; Whittingham, 1968), uterine transfer of flushed in-vivo fertilized and cultured embryos had been more successful, and had been achieved in rabbit, goat, sheep, ferret, rat, mouse, cow, and pig (Betteridge, 1981; Hammer, 1998; Alexandre, 2001). These achievements had opened up the early mammalian embryo to experimental manipulation, an opportunity seized most strikingly by Andrzej Tarkowski and Beatrice Mintz during the 1960s (Graham, 2000). Human chimaeras, genetic selection, and modification, and even cloning, were all contemplated. In the general press and popular literature, therefore, human IVF presaged a near-future brave new world, a science-fiction vision of dystopia (Squier, 1994; Henig, 2004).

However, it was not only the press that was antagonistic. Several scientists expressed doubts about the validity of the work (Rothschild, 1969; Mastroianni and Noriega, 1970; Brackett et al., 1971), but these doubts were soon dispersed by the rapid subsequent success in developing human embryos in vitro (Edwards et al., 1970; Steptoe et al., 1971; Elder and Johnson, 2015a,b). Encouraged by their success, Edwards and Steptoe decided to approach the Medical Research Council (MRC) for long-term support. They wished, particularly, to bring Steptoe from his base in Oldham (near Manchester) to Cambridge so that Edwards and his nurse-assistant Jean Purdy would not have to travel to and from Oldham (Edwards and

Steptoe, 1980, pp. 97–98; 1985, p. viii). So in mid-1970, Bob and Patrick Steptoe applied to the MRC for funding for their research, and the way that the application was handled, and declined funding, illustrates neatly the level and range of professional antagonism to them and their work and provides insight into the then dominantly sceptical attitudes of reproductive scientists and clinicians towards human IVF research (Johnson et al., 2010). Thus the application was handled by Sheila Howarth (Lady McMichael; Owen, 2000), who was initially sceptical: Was the area "really ready for a full-scale clinical development as a priority area? It is certainly not 'population control,'" which had been identified as high priority. The proposal "bristles with difficulties practical, ethical and financial," and "Dr Edwards is not medically qualified, yet virtually all of what he is requesting relates to providing clinical facilities for patients. I would have thought that a unit of this size, without the active involvement of somebody who is already part of the current Cambridge clinical scene, would run into all sorts of problems." Also, they did not get support from the clinical school in Cambridge University, Theo Chalmers (the Medical School Dean) responding negatively to an enquiry from Howarth that it was "the view of the clinicians that any clinical appointment for Mr Steptoe would not meet the needs of the University for an academic obstetric teacher within the new medical school." Indeed, Steptoe had, as recently as 1968, failed to get appointed to a consultant's post in Cambridge because, as described by Turnbull, "he is now 56 or 57, I think, and it was decided to appoint a younger man." Ralph Robinson was that younger man and had been appointed on January 1, 1969 (Johnson et al., 2010).

The Referees' Reports

However, it is in the referee's reports on the final grant proposal submitted on February 10, 1971, that the most illuminating statements of professional attitudes emerge. As referees, Howarth chose Norman Jeffcoate (Professor of Obstetrics and Gynaecology at Liverpool, and President of the RCOG), Roger Short (then a veterinary lecturer at Cambridge), Geoffrey Harris (Professor of Anatomy at Oxford), H. John Evans (director of the MRC Clinical and Population Cytogenetics Unit in Edinburgh), Tony Glenister (Anatomy, Charing Cross Hospital Medical School ,London), and Stanley Clayton (Obstetrics and Gynecology, King's College London). It is clear from reading the reports that both

Jeffcoate and Short are essentially hostile to the bid. Thus Short begins his report with an amazingly prejudicial if honest statement: "Dr Edwards feels the need to publicise his work on radio and television, and in the press, so that he can change public attitudes. I do not feel that an ill-informed general public is capable of evaluating the work and seeing it in its proper perspective. This publicity has antagonised a large number of Dr. Edwards' scientific colleagues, of whom I am one." And Jeffcoate was almost as scathing, saying: "Indeed, both Mr Steptoe and Mr Edwards are, with the best of intentions, becoming over enthusiastic so that some of their work has attracted much publicity and also adverse criticism from the standpoint of medical ethics." In 1971, unlike today, medical professionals were still strongly discouraged from "self-promotion," including talking to the media (Loughlin, 2005; Nathoo, 2008, pp. 33–56).

Press interest had been an inevitable feature of their work (Anon, 1965, 1968; Byrne, 1965; Leach, 1966; Maddox, 1968; Wright, 1970) and Edwards, and to a lesser extent Steptoe, took a principled decision to engage with and educate the public in this controversial field (e.g. Edwards and Gardner, 1968; Edwards and Steptoe, 1980, pp. 101–102; Edwards, 1989, 2001, 2005a, b). Edwards was a visionary, who saw progress in this field as dependent on activism for social reform of the kind that had recently liberalized laws on abortion and homosexuality, but he also recognized the risk, writing in 1971: "Scientists may have to make disclosures of their work and its consequences that run against their immediate interests; they may have to stir up public opinion, even lobby for laws before legislatures." He saw the necessity to prepare society so it could "keep pace" with "the transition of scientific discovery into technological achievement" (Edwards and Sharpe, 1971). Taking this stand, which was later adopted by others in the 1980s (Mulkay, 1997; Braude, 2009), clearly harmed his case then with the MRC.

But problems with the press were not the main reason that their bid failed. There was a widespread view at that time that infertility was not a problem in which it was worth investing. Thus the 1960s and 1970s were socially and scientifically obsessed with world overpopulation, and this dominated UK and global policies on reproduction (Ehrlich, 1968; Pfeffer, 1993; Clarke, 1998, pp. 202–203; Connelly, 2008). Moreover, population-control interests also funded much reproductive research, including the Ford and Rockefeller Foundations, the Population Council, and the

International Planned Parenthood Federation (Clarke, 1998, pp. 207–230; Connelly, 2008, pp. 195–236). The United Nations Fund for Population Activities was established in 1968, and led in 1972 to the influential Human Reproduction Programme of the World Health Organization, with its focus on population control (Connelly, 2008, pp. 232ff). Indeed between 1965 and 1972, worldwide support for contraceptive research rose from $31 to $110 million (Marks, 2001, p. 31; Connelly, 2008, p. 233). Against this background, IVF for infertile patients was not considered seriously. Indeed, Edwards himself had initially seen IVF as providing primarily a way to study the origins of genetic disease in humans (Johnson, 2010). It was only after meeting Steptoe in 1968 that Edwards was converted to the view that infertility was a problem worth solving by IVF, and thereafter he was galvanized into action by the many heart-rending letters he received from couples "abandoned by the medical profession to their infertility."

This fashion for contraception had three unfortunate consequences for Edwards, Steptoe, and Purdy's work. First, since the most obvious use of IVF was to circumvent blocked tubes, it generated immediate opposition from those surgeons who were then treating this condition surgically, such as Robert Winston, who was later to apologize to Edwards for taking this stance. Since it also involved laparoscopic recovery of eggs, the considerable opposition to laparoscopy that had greeted Steptoe's advocacy since the mid 1960s of this revolutionary surgical approach (Steptoe, 1967; Edwards, 1989) was also marshalled against the three of them, and one of the leaders of the opposition was Jeffcoate, who describes Steptoe as "almost obsessed with the procedure," and "exaggerat[ing] its importance." "Knowing how obsessive is Mr. Steptoe's approach I think he would find it difficult to keep the reins on himself and remain critical and detached; the same too applies to Mr. Edwards." Expressing skepticism about Steptoe's accomplishments, Jeffcoate alleged that the technique is "easily learned and carried out by any competent gynaecologist," but then went on to say it was also risky: "no matter how expert the surgeon, laparoscopy is not without risks and, in this country in recent years, women have died as the result and have suffered serious injuries leading to medico-legal problems." In making this latter claim, Jeffcoate did not claim that any of these problems were associated with Steptoe himself, for which there is no good evidence, most hazards coming from diathermy using high-frequency currents to produce heat. Steptoe did not employ this approach and in more than 3000 cases had had no mortality and only occasional minor complications (Johnson et al., 2010). Jeffcoate also expressed concerns that Steptoe would lack the support of colleagues, claiming that he had "learned in confidence that none of the senior local gynaecologists have been consulted [about a local attachment for Steptoe] and, if they were, they would not be agreeable." It will be obvious that there is a lot of damning, if opinionated, innuendo in this report from Jeffcoate.

Second, the opposition used an argument still used spuriously today by some critics that, since we have a population problem, why make it worse by solving infertility? Thus Short's comments "it would be wrong to place a major emphasis on techniques for augmenting fertility in infertile patients when we desperately need methods for limiting fertility in the normal population." Both Edwards and Steptoe argued strongly against this view that the few infertile should be penalized for the profligacy of the many fertile.

The third and most serious consequence was that, because infertility was not seen as a problem worth solving – or able to be solved – by IVF, all the patients involved were seen as experimental subjects and not as patients undergoing an experimental treatment. This distinction had become important (Landsborough Thomson, 1975, p. 29), because of the atrocities committed by Nazi scientists and doctors during World War II (Valier and Timmerman, 2008), a distinction that had been set out by the MRC in 1964: "A distinction may legitimately be drawn between procedures undertaken as part of patient-care which are intended to contribute to the benefit of the individual patient, by treatment, prevention, or assessment, and those procedures which are undertaken either on patients or on healthy subjects solely for the purpose of contributing to medical knowledge and are not themselves designed to benefit the particular individual on whom they are performed. The former fall within the ambit of patient-care and are governed by the ordinary rules of professional conduct in medicine" (MRC, 1964, p. 178). Thus, the treatment component of the proposal was not registered by referees as relevant, and the women are generally described as though "purely" research subjects. "In my view it is also unethical to subject women, even volunteers, to laparoscopy for *purely experimental purposes* such as to obtain follicular fluid and granulosa cells. These procedures are not without hazard and, unless clearly in the interests of the women

concerned, cannot be justified" (Jeffcoate; my bold italics). Clayton envisaged "ethical difficulties" with ovulation induction and laparoscopy performed for "purposes of *research alone*." "The proposals are not entirely clear, but imply that some laparoscopic examinations would be *purely for research*." Short put it in a nutshell: "From the ethical viewpoint, it is one thing to subject a woman to a course of gonadotrophin therapy and a laparoscopy in order to treat her infertility. But is it justifiable to carry out these procedures solely for the *purposes of obtaining ova for in vitro experiments, which in themselves offer no immediate benefit to the patient?*" (Johnson et al., 2010).

Any novel treatment confronts the issue of risk and safety versus positive benefits. The problem for Edwards, Steptoe, and Purdy was that the only reference to potential benefit from the IVF procedure found in all the examined papers was in a pre-submission report from Turnbull, who raised, but immediately qualified, an ethical issue: "There might be worries about the normality of the children which were born if successes were ever achieved. On the other hand, I think these theoretical considerations might tend to be outweighed by the tremendous pressure which would be created by infertile women themselves, even if slight success could be achieved. When the first reports of this possible method of treating infertility appeared in the press, I had letters from a large number of women in Wales asking if there was any possibility if they could have 'test tube' babies. There is a relatively small number of women . . . who would be desperately anxious to conceive . . . ." Not only is the only statement found in the MRC archive of possible benefits to the infertile, but also even here these benefits are qualified as a minority interest.

It was not just British medico-scientists that criticized them and their work, but Americans too. Notably at a meeting in Washington, DC in October of 1971, when Nobel laureate James Watson of Harvard and others attacked Edwards saying that monsters would be born. Max Perrutz, British Nobel laureate, when asked to comment on Watson's remarks, supported them (Edwards and Steptoe, 1980, pp. 112–116; see also Kass and Glass, 1971; Watson in Anon, 1971a; Perutz in Anon, 1971b, c). Similarly, at an NIH meeting on gene therapy in the USA, a prominent, but unidentified, American mammalian developmental biologist is reported to have said that in her opinion the blastocysts grown in vitro were definitely abnormal and if implanted into a human uterus would almost certainly develop into monsters. Indeed, at the Washington meeting the British embryologist Anne McLaren stated: "I fear Dr Edwards will go too far, too fast. I am worried by the possibility that the desire to be first in the field will bias the judgment of those in a position to carry out egg transfer.... However, babies produced in a test-tube ... will be routine procedure within twenty years" (Johnson et al., 2010).

The MRC Takes a Stand

It is not therefore surprising that in April 1971 the MRC turned down the grant application, including the statement that in their judgment "Board members and referees however, all had serious doubts about the ethical aspects of the proposed investigations, especially those relating to the implantation in women of oocytes fertilized *in vitro*, which was considered premature in view of the lack of preliminary studies on primates and the present deficiency of detailed knowledge of the possible hazards involved. Reservations were also expressed about the procedure of laparoscopy for purely experimental purposes..." More seriously, this negative attitude towards IVF persisted until 1980. Indeed we have evidence that the MRC, contrary to an assurance given to Edwards that "Council leaned over backwards in trying not to influence decisions by other bodies," pressured local hospitals not to support his work and also informed the NIH (National Institutes of Health) in USA of their decision (Johnson et al., 2010). At a press conference on July 23,1974, the Secretary of the MRC, Sir John Gray said of human IVF work: "The Council would not fund research in the field unless they were provided with satisfactory evidence that there would be no increased risk of abnormal offspring." And although the MRC did subsequently award Edwards two project grants, neither was for human work: one in 1975 on "the growth and differentiation of graafian follicles in the ovary (rodents)," although a request "to extend the study to human follicles was declined," and a second in 1976 to "Dr Edwards and [Azim] Surani for work on the cellular and molecular aspects of blastocyst–uterine interactions at implantation (rodents)" (Johnson et al., 2010). Fortunately, the Ford Foundation, Oldham Area Health Authority, a private American donor, and the staff working on the project provided sufficient funds and support in kind, to keep the research going (Johnson and Elder, 2015c).

Moreover, this critical stance did not end immediately when Louise Brown was born in 1978 (Steptoe and Edwards, 1978). Thus, although at the time of her birth, the press generally was positive initially about IVF and the birth, hailing it as a major and heroic breakthrough for British science achieved in the face of considerable adversity (Dow, 2017), professional hostility only wavered. However, the MRC did change its stance towards IVF, largely due to the massive international publicity surrounding Louise Brown's birth. Thus, a report in *The Times* complemented "[t]he personalities of Mr Patrick Steptoe and Dr Robert Edwards" for the "way they perfected the method of *in vitro* fertilization against enormous odds. In all probability most other people would have found them insurmountable." The paper commented that "their fields of study do not figure on the Medical Research Council's and the Department of Health and Social Security's priority lists for the allocation of their overstretched resources" (Anon, 1978). This report clearly prompted David Ennals, the new Labour Secretary of State at the Department of Health and Social Security, on the same day that the article was published in *The Times*, to ask the new MRC Secretary, James Gowans, for a report on why the MRC had not supported the work, because "He feels vulnerable from a public relations point of view." Howarth provided a history on July 28, 1978. Then the MRC set up a small working group to review policy on human IVF. Given the proof of principle provided by two healthy births, one 11-week ectopic pregnancy, two chemical pregnancies (positive for pregnancy hormones, but no evidence of a sustained implant), one premature loss of a normal fetus at 21 weeks, and one miscarried triploid fetus (Elder and Johnson, 2015a,b), the MRC reconstructed IVF as an experimental treatment and no longer as purely a research procedure, and decided: (i) to endorse "scientifically sound research involving both human and non-human gametes, where there is no intention to transfer the embryo to the uterus ... and if the aim of the research is clearly defined and ethically acceptable"; (ii) "that consent... should be obtained... from the donor of both ovum and sperm"; and (iii) that "human IVF with subsequent embryo transfer should now be regarded as a therapeutic procedure covered by normal doctor/patient ethics" (Johnson et al., 2010). This change of policy, announced in the 1978/1979 Annual Report, not only provided all that Edwards and Steptoe had previously been denied, but also sanctioned the production of human–animal hybrids for research purposes, probably because Short wanted to use the hamster egg test to assess human sperm fertility.

41

This decision made the MRC a major supporter of research on human IVF and human embryo research (Gunning and English, 1993). Thus, they supported Angell's work showing that many human embryos were chromosomally abnormal (Angell et al., 1983), and also awarded a major program grant to Johnson, Braude, and Pratt in 1983 to "establish criteria of normal development in the human embryo" (MRC, 1983). However, when Edwards and Steptoe had again applied to the MRC for funding in 1981, again they were refused. And, moreover, they were criticized publically by Ian Craft in a 1981 article in *The Sunday Telegraph* (repeated in the *New Scientist* in July 1981 in a piece written by Donald Gould), which claimed that if Edwards, Steptoe, and Purdy had been more open about their methods then more IVF babies would have been born in the UK since 1979, a claim that Edwards strongly rejected, as they set up their new clinic at Bourn Hall.

The Opposition to Edwards, Steptoe, and Purdy Moves to Parliament

Thus, with the MRC onside, some of the hostility abated, but not in Parliament, which in 1984 debated the Warnock Committee Report, where for the first time in the conflict faced by Edwards, Steptoe, and Purdy the moral status of the embryo became the focus of concern. This committee had been set up by the government in 1982 to produce proposals for the regulation of IVF. It produced a report that recommended a body be set up to supervise IVF and the use of human embryos in research. In the Parliamentary debates immediately following the publication of the Warnock Report (July 19; Warnock, 1984), the majority of Lords (October 31, 1984) and Commons (November 23, 1984) who spoke were firmly against human embryo research (Theodosiou and Johnson, 2011). Alarmed by the anti-research rhetoric, scientists reacted. The MRC responded to a letter from Norman Fowler (then Secretary of State for Social Services, 1981–1987), who was worried about the pressure for a moratorium on research, and who proposed that the MRC and the RCOG set up a voluntary self-regulatory system. In reply, James Gowans confirmed that he was taking forward discussions on what would later (in March 1985) become the Voluntary Licensing Authority. Moreover, earlier in 1984, Peter Braude (clinician), Martin Johnson and Hester Pratt (scientists) at the University of Cambridge had embarked on a five-year program of research on human and animal embryos funded by the UK Medical Research Council (MRC Annual Report for 1983/4), much of which risked becoming prohibited. During November and December 1984, they initiated a pro-embryo research campaign, contacting sympathetic MPs, including Leo Abse, David Crouch, Frank Dobson, Willie Hamilton, Jo Richardson, Peter Thurnham, and Daffyd Wigley, and contributing letters and articles in the media. Then, on December 5 of that year, Ulster Unionist MP Enoch Powell introduced a Private Members' Bill to ban all production and use of human embryos, other than to help an infertile woman to become pregnant. This Bill, which if enacted would have prohibited all research on human embryos, galvanized further campaigning, Braude and his colleagues expanding their media activities, and organizing an "all party discussion on embryo research in the House of Commons" (Theodosiou and Johnson, 2011). Joining forces with Joanna Chambers, the General Secretary of the Birth Control Campaign, a lobbying group with well-established political contacts and the Women's Reproductive Rights Centre that, by November 1985, had consolidated formally into the campaign group Progress, they nonetheless failed to prevent a large Commons majority of 238:66 at the second reading of Powell's Bill on February 15, 1985 (Hansard, 1985). Shortly thereafter, Braude and Johnson wrote to Callum Macnaughton (President of the RCOG) and Gowans (copied to Anne McLaren and David Whittingham, both heads of MRC Units), asking for more direct administrative support for the campaigning. The MRC responded by assigning Dr Keith Gibson to help with the lobbying (Theodosiou and Johnson, 2011). Thus, the hostile Parliamentary responses to the Warnock Report together with the Powell Bill were both threatening medical research. Powell did not want to stop IVF as a treatment for the infertile: it was the use of embryos in research to which he objected as being both unethical and unnecessary. This objection to research provided the focus around which a coalition of his supporters rapidly formed to generate a powerful Parliamentary opposition, who, like Powell, appeared impervious to the fact that IVF was based on human embryo research. Fortunately, the pro-research coalition managed to fight successfully this attempt to prevent research, the Bill being talked out on June 17, 1985 (Theodosiou and Johnson, 2011). However, the BMA was to revive the issue of embryo research in a way that prompted Edwards to sue it for defamation.

Edwards, Steptoe, and Purdy versus the BMA

Edwards had agreed to give a talk by way of a telephone link-up at a meeting of the Medical Journalists Association at the Hilton Hotel, Gatwick on September 26, 1982, which he duly did and answered some questions afterwards. That evening, the Press Association put out a statement that started "Test tube baby pioneer, Dr Robert Edwards, disclosed today that he had carried out experiments on between 14 and 15 spare human embryos and he calls for this kind of research to continue . . ." and concluded "British Medical Association Secretary Dr John Harvard said later that Dr Edwards experiments were 'way ahead' of present day thinking." "For the time being we are not in favour of freezing and cloning human embryos, he said." The following day this report was carried in *The Times*, *The Guardian* and *The Daily Telegraph*, and Harvard was asked to appear on the World at One and News Night, where he said that the BMA's advice to its members was that they should not supply any embryos to Dr. Edwards. This remark led the following day to the *Daily Express* leading with a front page headline: "Test tube baby warning DON'T WORK WITH THIS MAN." Edwards' patience was exhausted by these events and on September 28, he initiated legal actions against several parties for defamation. The cases against the *Daily Express*, *The Times*, and the Press Association were all settled fairly rapidly in Edwards' favor, but that against the BMA dragged on until July 1985 when the BMA also admitted it had been wrong and agreed to pay Edwards' costs and damages. During this protracted period, it is clear that Edwards regarded the BMA's attitude as being high handed and arrogant.

Conclusions

It is often not now understood by the current practitioners of ART just how many socio-legal difficulties the early pioneers of IVF had to confront and overcome, in addition to the many technical difficulties they had to surmount (Elder and Johnson, 2015a,b). This applies not only to Edwards, Steptoe, and Purdy but also to Johnston, Wood, Lopata, and Trounson in Australia, and to the Joneses in the USA. This chapter has attempted to give a flavor of some of the medico-scientific opposition experienced by Edwards, Steptoe, and Purdy in the early days of ART. Of necessity, it is not exhaustive and neither does it acknowledge that a few individuals were not opposed to the three pioneers.

Thus, at the MRC, Malcolm Godfrey (Howarth's superior) and Graham Bull (director of the MRC Clinical Research Centre at Northwick Park (BMJ, 1969, 1970) were both sympathetic to their case, as was Graham Cannon (the secretary of the United Cambridge Hospitals Board), although for the latter two possibly more for reasons of self-interest, than sympathy with the aims of the three (Johnson et al., 2010). More positive and active support came from Bunny Austin, Bob Edwards' immediate superior in Cambridge, who defended their work in the press, and from Ivor Mills, who was prepared to be named as a collaborator on the 1972 grant application. However, undoubtedly the strongest and most crucial professional support came from the dedicated team of nurses and doctors at Oldham General Hospital, led by Muriel Harris, who gave their time and labor for free, usually at very antisocial hours outside of their normal working hours, to see the work through to the birth of Louise Brown (Johnson and Elder, 2015c). Notwithstanding this support, the overwhelming professional opposition to the work of Edwards, Steptoe, and Purdy was deeply isolating and depressing for the three of them, who were largely sustained by the many letters of support that they received from couples who themselves ironically had also experienced the isolation and misery to which their infertility had for so long exposed them.

Acknowledgments

I wish to acknowledge my thanks to the Edwards family for allowing me privileged access to the files relating to the legal cases, now deposited in the Churchill College archives. I also wish to acknowledge support from the Wellcome Trust (via grants 088708, 094985 and 100606), which otherwise had no involvement in the research or its publication.

References

Alexandre H. A history of mammalian embryological research. *Int J Dev Biol* 2001; 45:457–467.

Angell RR, Aitken RJ, van Look PF, Lumsden MA, Templeton AA. Chromosome abnormalities in human embryos after in vitro fertilization. *Nature* 1983; 303(5915):336–338.

Anon. Culture of early human embryos is imminent. *World Med* 1965; 1:19–21.

Controlling the sex of offspring. *The Times* 1968; April 26:4.

Test-tube baby work likely to go on despite U.S. criticisms. *Cambridge Evening News* 1971a; October 18:10.

Scientist warns on test-tube babies research. *Cambridge Evening News* 1971b; October 19:11.

Deformity fears over test-tube babies. *The Times* 1971c; October 20:2.

Men in the news: Mr Steptoe and Dr Edwards: birth is the fruit of years of study. *The Times* 1978; July 27:5.

Betteridge KJ. An historical look at embryo transfer. *Reproduction* 1981; 62:1–13.

BMJ. Northwick Park Hospital and Clinical Research Centre. *Brit Med J* 1969; 4 (5675) October 11:105.

Northwick Park Hospital and Clinical Research Centre. *Brit Med J* 1970; 3 (5722) September 5: 576–580.

Brackett BG, Seitz HM, Mastroianni L. In vitro fertilization: animal and human. *Adv Plan Parent* 1971;7:157–166.

Braude PR. Learning from history: the clinician's view. In: Watts G. (ed.) *Hope, Hype and Hybrids: Science Policy and Media Perspectives of the Human Fertilization and Embryology Bill*. London, UK: Science Media Centre, 2009, pp. 36–37.

Byrne A. Births by proxy: a brave new world in motherhood is near. *The Sunday Times* 1965; November: 7.

Chang MC. Fertilization of rabbit ova in vitro. *Nature* 1959; 184:466–467.

In vitro fertilization of mammalian eggs. *J Anim Sci* 1968; 27:15–21.

Clarke AE. *Disciplining Reproduction: Modernity, American Life Sciences, and 'the Problems of Sex'*. Berkeley, California: University of California Press, 1998.

Connelly M. *Fatal Misconception: The Struggle to Control World Population*. Cambridge, USA: Harvard University Press, 2008.

Dow K. 'The men who made the breakthrough': How the British Press represented Patrick Steptoe and Robert Edwards in 1978. *Reproductive BioMedicine and Society* 2017; 4:59–67.

Edwards RG. Maturation in vitro of human ovarian oocytes. *Lancet* 1965; 2:926–929.

Tribute to Patrick Steptoe: beginnings of laparoscopy. *Human Reprod* 1989; 4(Suppl.):1–9.

Edwards RG. The bumpy road to human in vitro fertilization. *Nature Med* 2001; 7:1091–1094.

Edwards RG. An astonishing journey into reproductive genetics since the 1950s. *Reprod Nutr Devel* 2005a; 45:299–306.

Introduction: the Beginnings of In-Vitro Fertilization and its Derivatives. Cambridge, UK: RBMOnline Publications, 2005b, pp. 1–7.

Edwards RG, Gardner RL. Choosing sex before birth. *New Scientist* 1968; 38:218–220.

Edwards RG, Sharpe DJ. Social values and research in human embryology. *Nature* 1971; 231:87–91.

Edwards RG, Steptoe PC. *A Matter of Life*. London, UK: Hutchinson and Co. Ltd, 1980.

Preface. In: Edwards RG, Purdy JM, Steptoe PC (eds.) *Implantation of the Human Embryo*. London, UK: Academic Press, 1985, pp. vii–viii.

Edwards RG, Bavister BD, Steptoe PC. Early stages of fertilization in vitro of human oocytes matured in vitro. *Nature* 1969; 221:632–635.

Edwards RG, Steptoe PC, Purdy JM. Fertilization and cleavage in vitro of preovulatory human oocytes. *Nature* 1970; 227:1307–1309.

Ehrlich PR. *The Population Bomb*. New York, USA: Ballantyne Books, 1968.

Elder K, Johnson MH. The Oldham Notebooks: an analysis of the development of IVF 1969–1978. II. The treatment cycles and their outcomes. *Reproductive BioMedicine and Society* 2015a; 1:9–18.

The Oldham Notebooks: an analysis of the development of IVF 1969–1978. III. Variations in procedures. *Reproductive BioMedicine and Society* 2015b; 1:19–33.

Franklin S. Interview transcript with Martin Johnson, the history of mammalian developmental biology interviews, The British Library, C1324/14, 2008.

Gould D. Private medicine. *New Scientist* 1981; July 2 91(1260):40.

Graham CF. Mammalian development in the UK (1950–1995). *Int J Dev Biol* 2000;44:51–55.

Gunning J, English V. *Human in Vitro Fertilization. A Case Study in the Regulation of Medical Innovation*. Aldershot, UK: Dartmouth Publishing, 1993.

Hammer RE. Egg culture: the foundation. *Int J Dev Biol* 1998;42:833–839.

Hansard. Unborn Children (Protection) Bill. HC Deb 15 February 1985; 73:cc637–702.

Henig RM. *Pandora's Baby: How the First Test-Tube Babies Sparked the Reproductive Revolution*. New York: Houghton Mifflin, 2004.

Johnson MH. Robert Edwards: the path to IVF. *Reprod BioMed Online* 2011; 23:245–262.

Johnson MH, Elder K. The OldhamNotebooks: an analysis of the development of IVF 1969-1978. IV. Ethical aspects. *Reproductive BioMedicine and Society* 2015a; 1: 34–45.

The Oldham Notebooks: an analysis of the development of IVF 1969–1978. V. The role of Jean Purdy reassessed. *Reproductive BioMedicine and Society* 2015b; 1:46–57.

The Oldham Notebooks: an analysis of the development of IVF 1969–1978. VI. Sources of support for, and expenditure on, the work. *Reproductive BioMedicine and Society* 2015c; 1:58–70.

Johnson MH, Franklin SB, Cottingham M, Hopwood N. Why the Medical Research Council refused Robert Edwards and Patrick Steptoe support for research on human conception in 1971. *Hum. Reprod.* 2010; 25:2157–2174.

Kass LR, Glass B. What price the perfect baby? *Science* 1971; 173:103–104.

Landsborough Thomson A. *Half a Century of Medical Research, Volume 2: The Programme of the Medical Research Council (UK)*. London, UK: Medical Research Council, 1975.

Leach E. Test-tube babies. *New Statesman* 1966; March 4:293–294.

Loughlin K. Spectacle and secrecy: press coverage of conjoined twins in 1950s Britain. *Med Hist* 2005; 49:197–212.

Maddox J. Test-tube babies—the hazards and the hopes. *The Times* 1968; February 26:11.

Marks LV. *Sexual Chemistry: A History of the Contraceptive Pill*. New Haven, USA: Yale University Press, 2001.

Mastroianni L, Noriega C. Observations on human ova and the fertilization process. *Am J Obs Gynec* 1970; 107:682–696.

MRC. Responsibility in investigations on human subjects: statement by Medical Research Council. *Br Med J* 1964; 2 (5402) July 18:178–180.

The MRC Annual Report for 1983–84, 1983.

Mulkay M. *The Embryo Research Debate: Science and the Politics of Reproduction*. Cambridge, UK: Cambridge University Press, 1997.

Nathoo A. *Hearts Exposed: Transplants and the Media in 1960s Britain*. Basingstoke, UK: Palgrave Macmillan, 2008.

Owen G. Sheila Mary Howarth. *Brit Med J* 2000; 321:964

Parkes AS. Francis Hugh Adam Marshall. 1878–1949. *Obituary Notices of Fellows of the Royal Society* 1950; 7:238–251.

Pfeffer N. *The Stork and the Syringe: A Political History of Reproductive Medicine*. Cambridge, UK: Polity Press, 1993.

Rothschild. Did fertilization occur? *Nature* 1969; 221:981.

Squier, S. *Babies in Bottles: Twentieth-Century Visions of Reproductive Technology*. New Jersey, USA: Rutgers University Press, 1994.

Steptoe PC. *Laparoscopy in Gynaecology*. Edinburgh, Scotland: Livingstone, 1967.

Steptoe PC, Edwards RG. Birth after the reimplantation of a human embryo. *Lancet* 1978; 2:366.

Steptoe PC, Edwards RG, Purdy JM. Human blastocysts grown in culture. *Nature* 1971; 229:132–133.

Theodosiou AA, Johnson MH. The politics of human embryo research and the motivation to achieve PGD. *Reprod BioMed Online* 2011; 22:457–471.

Valier H, Timmermann C. Clinical trials and the reorganization of medical research in post-Second World War Britain. *Med Hist* 2008; 52:493–510.

Warnock M. *Report of the Committee of Inquiry into Human Fertilisation and Embryology*. London, UK: HMSO, 1984.

Whittingham DG. Fertilization of mouse eggs in vitro. *Nature* 1968; 220:592–593.

Wright P. Progress towards 'test-tube' baby. *The Times* 1970; February 24:1.

Yanagimachi R, Chang MC. Fertilization of hamster eggs in vitro. *Nature* 1963; 200:281–282.

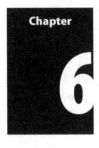
The Development of In-Vitro Fertilization in Australia

Alex Lopata and Gabor Kovacs

Introduction: 1971–1980 – Alex Lopata

In Australia, the development of in-vitro fertilization for the treatment of infertility began at the Monash University Department of Obstetrics and Gynaecology, at the Queen Victoria Medical Centre. This was a hospital in central Melbourne that had a compelling history in the primary care of women's health and welfare. It was initially established in 1896 as a Women's Clinic in St David's Hall, Latrobe Street, by Dr. Constance Stone and some of the first women medical graduates in Melbourne. By 1900 the clinic moved to a new site and became the Queen Victoria Hospital, located at the School for Working Women. After the death of Queen Victoria in 1901, the hospital added Memorial to its name. In 1946 the hospital moved to its main location, previously used by the Royal Melbourne Hospital. At this stage the Queen Victoria Memorial Hospital cared exclusively for women and was managed entirely by women doctors. It was not until 1965, when it became a teaching hospital linked to Monash University, that it became a general family hospital, and its name changed to Queen Victoria Medical Centre (QVMC). Professor Carl Wood became the founding head of Obstetrics and Gynaecology at the hospital. In 1971, Professor Wood appointed Dr. Alex Lopata to begin work on human in-vitro fertilization (IVF) in his Department.

Background

What type of information was available in 1971, on the fertilization of human oocytes in tissue culture, at the time when Carl Wood decided to start a program of IVF in his department? In 1965 Robert Edwards and Howard Jones, at Johns Hopkins Hospital, resumed the studies on human IVF that were abandoned by Menkin and Rock (1948). When Edwards began attempts at human IVF, it was known that sperm needed to undergo capacitation and he used various attempts to induce this process, both *in vivo* and in vitro. Despite various creative methods to achieve sperm capacitation, it is unlikely that fertilization was obtained in the 191 follicular oocytes that were matured and inseminated in vitro (Edwards et al., 1966). In 1968 Edwards met Patrick Steptoe, who was using laparoscopy for gynecological procedures, and both realized that this technique could be used for collecting oocytes that were maturing in pre-ovulatory ovarian follicles. By 1971 two other groups made partly successful attempts to fertilize human follicular eggs that were matured in vitro and inseminated with presumed capacitated sperm (Jacobson et al., 1970; Seitz et al., 1971).

Beginning of IVF in Melbourne

At the QVMC in 1971, Lopata occupied an office connected to a room that he transformed into the first IVF laboratory in Australia. The laboratory and some of the equipment are shown in Figure 6.1. In the photograph, Carl Wood and John Leeton, who aspirated oocytes from infertile patients, are seated on either side of Lopata, who performed oocyte cultures, sperm preparations, in-vitro inseminations, and the culture of fertilized eggs in preparation for embryo placement in the uterine cavity of the patients. When the project started, oocyte recoveries for testing IVF procedures began slowly because of the low number of patients available in 1972. Lopata proposed that the developmental work would be enhanced considerably if our group combined with the Infertility Clinic headed by Dr. Ian Johnston at the Royal Women's Hospital (RWH), which was located close to the QVMC. Carl Wood readily agreed with this proposal and Dr. Johnston enthusiastically accepted the idea of setting up an IVF program at RWH. Lopata recalls that when he outlined the purpose of his visit to RWH, Johnston's immediate response was "How the hell did you know that I wanted to set up an IVF clinic here?"

At the RWH, the only space that could be found for an IVF laboratory, near the operating theaters, was

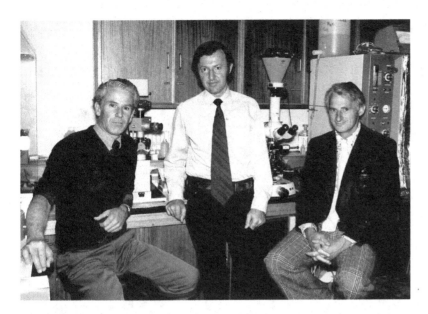

Figure 6.1 John Leeton (on left), Alex Lopata (center), and Carl Wood (on right) in the newly established IVF laboratory, in the Monash University Department of Obstetrics and Gynaecology, at the Queen Victoria Medical Centre.

Table 6.1 A comparison of oocyte recovery and fertilization rates in stimulated and un-stimulated cycles

Patients	Pre-ovul. oocytes	Non-ovul. oocytes	Inseminated	Degen	One-cell stage	Cleaved
Clomiphene + HCG group						
13	10	7	17 (1.3 / patient)	6	9	2* (11.8%)
No ovarian stimulation						
4	4	6	10 (2.5 / patient)	4	3	3 (30%)

a janitor's storage room. After constructing benches and installing scientific equipment, this newly refurbished IVF laboratory had room for only two people. Visitors who inspected the cramped space claimed that they have never encountered a smaller laboratory. Nevertheless, this became Australia's second IVF laboratory and the collaborative work with the QVMC more than doubled the patients participating in the project. With two groups working on the project, by the end of 1973, effective equipment and conditions were developed for aspirating ovarian follicles at laparoscopies and laparotomies. When results were combined from the two IVF groups, 45 laparoscopies had yielded 109 oocytes and 25 laparotomies produced 108 oocytes. It was also realized that oocytes may have been damaged when laparoscopies were performed using 100% carbon dioxide (CO_2) or nitrous oxide for the pneumo-peritoneum. Both groups agreed to employ a gas phase of 5% CO_2 in air, or even 5% CO_2 + 5% O_2 + 90% N_2. The results of these early studies were published jointly (Lopata et al., 1974).

First Human Embryos

In 1973, at the QVMC, a small trial was conducted to evaluate the recovery of oocytes, as well as their ability to be fertilized, after treating women with clomiphene and HCG, when compared with eggs obtained from untreated reproductive cycles. The results are summarized in Table 6.1. Eggs from both groups were fertilized in vitro and produced embryos that showed cell divisions in tissue culture. These were the first embryos that we observed in our IVF program. One of the embryos, derived from a woman treated with clomiphene and HCG, developed eight very regular cells that looked as if they would continue to divide. As we were inexperienced in judging embryos, Carl Wood invited a veterinary embryologist, R. A. S. Lawson from the Werribee Research Institute, to provide an

47

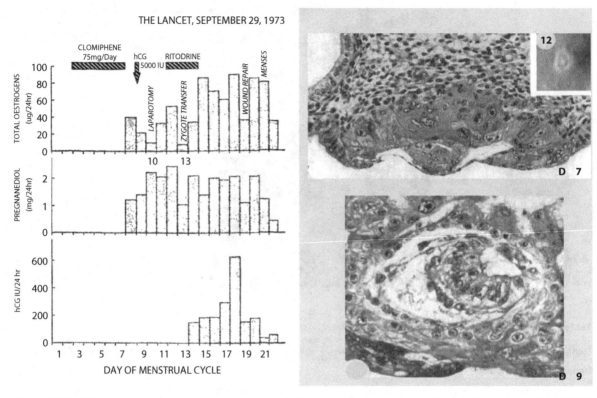

THE LANCET, SEPTEMBER 29, 1973

Figure 6.2 The histograms show the time sequence of ovarian stimulation and the daily urinary levels of estrogens, pregnanediol, and HCG in relation to the transfer of an embryo into the uterus on day 13 of the treatment cycle. The micrographs next to the histograms show the expected day 7 and day 9 stages of blastocyst implantation in the endometrium, based on the specimens described by Hertig et al. (1956).

opinion. Dr. Lawson considered that the embryo had normal morphology and agreed with our opinion that it should be transferred into the patient's uterine cavity.

A Promising Early Success

The time sequence of events that gave rise to a viable embryo, which was placed in the uterus to produce an early pregnancy, is shown in Figure 6.2. The woman received an injection of 5000 IU of HCG on day 9 of her cycle and 24 h later, on day 10, she had a laparotomy for clearing pelvic adhesions and aspirating ovarian follicles. An oocyte surrounded by cumulus cells was aspirated from a 9 mm follicle. The egg was incubated in its own follicular fluid for 4 h, at 37 °C in a humidified atmosphere of 5% CO_2 + 5% O_2 + 90% N_2. During this interval her husband's semen was diluted in modified Tyrode's solution and centrifuged, the sperm pellet was diluted again and centrifuged to obtain washed sperm pellet that was free of seminal plasma. A final sperm pellet dilution provided about 600,000 motile sperm in 1 ml of Tyrode's, supplemented with

albumin, was used for inseminating the oocyte. After 20 h in the sperm suspension the oocyte was transferred into a culture medium, known as Ham's F10 supplemented with 20% foetal-calf serum. By 74 h after insemination an eight-celled embryo was observed in the medium. This corresponded to day 13 of the cycle, when the embryo was gently drawn into the tip of a narrow polyethylene tube, which was passed through the patient's cervix, and the embryo released into her uterine cavity. The woman's urine was collected daily starting before oocyte retrieval and continuing after her embryo was placed in the uterus, to measure the output of estrogens and progesterone from her ovaries, as well as HCG to detect the possibility of an early pregnancy. Since the woman was given an injection of HCG on day 9 of her cycle, the level of this hormone in her urine should have decreased over the next few days. But instead of diminishing, her HCG levels began to rise over the next five days, attaining levels seen in early pregnancy. This HCG output suddenly stopped, on the day when her surgical wound burst open and she had to

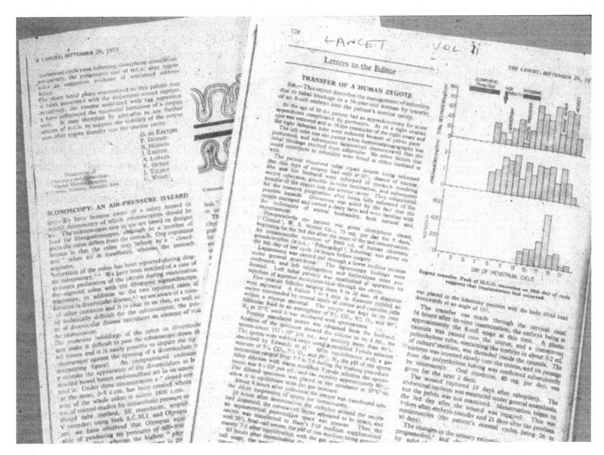

Figure 6.3 The report in *The Lancet*, 1973 (de Kretzer et al., 1973).

have emergency repair of her abdomen. These changes in urinary hormone levels are shown in Figure 6.2. In addition, the stages of embryonic development, possibly attained inside the uterus, which may have produced the increasing levels of HCG, are also illustrated in this figure.

A Report of Early Success

An article describing the early pregnancy, resulting from our work in the newly established IVF laboratory at the QVMC, was written jointly by Carl Wood and Alex Lopata. The novel laboratory work, leading to this early, but preliminary, success, was acknowledged unanimously by our team and a decision was made that Alex Lopata should be the first author. Carl Wood then asked John Leeton to submit the article for publication in *The Lancet* (Figure 6.3). Inexplicably, Leeton disregarded the team's decision, and chose to change the list of authors to an alphabetical order (De Kretzer

et al., 1973). The surnames of two project consultants and the biochemist responsible for routine urine tests, were placed at the front of the author list, whereas the team members contributing to the creative work, were relegated to the end of the list. After the article was published, Lopata was shocked by this betrayal of trust. Thirty years later, in a talk that John Leeton gave at a meeting of the Fertility Society of Australia in 2003, he publicly apologized to Lopata for rearranging the authors of the paper. In his apology, Leeton did not explain why he decided to change the order of authors, but he admitted publicly that he had made a mistake.

Attempts to Improve Outcomes

During the mid 1970s our main objective was to increase the number of mature oocytes that could be aspirated from the ovaries of infertile patients undergoing laparoscopies in both IVF programs. We predicted that collecting more oocytes from each patient

Table 6.2 A comparison of three methods used to stimulate the ovaries of infertile patients in preparation for oocyte collections

Stimulation Method	Treatment cycles	Recovery of mature oocytes	Oocytes per patient
HPG[a]	27	108	4.0
Clomiphene citrate (CC)[b]	35	54	1.5
CC + HPG	25	64	2.7

[a]HPG = Human pituitary gonadotrophin.
[b]HPG vs. CC: $X^2 = 9.07$, $P = 0.003$; other comparisons not significant.

oocytes that were capable of developing into implanting blastocysts that produced early pregnancies. This encouraged us to embark on a program of refining ovarian stimulation with clomiphene and HCG (Lopata et al., 1978a). The report evaluates three protocols, using 50–100 mg of clomiphene daily for five days, followed by either a single or double dose of HCG, and in one protocol further HCG was given to support the luteal phase. All of these protocols yielded embryos that were transferred into the uterine cavity of patients, but none produced a lasting pregnancy. Nevertheless this study set the scene for effective ovarian stimulation with clomiphene and HCG, but the remaining challenge in 1977, the establishment of ongoing pregnancies, still needed to be solved.

was essential for improving and optimizing the laboratory procedures. Lopata also postulated that a more physiological method for sperm preparation could improve IVF outcomes. Combined with these ideas we also believed that it is important to gain insight into the composition of human tubal fluid, the natural milieu in which fertilization occurs, to maximize sperm penetration into mature eggs. All of these ideas were included in our research and are briefly described in the paragraphs that follow.

Monitoring Ovarian Follicles

From 1976 to 1978 Dr. John McBain, a gynecological endocrinologist, became directly involved with the ovarian stimulation program both at the QVMC and at RWH. Professor James Brown, at the University of Melbourne Department of Obstetrics and Gynaecology, donated human pituitary gonadotrophin (HPG) for ovarian stimulation, and arranged urinary estrogen assays to monitor the ovarian responses, at both centers. Under McBain's guidance, ovarian stimulation with HPG, as well as clomiphene with HPG, significantly improved oocyte recovery at both IVF Units (Table 6.2). The increased yield of oocytes per patient was particularly marked when the ovaries were stimulated with HPG alone. Some of these results were published as preliminary reports (Talbot et al., 1976).

Improving Ovarian Stimulation

We knew from our work in 1973 that a five-day course of pre-ovulatory clomiphene, combined with an ovulatory injection of HCG, could produce fertilizable

Novel Sperm Preparation

When semen is ejaculated into the vagina during intercourse the seminal plasma comes into contact with the mucus in the external opening of the cervix. Almost immediately sperm begin to swim into the mucus that fills the canal of the cervix. Within about 10 min the fastest sperm enter the uterine cavity and by about 30 min sperm enter the Fallopian tubes. This is the natural mechanism that separates motile sperm from the seminal plasma in the vagina, beginning the journey during which spermatozoa become capacitated, and reach the site of fertilization within a Fallopian tube. In 1975 we devised a laboratory method that imitates the process of sperm migration out of the seminal plasma (Lopata et al., 1976). The simple method consisted of several sterile Pasteur pipettes with wide tips, filled with culture medium, and vertically dipped into semen. By 30 min highly motile sperm migrated to the top of the liquid column. The lower half of the medium was discarded in case some seminal plasma diffused a short distance into the liquid. The upper half of the medium contained very active sperm suspensions that produced better fertilization rates than sperm washings prepared by two centrifugations (Table 6.3). In the 1980s, newly established IVF groups adopted a combination of centrifugation of diluted semen followed by a swim-up procedure from the sperm pellet, after the medium over the pellet was replaced with fresh medium.

The Tubal Environment

The composition of human tubal fluid was determined from tiny samples obtained by means of fine catheters, inserted into the lumen of Fallopian tubes, at

Table 6.3 A comparison of oocyte recovery and fertilization rates following ovarian stimulation using Human Pituitary Gonadotrophin (HPG)

Patients	Follicles aspirated	Follicles per patient	Pre-ovulatory oocytes	Oocytes inseminated	Embryos cultured	ETs[a]
Royal Women's Hospital						
71	323	4.6	79 (1.1 / patient)	48	27 (56.3%)	15
Queen Victoria Medical Centre						
12	63	5.3	32 (2.7 / patient)	26[b]	20 (76.9%)	8

[a]ETs = embryo transfers.
[b]Insemination suspensions from sperm swim-up into culture medium.

laparoscopies in patients treated with HPG for oocyte recovery. The physiological tubal fluid was remarkably similar to the media used for washing sperm and for the fertilization process. The main differences were the much lower level of lactate and higher levels of iron, copper, and zinc in the real tubal fluid. In the years that followed, during the period of rapid establishment of IVF clinics, commercial companies used the results of our studies on the composition of tubal fluid to manufacture culture media for the fertilization process.

In 1977 attempts were made to transfer washed sperm together with a mature egg into a Fallopian tube during several laparoscopies. When this failed to produce a pregnancy, we transferred eggs fertilized in vitro, at the pronucleate stage, into the tubal environment, hoping they would develop within their natural milieu. These endeavors also failed to produce pregnancies.

Viewing the Fertilization Process

Our combined group demonstrated for the first time all the definitive parameters of in-vitro fertilization by using pre-ovulatory oocytes obtained from ovarian follicles during natural menstrual cycles (Lopata et al., 1978b). Within 3 h after insemination, fertilization was authenticated in serially sectioned oocytes. These oocytes contained a decondensing sperm head and mid-piece in the cytoplasm, together with an extruding second polar body. A cortical granule reaction had also occurred, confirmed by the absence of these dark granules from the surface of the egg. By 6 h after insemination, early female and male pronuclei were present in the vicinity of two polar bodies that were in the perivitelline space. These studies

established clearly that sperm capacitation occurred in 3 h, or sooner, after sperm preparation in vitro. Very similar results were obtained in studies examining the ultrastructure of pre-ovulatory oocytes, obtained at laparoscopies, from infertile patients treated with clomiphene and HCG, that were inseminated in vitro (Lopata et al., 1980a). In these studies, electron microscopy was used to reveal additional information on the cytoplasmic organelles, cell membrane changes, and meiotic chromosome distribution involved in the dynamics of fertilization.

Changes in the IVF Team

In 1977 Dr. Alan Trounson joined the group that was working on IVF at the QVMC. In the early 1970s Trounson specialized in animal embryology, and general reproductive biology, in Jerilderie NSW and Cambridge UK, producing results that were highly relevant for human IVF (Trounson et al., 1976). Lopata recalls that this was an eventful advance of expertise for the IVF team. Exchanging valuable information boosted the morale of the evolving project. Unexpectedly, all of this optimism ended abruptly in 1978. Carl Wood, perhaps encouraged by Leeton and Trounson, made a decision that required Lopata and Trounson to work separately, as if they were competing teams. All collaboration ceased, sharing of ideas ceased, mutual problem solving ceased, even conversation ceased. We were excluded from each other's laboratories, so that when Lopata performed IVF work, Trounson was excluded, and when the latter was involved with IVF, Lopata was shut out. As a united team, we may have been able to produce the world's first IVF births, but a lack of vision destroyed this opportunity.

51

Birth of an IVF Baby in England

In 1978 Robert Edwards and Patrick Steptoe reported the birth of Louise Brown, their first IVF baby, in Oldham. We were avid for insights into the changes the English team had made that led to their first successful IVF pregnancy. Steptoe and Edwards declined to share their novel protocol with us and with their English colleagues. Hoping that proximity might encourage a more generous sharing of vital information, Ian Johnston arranged first-class air tickets for Steptoe and his wife Sheena to visit Melbourne from late October 1978, with the further inducement of prime seats at the Cox Plate, Australia's prestigious horse race. Unfortunately, at meetings attended by the QVMC and RWH teams, Steptoe was unable to shed any light other than that successful IVF could only be attained during natural, unstimulated cycles, which we already used. He also hinted broadly that luteal phase support might be an important element for success. Overall, we were left none the wiser.

Expanding Efforts to Succeed

In 1979 the RWH Senior Medical Staff and hospital administration strongly supported the establishment of a clinical Reproductive Biology Unit, directed by Ian Johnston. Funding was allocated for converting a labor ward into an operating theater, exclusively for collecting oocytes from infertile patients. At the same time, an adjacent labor ward was converted into a modern IVF laboratory that was directly connected to the operating theater. These essential facilities increased markedly the throughput of patients having IVF procedures. In addition, the team at RWH expanded by introducing the application of ovarian ultrasound for measuring the growth of pre-ovulatory follicles in preparation for oocyte collection (O'Herlihy et al., 1980). Before the use of ultrasound, the response to follicular stimulation for IVF was inferred from daily oestrogen measurements. At RWH, the first application of ultrasound was not for monitoring follicle numbers and their growth, but for the assessment of follicle presence or absence in timing oocyte recovery at laparoscopies. Oocyte aspirations were performed about 26 h after detecting the urinary LH rise when ultrasound confirmed the presence of intact follicles. A 24 h service became available for this critical timing by the use of ultrasonography by Drs. Hugh Robinson, Lachlen de Crespingy, and Colm O'Herlihy (O'Herlihy et al., 1980; Hoult et al., 1981). This backup for effective oocyte retrieval at RWH halved the incidence of "ovulated follicles" which Ian Johnston and Andrew Speirs encountered, compared with higher "follicle loss" at QVMC where this ultrasound service was not available. Andrew Speirs designed an embryo transfer catheter that traversed the cervical canal more easily and gently, enabling a precise and quick embryo placement in the uterus.

Australia's First IVF Birth

By October 1979 this impetus to obtain better clinical outcomes resulted in the establishment of the first ongoing pregnancy at RWH. The pregnancy was tracked using ultrasound, as well as an amniocentesis, to ensure that the baby's growth and chromosomal constitution were normal. The exciting normal birth of Australia's first test-tube baby occurred on June 23, 1980. Ian Johnston delivered the baby girl (Figure 6.4), in the presence of her father as well as a crew of filmmakers and photographers from the media. The team involved with this successful IVF birth, as well as mother and baby, are shown in Figure 6.5.

Information about the successful pregnancy, with detailed description of the methods used, was published before the birth of the baby (Lopata et al., 1980b). The authors of this paper are shown in Figure 6.5. It is indisputable that John McBain should have been a co-author in the paper. He had been a stalwart person in establishing and refining the ovarian stimulation for the IVF program. He was also deeply involved in managing IVF patients and in obtaining some of the early pregnancies. Carl Wood should also have been listed as a co-author on the paper dealing with Australia's first IVF birth. Although he was not a member of the RWH team, he generously gave Lopata the opportunity and support to work with both teams. In retrospect it is difficult to understand why the authors of the paper neglected to include these two valuable contributors who played an important part in the early development of IVF in Melbourne.

After the publication of the RWH paper on Australia's first IVF pregnancy, John Leeton and Alan Trounson complained about their names not being included as co-authors. They both maintained that there was an agreement to include all names of the QVMC group with the RWH group. Ian Johnston, who was a highly moral individual and scrupulous about good relationships, would have definitely honored any existing agreement on authorship. McBain, Speirs, and

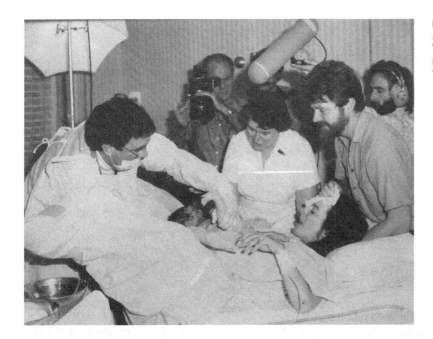

Figure 6.4 Dr. Ian Johnston delivering Australia's first IVF baby at the Royal Women's Hospital in Melbourne. The parents, Linda and John Reed, are watching expectantly.

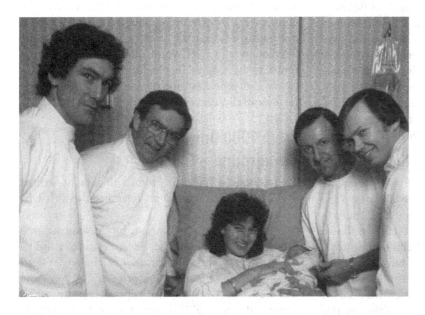

Figure 6.5 The team at the Royal Women's Hospital, involved with the first successful IVF pregnancy and birth in Australia. Starting from the left the people are Dr. Ian Hoult, Dr. Ian Johnston, Mrs. Linda Reed holding her baby (Candice), Dr. Alex Lopata, and Dr. Andrew Speirs.

Lopata are certain that a joint authorship agreement never existed between the two groups.

A second pregnancy was established at RWH before the end of 1979. At 19 weeks' gestation a routine amniocentesis was performed to evaluate the chromosomal status of the normally growing foetus. Unfortunately the sampling needle penetrated a loop of bowel that was adherent to the surface of the uterus. The amniotic fluid became infected resulting in chorioamnionitis and the miscarriage of a completely normal male foetus close to 20 weeks of gestation. As a result, the RWH team decided to abandon routine amniocentesis, particularly in uncomplicated IVF pregnancies.

Table 6.4 Outcome of IVF pregnancies at RWH from 1980 to 1983

Pregnancy Outcome	1980	1981	1982	1983
Biochemical	6	12	19	28
Ectopic	0	1	6	15
Abortion	5	12	21	41
Live-birth	1	11	30	97
Still-birth	0	0	0	4
All pregnancies	12	36	76	185
Live-birth %	**8.3**	**30.6**	**39.5**	**52.4**

Table 6.5 Chronology of IVF births achieved in different countries and the names of the teams that accomplished the clinically successful IVF

Country	Birth dates	Baby sex / name	IVF team
England	July, 1978	F (Louise)	Edwards, Steptoe
Australia	June, 1980	F (Candice)	Lopata, Johnston
USA	December, 1981	F (Elizabeth)	Jones, Veek
France	February, 1982	F (Amandine)	Testart, Frydman
Germany	April, 1982	M (Oliver)	Kniewald, Trotnow
England	April, 1982	M,M (twins)	Craft, Green
Austria	August, 1982	M (Zaltan)	Feichtinger, Szalay

Progress in IVF Births and Sharing Information

It became clear in 1980 that successful methods for treating infertility had started in Australia. The subsequent rapid progress in IVF, with improving pregnancy rates each year at RWH, is recorded clearly in Table 6.4.

Two months after the IVF birth, Lopata resigned from the QVMC team and commenced a full-time position at the University of Melbourne Department of Obstetrics and Gynaecology, headed by Professor Roger Pepperell. A close and valuable collaboration was established with the Reproductive Biology Unit directed by Ian Johnston, with the indispensable endocrine laboratory run by Professor James Brown, and with the ovarian ultrasound services of Hugh Robinson's team. The scene was set to share our information with other Australian and overseas groups planning to set up IVF clinics. Several groups visited our IVF laboratory and subsequently became the first successful IVF teams in their countries (Table 6.5). It is of interest that Professor Ian Craft, who was setting up an IVF clinic at the Royal Free Hospital in London, was one of our first visitors to benefit from the open sharing of IVF information in Melbourne. Also, Dr. Howard Jones acknowledged the input from our team following the birth of the first IVF baby in the United States (Figure 6.6).

Carl Wood's Invitation to Write

Close to the end of 1980, Carl Wood contacted Lopata and proposed sharing the writing of a joint paper on IVF for the *Oxford Reviews of Reproductive Biology*. Lopata immediately accepted the offer and suggested a visit to Carl's office to plan the review. Carl rejected this idea and said that he wanted to work on the writing at the RWH. Lopata could not fathom why Carl did not partner with someone from his own team, nor why he chose to make repeated visits to the RWH to write the joint review. Despite these unsolved enigmas, Lopata once again enjoyed the stimulating and challenging interaction with Carl Wood. On this occasion, Carl's return to the hospital that had launched his illustrious career had produced one of the first comprehensive reviews on clinical IVF (Lopata and Wood, 1982).

From 1980 Onwards with a Bit of Background – Gab Kovacs

The section in italics is from a document written by Carl Wood – non-italics have been inserted by Kovacs.

IVF research was started by Melbourne and Monash Universities at the Queen Victoria Hospital under the guidance of a committee chaired by Carl Wood in 1970, called "The egg project." The core team included Wood, Leeton, and Lopata (Lopata was not appointed until 1971) *from Monash University, to recruit more patients, and subsequently at The Royal Women's with Johnston* (Johnston was not involved until 1972) *and Brown from Melbourne University and Royal Women's Hospital (RWH). John McBain became involved and supervised stimulated cycles with gonadotrophins in 1977.*

The team achieved the world's first human IVF pregnancy (albeit a biochemical one) in 1973, with the report published in The Lancet (Figure 6.3).

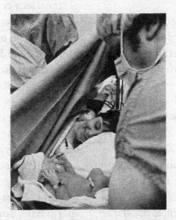

Elizabeth Jordan Carr

and her parents

Roger and Judy Carr

and

The Entire In-Vitro Team

THANK YOU

For your part in making possible the first birth
by in-vitro fertilization in the United States,
at
Norfolk General Hospital
December 28, 1981

Figure 6.6 Certificate received from the Jones Institute for Reproductive Medicine, Eastern Virginia Medical School, Norfolk, after the birth of the first IVF baby in the United States.

Despite continuing attempts, no further pregnancies were obtained.

In 1977, "The Melbourne Family Medical Centre" Trust was established to run the Donor Insemination and IVF research, and later the "Infertility Medical Centre Trust," to have the program at arm's length from the University.

Direct funding from NHMRC and other grants, and from the University were small.(In 1977 Lopata obtained a three-year NHMRC grant for the salary of an electron microscopist. Deborah Kohlman was appointed to do research on the electron microscopy of human fertilization and embryo development supervised by Lopata). *In 1977, a $750,000 grant from the Ford Foundation (who were keen to support the project as they thought that the basic scientific information obtained may help the development of new contraceptives), but did not want to be acknowledged if an IVF birth occurred. This highlights the difficulties that organisations such as Monash University or the Ford Foundation had in openly supporting such unusual research in the 1970s. By using the trusts and not the Monash name, the university felt at arm's length if the system failed, or worse, resulted in abnormal children, so that the criticism would be leveled at the clinical research team rather than the University.*

The Ford Foundation Grant enabled Carl Wood to recruit Alan Trounson, who he first met at an Australian Society of Reproductive Biology meeting in the 1960s and later in 1970 when Alan was working with Neil Moore on sheep embryo culture and transfer in Jerilderee. After graduating in agricultural science, Alan took a job as a "professional officer" at the research station in Hay NSW and did his Masters at the same time. There he met Neil Moore who was Professor at the McCaughey Memorial Institute. Alan decided to do a PhD with Neil Moore, although their relationship was described by Alan as "stormy." It was while at Jerilderee that Alan met Carl again. Alan was doing sheep embryology, embryo culture, and embryo micromanipulation, and Carl went to Jerilderee to observe, because of his desire to apply IVF to humans. Alan remembered Carl as "an interesting person but a little bit off the planet." Carl believed that Alan could apply the principles of animal embryology to humans and would be able to work with Lopata to advance the project. Carl asked Alan to join the egg project after his PhD, but Alan was awarded a Dalgetty Fellowship to work in Cambridge with Professor Chris Polge, who was a pioneer of cryopreservation, and was the first to use glycerol as a cryoprotectant.

When Carl obtained the Ford Foundation Grant, he was able to offer Alan a salary and bring him back to Melbourne, aided by the fact that Alan's first wife, Sue, wanted to return to her family there.

However, it was not easy for Alan to enter the system. Alex Lopata, who had been there for years, had established his research processes. Alan found that Lopata's method of research was different to what he was used to. Lopata's recollection was that Alan was involved in "The egg project" from 1977, but Alan remembers differently. Alan remembers that he concentrated on other projects. Most important was establishing a frozen sperm bank and showing that the outcome for thawed stored frozen sperm was as good as for fresh sperm.

Edwards had presented The Duphar Lecture at the Royal College of Obstetricians and Gynaecologists in Regents Park, London, on April 10, 1976, (Figure 6.7), 15 weeks prior to Louise Brown's birth, but made no mention of their success.

Three months later, the first human IVF birth was reported by Steptoe and Edwards in the UK, with a second birth in January 1979.

Following this, the Melbourne team approached IVF with more vigor, and Carl decided that it was time for Alan to get involved. At the same time he also decided that he would personally get involved with a "hands on" approach. He said to Alan that he would give it two years, and if it did not work, they would move on to other projects.

In March 1979 a meeting was held at Alex Lopata's house in Hawthorn to discuss how to move forward. Attendees included Lopata, Trounson, Wood, Leeton, Johnston, Speirs, McBain, and Kovacs. At the meeting a seven-page summary of the talk given by Bob Edwards at the RCOG in London, written by David Baird to Alan, was reviewed.

Wood, Leeton, Trounson, and Kovacs recall that: "It was agreed, that if we had a success the whole team would be named on the paper, with the scientist who did the laboratory work being the first author, the clinician whose patient it was, would be second." According to McBain, Speirs, and Lopata no such agreement involving the RWH group was made. Lopata remembers that when he and Trounson started to work separately at the QVMC there was a tacit agreement that if one of the embryologists produced an ongoing pregnancy then the whole QVMC team would be co-authors of the paper describing the success.

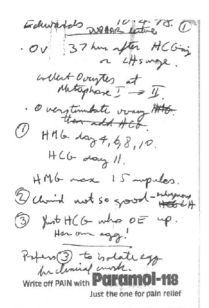

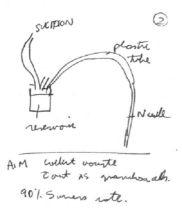

Figure 6.7 G. Kovacs' handwritten lecture notes from The Duphar Lecture, 1976.

Carl Wood decided that Alan Trounson and Alex Lopata would work better if they did not work together, but competitively; he decided to have a two-weekly rotation. When Alex was not on duty at QVMC, he could spend his time at the RWH. At the QVMC, Alan organized the endocrinology, and as we were running natural cycles with spontaneous ovulation, we needed to detect the LH rise. Alan miniaturized the assays, so that we could get results in 6 h, instead of 24 h. He did this in the "off weeks" when Alex was doing embryology, then did both biochemistry and embryology in the

"on weeks." His first technician was Janice Webb (subsequently Mrs. Lutjen).

Sister Jillian Wood (unrelated to Carl) who was employed as an insemination nurse, decided to help out with "The egg project" out of the goodness of her heart. She helped Paul Shekleton (senior registrar) co-ordinate the patients, and came in for all the egg collections around the clock, even during the night. She was very supportive of Alan, and they developed a close working relationship. She also had her name on the *Science* paper reporting the first five pregnancies. She moved over

57

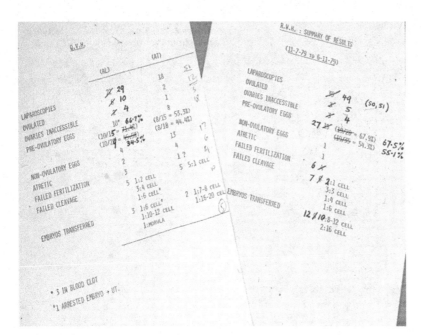

Figure 6.8 Summary of 1979 results at both hospitals.

to full-time IVF senior nurse co-ordinator when we could afford her salary. As we grew, we employed two other IVF nurses, Kim Breheny and Jillian McDonald. This established the important role of IVF nurse co-ordinators, which exists to the present day.

The year 1979 was a disappointing one, especially for the QVMC team. A meeting chaired by the late Bryan Hudson was held to review the year's results. These were presented as RHW results, QVH AL results, and QVH AT results. (Figure 6.8). Candice Reed was born on June 23, with conception around September 30, so Mrs. Reed would have been about 7 weeks at the time - one pregnancy out of 12 embryo transfers, but this was not discussed at the meeting.

The QVH team had no successes.

The world's third IVF birth (or fourth if the Indian pregnancy is counted) was achieved in June 1980. The pregnancy was at the RWH, the clinician was Ian Johnston, the embryologist Alex Lopata. Another pregnancy was also achieved at RWH, but it aborted after amniocentesis. The teams then split, RWH with Johnston, Lopata, Spiers, and McBain, and the Monash team with Wood, Leeton, Trounson, and Kovacs. Mac Talbot who had worked with John Leeton in the early days of IVF, and was a pioneer with laparoscopic egg collections, had an honorary appointment in the Infertility Clinic at QVH later rejoined the team.

The only two full-time University employees were Trounson and Wood.

Although the University department was located at the Queen Victoria Memorial Hospital, the team received virtually no support, and a lot of obstruction, from the hospital. The Medical Director was quoted as saying "stop wasting the time of the hospital and resident staff with IVF experiments." The Monash team then moved to St. Andrew's Hospital in 1980 where Kovacs already had a regular operating list, and started using stimulated cycles using the hormone clomiphene citrate, at the instigation of Alan Trounson. He insisted that stimulated cycles worked in animals, so must work in women. This was in strong disagreement with Bob Edwards, whose two births were obtained in spontaneous natural cycles, as was the Lopata/RWH pregnancy.

Three changes - location, stimulated cycles, and the development of a new Teflon-lined needle with no junctions for the eggs to get caught in, designed by Peter Renou - resulted in a total change of fortune, with the first conception (Baby Victoria - surname kept secret) in June 1980, followed by many others.

During 1980 we achieved 15 pregnancies resulting in nine births, all conceived at St. Andrew's Hospital, but delivered at the QVH. This included the world's first IVF twins (the Mayes twins). The pregnancies were reported in a paper in *Science*, and presented by

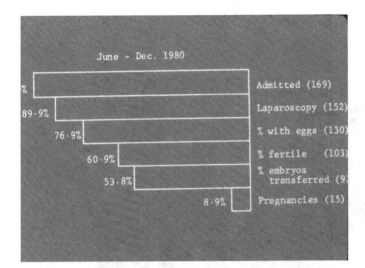

June – Dec. 1980

%   Admitted (169)
89.9%   Laparoscopy (152)
76.9%   % with eggs (130)
60.9%   % fertile   (103)
53.8%   % embryos
                                              transferred (9
8.9%   Pregnancies (15)

Figure 6.9 The Monash–QVH–St. Andrew's results, June to December 1980.

Alan at a number of international meetings (Trounson et al., 1980). The world's attention then became focused in Melbourne, and, in particular, on Trounson and Wood. The results using stimulated cycles were much more encouraging, with 15 pregnancies achieved from 152 laparoscopies between June and December 1980 (Figure 6.9).

There were a number of international visitors who each added their expertise and opinion. There was John Buster, who helped with the estrogen assays; Pierre Soupart from Tennessee, who had some human IVF experience, but whose work was rejected by the US Health Ethics Committee. Also David Whittingham, who was an expert in culture media. In those days all culture medium was made in-house, which made quality control difficult. Alan introduced mouse embryo culture as a form of quality control, previously not used. One of the early clinicians to visit both Melbourne teams was Professor Ian Craft, who was planning to establish an IVF program in the UK.

In 1981, just after the first Monash/St. Andrew's pregnancies were being established, Ed Wortham from Howard Jones' clinic in Norfolk, Virginia, came over to study the techniques used by the two Melbourne teams. After his return, Howard Jones' team achieved their first pregnancy – Ms. Elizabeth Carr, born on December 28, 1981. Howard generously expressed his thanks to the two Melbourne units, who had helped them in their program in his report in *Fertility and Sterility*. It was true that both Australian programs had an "open door policy," and had many international visitors.

My involvement with the team started in 1978 when I was Senior Registrar at the "Queen Vic," and resulted from an "over lunch" discussion with Carl; as I had very few patients, my role in egg collections was as a surgical assistant. My job was to disconnect the test tubes as they filled with follicular fluid, and replace them with empty ones. After the *Science* paper, and the birth of baby Victoria in March 1981, Carl, John Leeton, Alan and Jillian Wood, all headed off to international meetings, to spread the word. I was left behind with Janice Webb to do any procedures. During this time my first private patient Ann Stokes came along for egg collection. As both Carl and John were away, I got to do the egg collection, Janice did all the embryology, I did the transfer, and the positive pregnancy test came through on April 6 (my birthday – not a bad present!). Julian Stokes delivered on December 5, 1981, the world's thirteenth IVF baby, and the third boy.

We were so overwhelmed by visitors, both from Australia and overseas, that we decided to hold the world's first IVF Workshop in August 1982 (Figures 6.10 and 6.11).

In my job as "Clinical Administrator" of the program, it was my role to convene the workshop, which had theoretical, clinical and hands on laboratory components. We thought that we were very entrepreneurial, and charged $500 per registrant. We had 43 attendees, from every continent (Figure 6.10), and included some future IVF greats; Andre van Steirteghem, Paul Devroey (Figure 6.11), David Meldrum, Bud Keye, and Christopher Chen (first frozen egg pregnancy).

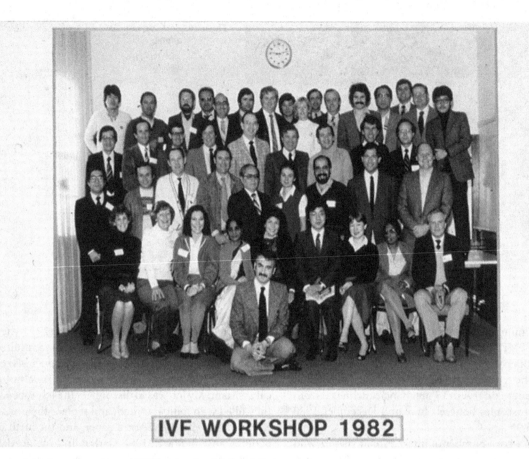

Figure 6.10 Attendees at Monash IVF Workshop (world's first). G. K. sitting in front.

In 1982, the team moved to Epworth, as St. Andrew's could not accommodate the increased demand (they limited the through-put at seven patients per week). By this stage the clinicians included Downing and Lolatgis, and Mac Talbot re-joined the roster. Beresford Buttery, Peter Renou, and Paul Shekleton joined to provide ultrasound expertise, Henry Burger and Jock Findlay endocrinology, and David deKretser as an andrologist. John McBain also worked for a while with the Monash team to introduce his expertise of using clomiphene citrate and HMG in combination to improve oocyte harvesting rates. The number of patients treated and the number of pregnancies steadily increased: 22 in 1981, 52 in 1982, 74 in 1983, and 95 in 1984.

Expanding the Horizons

Idiopathic Infertility

Although IVF was developed for the treatment of tubal infertility, Alan Trounson wanted a scientific approach to see if couples with unexplained infertility had problems with fertilization. Consequently a trial was established in parallel with "The egg project" to see what fertilization rates we could achieve. Ironically, the first paper published by Alan Trounson on human IVF related to its application to idiopathic infertility (Trounson et al., 1980).

Male Factor

A discussion with David deKretser about the number of sperm needed for IVF, led to David's suggestion that maybe some of his male factor patients could achieve in-vitro fertilization of their partner's eggs, where they could not do so in vivo. This led to David taking a sabbatical to look at "male factor IVF" and the establishment of the "male factor group" with David, Chris Yates (scientist), Jillian McDonald as nurse co-ordinator, and Kovacs as the IVF clinician. This is discussed in more detail in Chapter 22.

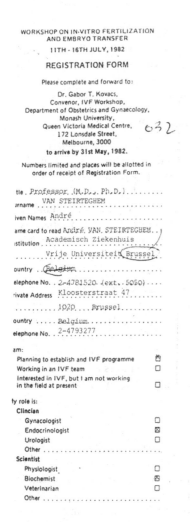

WORKSHOP ON IN-VITRO FERTILIZATION
AND EMBRYO TRANSFER
11TH - 16TH JULY, 1982

REGISTRATION FORM

Please complete and forward to:

Dr. Gabor T. Kovacs,
Convenor, IVF Workshop,
Department of Obstetrics and Gynaecology,
Monash University,
Queen Victoria Medical Centre,   032
172 Lonsdale Street,
Melbourne, 3000
to arrive by 31st May, 1982.

Numbers limited and places will be allotted in
order of receipt of Registration Form.

tle . Professor. (M.D., Ph.D.).........
urname   VAN STEIRTEGHEM
iven Names André
ame card to read André. VAN. STEIRTEGHEM..
istitution Academisch Ziekenhuis
.........Vrije Universiteit Brussel
ountry ..Belgium
elephone No. 2-4781520. (ext.. 5050)....
rivate Address Kloosterstraat 47
.........1020...Brussel.........
ountry .....Belgium..........
elephone No. . 2-4793277...........

am:
Planning to establish and IVF programme ☑
Working in an IVF team ☐
Interested in IVF, but I am not working
in the field at present ☐

ty role is:
Clincian
Gynacologist ☐
Endocrinologist ☒
Urologist ☐
Other . . . .
Scientist
Physiologist ☐
Biochemist ☒
Veterinarian ☐
Other . . . .

WORKSHOP ON IN-VITRO FERTILIZATION
AND EMBRYO TRANSFER
11TH - 16TH JULY, 1982

REGISTRATION FORM

Please complete and forward to:

Dr. Gabor T. Kovacs,
Convenor, IVF Workshop,
Department of Obstetrics and Gynaecology,
Monash University,
Queen Victoria Medical Centre,
172 Lonsdale Street,   031
Melbourne, 3000
to arrive by 31st May, 1982.

Numbers limited and places will be allotted in
order of receipt of Registration Form.

Title . . M.D.
Surname .DEVROEY
Given Names Paul
Name card to read Paul DEVROEY......
Institution .Academisch Ziekenhuis
.........Vrije Universiteit Brussel
Country ..Belgium
Telephone No. .2/478.15.20.(ext..3187)..
Private Address .De.Dammelaan.188
.........9330   Dendermonde
Country .....Belgium
Telephone No. ..52/21.41.44...........

I am:
Planning to establish and IVF programme ☒
Working in an IVF team ☐
Interested in IVF, but I am not working
in the field at present ☐

My role is:
Clincian
Gynacologist ☒
Endocrinologist ☐
Urologist ☐
Other . . . .
Scientist
Physiologist ☐
Biochemist ☐
Veterinarian ☐
Other . . . .

Figure 6.11 Paul and Andre's registration forms.

Donor Egg Pregnancies

The first donor egg pregnancy in 1982 resulted from the donated egg from a 42-year-old IVF patient who had a synchronous cycle with the 38-year-old recipient. Unfortunately the woman aborted at 11 weeks, the products of conception being found to be chromosomally abnormal. This was reported in the *British Medical Journal* (Trounson et al., 1983). The team received a lot of criticism because the donor was thought to be too old. Furthermore, as donor sperm was also used with the donor egg (double donation) the Ethics Committee of Queen Vic accused the team of breaching guidelines, although it was approved by the Epworth Ethics Committee. The IVF program now had opposition, not surprisingly from the Catholic Church, but also from the Anglican Church, as well as from a group of feminists. The Attorney General then called for a halt to the use of donor sperm and donor eggs in IVF. The Waller Committee was then set up (Chapter 28) to review IVF, and the use of donor gametes was re-introduced in late 1982.

However, due to pressure groups, a ban on donor eggs was again implemented in March 1983. Following lobbying, the ban on the use of donor sperm (but not donor eggs) was lifted in June 1982. During the few months that the donor egg program could continue, an Italian woman conceived with donor eggs, and delivered a healthy baby in November 1983. When the patients sued John Leeton and the Government for "discrimination" as sperm could be used but not eggs, the Equal Opportunities Court found in favor of the patients and the moratorium was lifted on December 15, 1983. The woman who conceived in the window of opportunity had congenital absence of her ovaries. She had an artificial cycle produced using estrogen and progesterone replacement with Jock Findlay from the Prince Henry's Institute helping to design the regime, with Peter Lutjen, then a PhD student (later Medical Director of Monash IVF), co-ordinating the cycle. Many other successful donor egg pregnancies followed.

Frozen Embryo Pregnancies

On April 4, 1981, Carl Wood and Alan Trounson were interviewed on the Australian Broadcasting Commission radio station's Science Show about IVF. Carl spoke about their plans to freeze embryos, which resulted in a very negative response from the media and the community. Nevertheless, Alan, who had experience with freezing cow embryos in Cambridge, took the proposal to the QVH Ethics Committee, who approved it. The committee, including both a Catholic priest and a Protestant minister, saw freezing as a better alternative than letting embryos die.

Alan was assisted in his work on freezing by Linda Mohr. The technique they used was similar to animal embryo freezing. In 1983, the team achieved the world's first human frozen embryo IVF pregnancy, but the baby aborted at 24 weeks due to infection and premature rupture of membranes. The Mohr/Trounson team achieved the world's first birth from a frozen embryo in 1984, of baby Zoe. The baby was normal at birth, and the parents sold the story to a popular women's magazine. Alan and Linda published the details in *Nature* (Trounson and Mohr 1983). They attributed the success to meticulous care throughout the process and to changing the timing of freezing to the four- to eight-cell cleavage stage. We have now gone the full circle, and freezing, using vitrification, is almost always at the blastocyst stage.

An early complication of embryo freezing was highlighted by Mario and Elsa Rios, a wealthy couple from the United States who came to Melbourne for treatment. Mrs. Rios's only child, by a previous marriage, had died and the couple came to Australia in 1981 to try to have a child of their own. Three embryos were fertilized at the clinic. One was implanted in Mrs. Rios but she later had a miscarriage. The two other embryos were frozen for possible future use. This was in the very early days of freezing, but the couple insisted they wanted to give it a go. Before a frozen embryo transfer could be performed, the couple were killed in 1983 in a plane crash in Chile, and there was much debate about the inheritance rights of any potential children produced from the frozen embryos.

In Britain there was a lot of opposition to embryo freezing. The Royal College of General Practitioners, and the Royal College of Nursing both said that such "experimentation" was unethical. Today it can be said that NOT providing embryo freezing is unethical!

Subzonal Sperm Injection (SUZI)

Alan Trounson together with Geoff Mann had devised a technique for the injection of several sperm under the zona pellucida of eggs (Lacham et al., 1989). As there was concern about possible chromosomal abnormalities, Wood and Trounson requested the Standing Review and Advisory Committee (SRACI), for permission to examine the chromosomes of eggs fertilized in this way. This was not allowed under existing legislation, but the Infertility Medical Procedures Act was amended to study these early fertilized eggs before syngamy. The studies showed no increase in chromosomal abnormalities. Owing to these delays, the technique (although pioneered in Melbourne) was taken back to Singapore, where the first birth occurred in 1988 by S. C. Ng. Although some pregnancies were achieved in 1991 by SUZI, the technique was superseded by ICSI (Chapter 9).

Embryo Biopsy

(This is discussed in detail in Chapter 23.)

The technique of embryo biopsy at the four- to eight-cell stage in mice was pioneered by Leanda Wiltson and Alan Trounson.

An application to SRACI to undertake this technique on human embryos was approved, but overruled by the Victorian Health Minister following an outcry from the anti-IVF lobby. Two members of SRACI resigned in protest, and Leanda Wilton moved to the UK, where she collaborated with Alan Handyside, who achieved the first human pregnancy using this new technique of Preimplantation Genetic Diagnosis (PGD).

Surrogacy

The first human IVF enabled surrogacy was reported from the USA in 1985. John Leeton was referred the Kirkmans in 1986. Maggie Kirkman had had a hysterectomy in 1978, with conservation of her ovaries, which were confirmed to be ovulating. Her sister Linda had finished her family and was a willing surrogate. A legal nightmare had to be negotiated, with opposing opinions from the State's Solicitor General and Attorney

General. Epworth Hospital Ethics Committee did not approve the process, and it was consequently carried out at Masada Hospital, whose Board, after detailed consideration, approved the process. A healthy female (Alice) was delivered, with both couples being present at birth, and as all fairy tales end, "lived happily ever after."

Commercialization in IVF/ART

The Monash University-owned clinic commenced trading as The Melbourne Family Medical Centre, then as Infertility Medical Centre, established in 1988. Monash IVF Pty Ltd was established in 1990. Donna Howlett, initially employed as an embryologist in 1984, who then established IVF Australia's (IVFA) laboratories in the USA, became manager in 1996, then Chief Executive Officer and later Managing Director of Monash IVF Pty Ltd, commercializing the company, with greenfield clinics and acquisitions.

In 2002, the University issued shares to the doctors' group and key personnel. In 2007 the University decided to divest itself of the company, and sold to ABN Amro, for over $220 million (*Australian Financial Review*).

The Rest of Australia

I don't want to give the impression that it only happened in Melbourne, but it happened in Melbourne first. Both Melbourne units had an "open door" policy, and both willingly taught our colleagues from other states or overseas.

New South Wales

The first Center to be established in Sydney was at The Royal North Shore Hospital, by Doug Saunders. Doug was introduced to IVF when Patrick Steptoe visited Sydney and gave a lecture at Crown Street Hospital for Women. In Doug's words "he was not too forthcoming," but was more interested in showing the video of the cesarean section, to prove the mother had no tubes. Doug was wondering how he could expand his established Fertility Clinic. When pregnancies happened in Melbourne he decided to join the race. Royal North Shore Hospital, a teaching hospital of Sydney University, already had ovulation induction, donor insemination, semen analysis, and sex steroid radioimmunoassay, and a full time fertility nurse, Diana Craven. He also had a "cash flow" from the hormone laboratory. Doug and his colleague John Kemp went to Melbourne, and he says "where they told us everything we needed to know." When Doug spoke with his Chairman, Rodney Shearman, he was told that Rodney did not consider that IVF would be part of fertility treatment (even great men can be wrong), but he did not oppose RNSH setting up IVF. Doug received support from the hospital and he recruited Ian Pike, who had grown mouse embryos for his PhD at Sydney University. Ian spent time in Melbourne and observed both clinics, and in his words "copied it back at RNSH." It took Ian a year to set up and have the equipment working to his satisfaction. Diana Craven (the fertility nurse) became the IVF co-ordinator.

When they achieved pregnancies in 1982, the first three came through on the same day! As the clinic outgrew the RNSH facilities it moved to Hunter Hill Private Hospital. It subsequently became part of IVFA in 2002, and ultimately Virtus, which also acquired Melbourne IVF, Queensland Fertility Group, Hunter IVF, and then floated on the Australian Stock Exchange in 2013.

The IVF unit at Westmead Hospital was set up by Geoffrey Driscoll in September 1983 – the second IVF unit in NSW. John Tyler had been recruited from the UK to work in the Donor Insemination Program, and he was the obvious choice for the IVF scientist.

In 1985 Geoff launched Integrated Fertility Services (IFS), later renamed City West IVF, as a separate but essentially parallel entity in the private sector, designed to be a "one stop" fertility service (the concept extended later with the building of a Day Surgery). City West IVF was the foundation stone for IVFA.

David Macourt, who ran a large Donor Insemination program in St. George, also was an early entrant into the IVF field. His embryologist and partner came to Epworth Hospital to learn IVF technology.

The Royal Prince Alfred Hospital/King George V Hospital was slow to get into IVF, despite its reputation as a center of excellence in gynecological endocrinology. This was probably due to Rodney Shearman's pessimism about IVF. Both Rob Jansen and Ian Fraser registered for the second Monash IVF workshop in 1983, but then withdrew. Rob Jansen subsequently established Sydney IVF (now known as Genea), with Alan Trounson as Scientific Director (whilst Alan was employed by Monash University) which became one of the leading IVF providers in Australia. It was also responsible for a number of firsts, including ultrasound guided-transcervical GIFT, a leader in PGD and cytogenetics. Each year 10% of profits have been re-invested in research, principally in stem cells. They developed culture media, embryo transfer catheters, and more recently incubators with time lapse photography and freezing machines.

Steven Steigrad and Graeme Hughes established an IVF unit at The Hospital for Women in Paddington. This was built on Steve's practice in donor insemination and Graeme's in ovulation induction. They became the Eastern part of IVFA.

Several smaller units were formed in the 1990s, for example Michael Chapman (IVFA South), and Ann Clarke at Fertility First (with a high percentage of single women using donor sperm). Next Generation IVF and Bondi Junction were commenced by David Knight and Joel Bornstein (both ex-City West doctors) after Geoff Driscoll retired. Primary Health has recently established a discounted IVF unit in Sydney.

West Australia

One of the earliest clinics to follow Melbourne was the PIVET IVF Program which was established by John Yovich in 1981. I remember having dinner with John in North London in January 1977, when he told me that Professor Craft was sending him to the library at Cambridge, to read and summarize all articles on IVF. John was thus introduced to IVF by Ian Craft in London. John established the clinic in Perth, with some collaboration with the Melbourne units. Carl Wood attended the opening of PIVET. The first IVF infant born in Western Australia, in July 1982, was through the PIVET program. John's wife, Jeane, attended the 1983 Monash IVF Workshop, and then worked as embryologist and clinic manager.

Other clinics in Perth also followed, with both Terry Thomas and Rob Mazzucchelli attending the 1982 workshop together with their nursing staff, and setting up subsequently at Avro Hospital.

Queensland

John Hennessey already had a busy infertility practice with donor insemination, in association with Professor Tim Glover, and in ovulation induction, when the first IVF babies were born. In 1982 with John Hynes and Warren deAmbrosis he attended the Monash workshop. On return to Brisbane the three gynecologists established the Queensland Fertility Group, also recruiting Doug Keeping and Gordon Kilvert. They were the major IVF group in Queensland, and pioneered satellite clinics in Mackay.

Other players have entered the arena in Queensland, including Monash IVF, City Fertility, as well as a number of independent units.

South Australia

Adelaide has always been a center of excellence in reproductive medicine. Lloyd Cox was one of the drivers for the Australian Human Pituitary Gonadotrophin Programme, and established a computerized register that recorded details of every woman, and every dose of FSH administered from 1967 till 1985 (when it was suspended due to Creutzfeld Jacob Disease). Together with Colin Matthews they were the first to establish a sperm cryobanking program in the mid 1970s. Bob Seamark a leading reproductive scientist was also collaborating.

Colin Matthews recalls (personal communication) that Lloyd Cox sent him to Melbourne in the early days of IVF, to assess whether they should start IVF. Colin's advice was that it was unlikely to work, and they should not start yet. They eventually did start an IVF program under the auspices of the University of Adelaide, with John Kerin, and produced their first baby in 1982. In 1987, Repromed Pty Ltd was formed as a spin-out company providing clinical and other services in reproductive medicine. This became one of the University's most successful ventures, contributing more than $30 million to the department for reproductive research. In 2006 Repromed was sold to a private concern, consisting of senior doctors and staff. The proceeds were used to establish the Robinson Institute in 2008. The sell-out resulted in some senior doctors, for reasons which are unclear, being unfairly excluded from the deal. This resulted in Rob Norman (Australia's leading reproductive gynecologist) and Ossie Petrucco (an outstanding reproductive surgeon) establishing Fertility SA, a highly successful private clinic.

Repromed was joined to Monash IVF after both companies were bought out by Healthbridge Pty Ltd. The company Monash IVF Pty Ltd was floated on the Australian Stock Exchange in June 2014.

Flinders University, under the leadership of Warren Jones, also established an IVF unit, with the first baby born in 1982. Warren's senior lecturer, Christopher Chen, reported the world's first frozen egg pregnancy in 1986, but this was not reproducible.

City Fertility from Queensland also established a clinic in Adelaide.

The final project that needs to be mentioned is the formation of The Fertility Society of Australia (FSA). This was based on the successful AID Workshops, begun by Ian Johnston in 1977. The group was multidisciplinary: doctors, nurses, scientist, and counselors. This principle was carried forward to FSA, with consumers also included.

Quite appropriately Ian Johnston was its first President, and is honored annually by the "Ian Johnston Memorial Lecture."

It continues as a vibrant society, and its annual meetings attract over 500 registrants.

References

De Kretzer D, Dennis P, Hudson B, et al. Transfer of a human zygote. *Lancet* 1973; Sept. 29: 728–729.

Edwards RG, Donahue RP, Baramki TA. Jones HW Jr. Preliminary attempts to fertilize human oocytes matured in vitro. *Am J Obst Gynec* 1966; 96: 192–200.

Hertig AT, Rock J, Adams EC. A description of 34 human ova within the first 17 days of development. *Amer J Anat* 1956; 98: 435–493.

Hoult IJ, De Crespigny L Ch, O'Herlihy C, et al. Ultrasound control of clomiphene-human chorionic gonadotropin stimulated cycles for oocyte recovery and in vitro fertilization. *Fertil Steril* 1981; 36: 316–319.

Jacobson CB, Sites JG, Arias-Bernal LF. In vitro maturation and fertilization of human follicular oocytes. *Int J Fertil* 1970; 15: 103–114.

Lacham O, Trounson A, Holden C, Mann J, Sathananthan H. Fertilization and development of mouse eggs injected under the zona pellucida with single spermatozoa treated to induce the acrosome reaction. *Gamete Res* 1989; 23: 233–243.

Lopata A, Wood C. In vitro fertilization and embryo transfer: its clinical application. *Oxford Reviews of Reproductive Biology,* Ed. Finn, CA. Clarendon Press, Oxford,1982; 4: 148–194.

Lopata A, Johnston IWH, Muchnicki D, Talbot JM, Wood C. Collection of human oocytes at laparoscopy and laparotomy. *Fertil Steril* 1974; 25: 1030–1038.

Lopata A, Patullo MJ, Chang A, James B. A method for collecting motile spermatozoa from human semen. *Fertil Steril* 1976; 27: 677–684.

Lopata A, Brown JB, Leeton JF, Talbot JMc, Wood C. In vitro fertilization of preovulatory oocytes and embryo transfer in infertile patients treated with clomiphene and human chorionic gonadotropin. *Fertil Steril* 1978a; 30: 27–35.

Lopata A, McMaster R, McBain JC, Johnston WIH. In-vitro fertilization of human preovulatory eggs. *J Reprod Fert* 1978b; 52: 339–342.

Lopata, A., Johnston, W. I. H., Leeton, J. and McBain, J. C. Use of in vitro fertilization in the infertile couple. *The Infertile Couple,* Eds. Pepperell RJ, Hudson B, Wood C. Churchill Livingston, Edinburgh, 1980a; 209–228.

Lopata A, Johnston IW, Hoult IJ, Speirs AL. Pregnancy following intrauterine implantation of an embryo obtained by in vitro fertilization of a preovulatory egg. *Fertil Steril* 1980b; 33: 117–120.

Menkin MF, Rock J. In vitro fertilization and cleavage of human ovarian eggs. *Am J Obst Gynec* 1948; 55: 440–452.

O'Herlihy C, De Crespigny L Ch, Lopata A, et al. Preovulatory follicle size: A comparison of ultrasound and laparoscopic measurements. *Fertil Steril* 1980; 34: 24–26.

Seitz HM, Rocha G, Brackett BG, Mastroianni L Jr. Cleavage of human ova in vitro. *Fertil Steril* 1971; 22: 255–262.

Talbot JM, Dooley M, Leeton J, et al. Gonadotrophin stimulation for oocyte recovery and in vitro fertilization in infertile women. *Aust NZ J Obstet Gynaecol* 1976; 16: 111–118.

Trounson A, Mohr L. Human pregnancy following cryopreservation, thawing and transfer of an eight-cell embryo. *Nature* 1983; 305: 707–709.

Trounson AO, Willadsen SM, Rowson LEA. The influence of in-vitro culture and cooling on the survival and development of cow embryos. *J Reprod Fertil* 1976; 47: 367–370.

Trounson AO, Leeton JF, Wood C, Webb J, Kovacs G. The investigation of idiopathic infertility by in vitro fertilization. *Fertil Steril* 1980; 34: 431–438.

Trounson A, Leeton J, Besanko M, Wood C, Conti. A pregnancy established in an infertile patient after transfer of a donated embryo fertilised in vitro. *Br Med J (Clin Res Ed)* 1983; 286: 835–838.

The Joneses and the Jones Institute

Charles C. Coddington III and Sergio C. Oehninger

The Beginnings

In the year 1978, Drs. Howard and Georgeanna Jones moved from Baltimore, Maryland, to Norfolk, Virginia. It was to be retirement time after long and productive careers at Johns Hopkins Medical School, where they had excelled in gynecological surgery and reproductive endocrinology. They were actively recruited by Dr. Mason C Andrews, Chairman of the Department of Obstetrics and Gynecology and co-founder of Eastern Virginia Medical School (EVMS), also a prior Johns Hopkins graduate. Dr. Andrews was a member of the Norfolk's City Council and at the time became Vice-Mayor for city redevelopment. He gave them the task of starting a new division of a subspecialty known today as reproductive endocrinology and infertility (REI), and provided encouragement and facilitated their continuing efforts to further develop the emerging technique of IVF. With support from local business-men including Henry Clay Hofheimer, Chairman of the board of EVMS Foundation, and in collaboration with the administration of Norfolk General Hospital, in addition to "serendipitous events" that Dr. Howard joyfully recalled (unsolicited donation of funds by infertility patients) the enterprise was started. The conditions were set to develop a unique undertaking, albeit fraught with challenges and controversies. As recently stated by Dr. Howard: "That there are several million IVF babies in the world today is proof enough that the public has opened its arms to controversial technology, because it has brought great happiness to so many" (Jones, 2014).

Dr. Howard had originally met Robert Edwards, PhD, at the time of his visit to Hopkins in 1965. Dr. Edwards was a scientist, pioneer in gamete and embryo biology, a visionary, who would later be awarded the Nobel Prize in Medicine in 2013 for his accomplishments in assisted reproductive technologies (ART). They immediately shared interests in reproductive topics and initiated informal collaborations.

In July 1978, while in the moving process to their new home on Shirland Avenue in Norfolk, Louise Brown, the first IVF baby "miracle" in the world, was born in Oldham, England, following the pioneering work of Drs. Edwards and Patrick Steptoe. This was invigorating news to the Joneses who decided to take in full speed with their aim to increase the so-far very low efficiency of IVF.

The Initial Team

Dr. Anibal Acosta, from Argentina, former Hopkins trainee of Dr. Georgeanna in reproductive endocrinology, and Dr. Jairo Garcia, from Colombia, were the first medical recruits. Recognizing the need for an embryology team (with the caveat that there were simply no prior experienced scientists or technicians with knowledge of human IVF at that time), Dr. Jack Rary, cytogeneticist from Johns Hopkins, J. W. Wortham Jr., PhD, from Old Dominion University in Norfolk, and Lucinda Veeck (later Veeck-Gosden), with certification in medical technology, were appointed. These initial embryology efforts followed productive interactions with the groups in Cambridge and Melbourne. Lucinda was on her way to becoming a superb clinical embryologist, based on her extreme dedication, fabulous technical skills, and superior mentoring competence manifested in the training of numerous embryologists who came to Norfolk from all over the world. In addition, Lucinda's warm and collegiate personality made her a long-term asset to the group. The team was set: Dr. Howard mastered the laparoscopic method of egg harvesting and developed the original embryo transfer catheter used in the program (the now historic "Jones catheter"), Dr. Georgeanna was responsible for the hormonal manipulations, Drs. Acosta and Garcia took care of patients and clinical procedures, and Lucinda became the chief embryologist.

Notwithstanding an initial political–religious climate of opposition, aggressive negative press, legal challenges, and bureaucratic hurdles in obtaining a certificate of need for opening new clinical operations in the hospital, eventually the IVF enterprise started. In spite of a handful of worldwide efforts, by early 1981 there were only two more IVF deliveries in the world, a second one in England and the third one in Australia. All these births were the result of natural cycles. Dr. Georgeanna had mastered ovulation induction in her practice, and had repeatedly argued that IVF results should be improved by administration of gonadotropins with the subsequent multifollicular development over the more erratic retrieval of a single oocyte in the natural cycle. Using the available human menopausal gonadotropin to stimulate multiple follicular growth followed by human chorionic gonadotropin to trigger ovulation, the Norfolk IVF team learned how to monitor folliculogenesis and time oocyte retrievals with newly developed controlled ovarian hyperstimulation (COH) protocols, and were thrilled to obtain mature and fertilizable oocytes (Jones, 2008).

After a few initial failed embryo transfer attempts, a courageous and determined infertility couple with tubal disease achieved a pregnancy following the transfer of a three-cell embryo on day 2 of culture. The pregnancy progressed uneventfully to term, and on December 29, 1981, a healthy baby, Elizabeth Carr, was born under strict attentive eyes from the medical team and others (Figure 7.1). She was the first IVF birth following use of gonadotropin stimulation. Three and a half decades later, gonadotropins (newly refined preparations) still constitute the state-of-the-art way of performing ovarian stimulation for IVF. In a classic paper, Dr. Howard and the IVF team reported in Fertility and Sterility on the first three-year experience of IVF at Norfolk (Jones et al., 1984). The relatively high pregnancy rates achieved were quite impressive considering that in those years the hormonal preparations were more impure, and embryo culture conditions (equipment, media, materials and supplies) were inferior compared to current standards. As a result, Norfolk quickly became a world reference center. Drs. Howard and Georgeanna openly shared results, techniques, and troubleshooting with colleagues that visited from all continents. This was always done in an academic yet transparent and honest way, by face-to-face teaching of clinicians and scientists visiting Norfolk, and through data presentation in the most prestigious national and international meetings as well as in peer reviewed journals in the field.

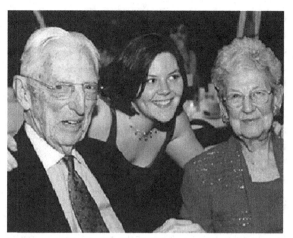

Figure 7.1 Elizabeth Carr at the time of a visit to the Joneses. Note: Elizabeth Carr delivered a healthy baby boy at age 29.

The Jones Institute

In the next few years, two other outstanding clinicians joined the team, Dr. Zev Rosenwaks from New York, and Dr. Suheil Muasher from Jordan. Dr. Rosenwaks became the Director of the REI Division, and Dr. Muasher was indeed the first REI graduate from the Norfolk REI fellowship. Both of them contributed superbly to the advances of assisted reproductive technologies particularly in the fields of COH, the design of novel stimulation protocols, and the initiation of the oocyte donation program. In parallel, Dr. Acosta developed what would become a uniquely qualified male infertility program, with state-of the art andrology and sperm cytology laboratories. The first experiences were summarized in landmark publications that became "classic" IVF books and articles detailing the whole IVF process and techniques (Jones et al., 1986), the unique and, at the time, novel morphological features of normal and abnormal human eggs and embryos (Veeck, 1986), and male infertility advances in assisted reproduction (Acosta et al., 1990). As IVF evolved, so did the Howard and Georgeanna Jones Institute for Reproductive Medicine, formally named after its founders in 1983. Two years later, in 1985, to assist with financial and advisory support of the Institute endeavors, the Howard and Georgeanna Jones Foundation for Reproductive Medicine was created.

There was still a missing link: Drs. Howard and Georgeanna were profound followers of the scientific method, always formulating questions on etiologic causes and mechanisms involved in reproductive disease. The need arose for assembling a basic science program that would be coupled to, and would work in a symbiotic way with, the clinical IVF team.

Gary D. Hodgen, PhD, had been engaged in research in the science of reproduction and the discipline of reproductive medicine for more than two decades. He had turned his focus to the study of ovarian physiology and the process of ovulation using the non-human primate monkey model and as a result redefined the physiology of the normal ovarian-menstrual cycle and the effects of COH (Hodgen, 1982; Goodman and Hodgen, 1983). In 1985, Dr. Hodgen relocated from the National Institutes of Health (NIH), where he was Chief of the Pregnancy Research Branch in Bethesda, to EVMS to become Scientific Director of the Jones Institute. With a clinical program well underway, the new addition of a renowned and energetic physiologist, and thanks to the tremendous effort of the newly established Jones Foundation, an incredible momentum was gained. The goals of the Jones Institute for Reproductive Medicine and its Foundation were then clearly delineated as follows: "The Jones Institute for Reproductive Medicine is dedicated to the education and training of developing physicians and scientists in the areas of reproductive biology/medicine, the scholarly pursuit and dissemination of new knowledge in the reproductive sciences, and their application for improvement of patient care in the treatment of reproductive problems, including female and male infertility, better methods of fertility control, post-menopausal women's health maintenance, and the prevention of heritable birth defects."

Although a cohesive functional unit, the Jones Institute was initially physically located in three neighboring areas of EVMS campus. The clinics were on the sixth floor of Hofheimer Hall, the IVF lab and operating suite were at Norfolk General Hospital, and an impressive science site was across Brambleton Avenue, a busy avenue in downtown Norfolk, that was fully functional under Dr. Hodgen's masterful direction. In 1991 the Jones Foundation was instrumental, with assistance from various business partners, in fulfilling the cherished desired dream of housing all activities under one roof in a modern and functional new building in EVMS campus, the new Jones Institute Building located now on the corner of Colley Avenue and Olney Road. In April 2006, Sergio Oehninger, MD, PhD, Director of the REI Division, brought the plan to fruition by securing the move of the IVF lab from Norfolk General Hospital into the Jones Building, and established an in-house

state-of-the-art laboratory and operating room suite. This set-up continues as of today, and has brought immense patient satisfaction (Figure 7.2).

In 1986 Dr. Hodgen became the founding principal investigator of the Contraceptive Research and Development (CONRAD) Program, funded by the United States Agency for International Development. In 1986 this five-year, $35 million program was the largest biomedical research award ever granted by a federal agency. He remained the CONRAD director until 1990, when he became the President of the Howard and Georgeanna Jones Institute for Reproductive Medicine Foundation. Dr. Hodgen's productivity was immense: he advanced our understanding of folliculogenesis, contraception, and preimplantation genetic

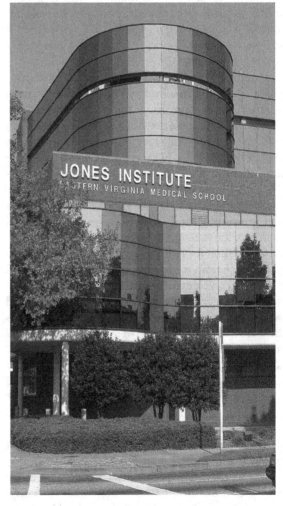

Figure 7.2 The Jones Institute Building, Norfolk, Virginia.

diagnosis, and therefore participated in the progress of the emerging assisted reproductive technologies, while at the same time mentoring a generation of clinical and basic investigators. To quote him: "Infertility and contraceptive research are nothing but two sides of the same coin," i.e., all information gained in one area surely can bring some application to the other. Within the Jones Institute, he founded the Technology Development Center in 1994 and focused the last years of his career on developing new technologies for reproductive medicine. He was assisted by two devoted collaborators, Robert Williams, PhD, and Andy Anderson, MD. During his 17 years at EVMS, Dr. Hodgen was the principal investigator on $258 million worth of sponsored research, and his inventions provided $34 million of patent licensing income. Serious and professional in his daily enterprises, Gary, as he liked to be called, was an imposing but fun person. He was also a motivated fisherman and a good golfer. We were fortunate to spend some time with him in these activities, either deep sea fishing, or golfing. In a way he was a unique golfer: he only managed the course with wood clubs, no irons, and had a single digit handicap, usually around 8. His dogma during these recreational activities was very simple: no talking about work, just enjoy the game of golf with the comradery.

During his tenure Dr. Hodgen surrounded himself with a unique group of qualified reproductive biologists and scientists. They included, among others, Nancy Alexander, PhD (expert in immunologic infertility and andrology), Drs. Robert Williams and Arnold Goodman (who participated in primate model studies and were recruited from NIH), Stephen Beebe, PhD (bringing expertise in molecular biology), Ted Anderson, PhD (knowledgeable in implantation), Keith Gordon, PhD (reproductive biologist and endocrinologist), Doug Danforth, PhD (who searched for the putative gonadotropin-surge inhibiting factor), Lani Burkman, PhD (who developed the original concept of sperm hyper activated motility), Susan Lanzendorf, PhD (dedicated gamete biologist then converted to an excellent clinical embryologist), Charles Coddington, MD, a prior Fellow of Dr. Gary Hodgen from the program at NIH (to work on sperm binding and oocyte micromanipulation), and Mary Mahony, PhD (andrologist). This amazing group of scientists attracted interactive collaborations with many other national and international colleagues, and brought dozens of research fellows and post-graduate PhD students that joined at different times and expanded horizons. It was indeed an exciting time. Some of us had mixed feelings about mandatory research seminars taking place at 6:00 am (too early for many of us) across Brambleton Avenue every Tuesday, attended by all clinicians and biologists of the Institute, but the scientific rewards of those early awakenings were superior. While the atmosphere, comradery, collegiality, and scientific depth of the gatherings were superior, at the same time they were always conducted in a jovial way. Many times one would come away from the meetings with an energized approach and new ways of investigating the biologic issues of the day. These types of interactions between practitioners and scientists were unique, and often resulted in illuminating new ideas to embark in new research projects and strategies.

Further Contributions that led to Significant Scientific Advances in ART

In the *In Vitro Fertilization – Norfolk* book that marked a turning point in ART (Jones et al., 1986), Dr. Hodgen schematically delineated the five principal steps in IVF therapy, from ovarian stimulation and optional ovarian stimulation protocols, to follicular aspiration, in-vitro fertilization and development of embryogenesis, to embryo transfer and pregnancy diagnosis. While three decades later these steps remain as a backbone of the treatment, a remarkable number of new strategies have been developed stemming from these initial concepts defined by the Joneses and Gary in those early days of ART. They have arisen from the "basic" IVF principles, and have been the results of dramatic advances in all areas of the process, from development of new optimized hormones, the serendipitous "discovery" of ICSI, to major improvements in lab equipment-material-supplies, culture media, optimized egg and embryo cryopreservation protocols (vitrification), and remarkable genetics new information and technologies, resulting in currently applied exact methods of preimplantation chromosomal and genetic screening of embryos. New purified gonadotropin preparations and development of GnRH analogs, as well as modified minimal and friendlier ovarian stimulations, have been utilized since. Continuing improvements of in-vitro maturation of prophase I oocytes, and births following ovarian transplantation tissue are other examples. The Jones Institute continued to strive on clinical outcomes, while at the same time contributing significantly to the scientific literature.

Clinical Contributions: High Points

Muasher et al. (1988) were the first ones to signal the value of the examination of serum gonadotropins and estradiol serum levels on basal cycle day 3 to determine ovarian response to gonadotropin stimulation. This landmark method is still used today, in addition to the measurement of AMH and ultrasound assessment of antral follicular counts as complementary ways to prospectively predict ovarian reserve. James Toner, MD, PhD, from the University of Pennsylvania completed his residency and REI fellowship in Norfolk and became an outstanding member of the clinical team. He was instrumental in assisting Dr. Howard in investigations on human implantation (Toner et al., 1991b) and also in elaborating on the concept of total reproductive potential, i.e., defining the combined cumulative impact of the transfer of embryos in fresh and frozen cycles deriving from one COH cycle (Toner et al., 1991a). William Gibbons, from Houston, joined the REI Division in 1990 the time at which he became Chair of the Department of Obstetrics and Gynecology, as successor to Dr. Mason Andrews. Teaming up with Dr. Hodgen, Sue Gitlin, PhD, and others achieved success with the first published healthy (unaffected) delivery of an IVF case augmented with preimplantation genetic diagnosis (PGD) in a couple who were carriers of the devastating Tay–Sachs disease gene mutation (Gibbons et al., 1995).

Charles C. Coddington, MD, who had completed his Navy service and had been in Dr. Hodgen's program in Bethesda, arrived at the Jones Institute in 1989 to direct the REI Fellowship. Dr. Coddington excelled in various areas of reproductive medicine, including organizing the ovulation induction program, reproductive surgery, and clinical research, directing clinical trials on GnRH analogues, adhesion prevention in reproductive surgery, and uterine fibroid therapy. Many mentoring sessions would occur when enjoying a round of golf with Gary who was very insightful in science as he was in life. Drs. Howard and Georgeanna were very proud of the Institute and when the time came to interview for fellowship they wanted to invite all the candidates and meet the "new" young people of our specialty and share their enthusiasm with them. Sergio Oehninger, MD, PhD, from Uruguay, completed a fellowship in REI at the Jones Institute in 1988, and

joined the faculty, and continues in the program until today. Together with the IVF team and the scientists of the clinical and research laboratories, he published extensively in all areas of ART. We have been privileged to learn from and work with many of the most illustrious names in our field, at the Jones Institute, and also through national and international collaborations and meetings (Figure 7.3).

Male Infertility Program

Research and clinical advances in the male gamete physiology and pathology were pioneered by Dr. Anibal Acosta. He worked together with members of the Department of Urology for a comprehensive evaluation of the infertile man, and established the andrology and sperm bank laboratories, which have become reference labs for the region (in the last several years directed by Mahmood Morshedi, PhD). He developed a very friendly and productive relationship with Tygerberg Hospital in Capetown resulting in numerous publications. In 2006 Fertility and Sterility published an article on citation classics (Yang and Pan, 2006). The authors identified the top 102 most frequently cited articles in the journal from 1975 to 2004 (Science Citation Index). At positions 2 and 3 on this list were two papers by Thinus Kruger and collaborators, one from Tygerberg, the other one from Norfolk (Kruger et al, 1986, 1988). Kruger and colleagues described the so-called strict Tygerberg criteria for assessment of sperm morphology in the basic evaluation of the semen. This work and subsequent validation papers had such a positive impact that the World Health Organization (WHO) has adopted this classification in 1999.

In those pre-ICSI IVF years (prior to the "boom" of ICSI), special emphasis was also given to the development of sperm function tests, i.e., bioassays of sperm–egg interaction under in-vitro conditions. Dr. Hodgen assembled a team to work on the idea of a "hemi-zona pellucida sperm binding assay," and Drs. Burkman, Coddington, and Oehninger, in collaboration with Daniel Franken, PhD (from Tygerberg), pioneered these studies that greatly advanced knowledge on sperm-zona pellucida interaction, induced-acrosome reaction, and involvement of carbohydrates-selectin types of interactions (Oehninger et al., 1989; Coddington et al., 1991; Clark et al., 1995). These studies were not only regarding fertility but learning about contraception as well. These tests are also now cited in the WHO manual as available research tests.

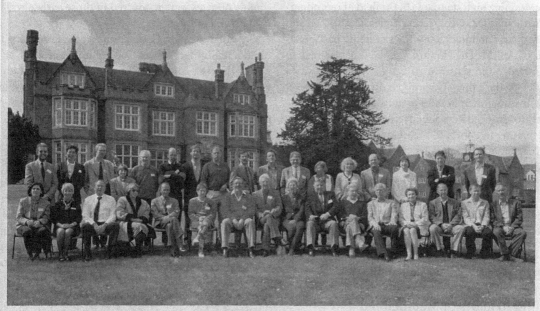

Bourn Hall Reunion Meeting 1995

Back Row: A. Handyside, Soon-Chye Ng, J. Carroll, J. Mandelbaum, A. Van Steirteghem, M. Wikland, E. Loumaye, S. Oehinger, P. Brinsden, R. Frydman, P. Devroey, K. Elder, L. Mettler, K. Diedrich, I. Stillger, T. Hillensjo, B. Siebold.

Front Row: V. Durante, S. Glenister, J. Webster, J. Belaish-Allard, J. Salat-Baroux, M. Plachot, I. Johnston, H. Jones, G. Jones, J. Cohen, R. G. Edwards, L. Hamberger, A. Eshkol, A. Lopata, A. Spears, C. Howles.

Figure 7.3 Bourn Hall meeting of IVF experts that took place in 1995.

Drs. Kruger and Oehninger extended this work with a follow-up updated book on male infertility diagnosis and treatment (Oehninger and Kruger, 2007).

Continuing Missions of Mentoring Clinicians, Scientists, and Embryologists, and Service in National Reproductive Societies

Clinical Training

The Jones Institute continues to have a prestigious REI Fellowship through the American Board of Obstetrics and Gynecology, now in transition to the Accreditation Council for Graduate Medical Education (ACGME). Past Fellowship directors include Drs. Georgeanna S. Jones, Charles Coddington, Jim Toner, and David Archer, and currently Laurel Stadtmauer, MD, PhD. Forty-two Fellows have graduated from the REI program, and are now at prestigious academic and private REI centers throughout the United States. Numerous international clinical fellows have trained too.

Basic Science and Embryology Training

With active participation of the clinical and research faculty, dozens of research fellows, PhD students, and postdoctorate PhD graduates have been mentored. Furthermore, Helena Russell has been instrumental in the establishment of a new very successful Reproductive Clinical Science Master's Program, initiated in 2003 with ongoing faculty leadership from the Jones Institute. This is an Internet-based graduate program in Clinical Embryology and Andrology that has now been expanded with the recent creation of a Clinical Embryology PhD program as of 2016.

National Organizations

Since its inception the Jones Institute has actively participated with the American Society for Reproductive

Medicine (ASRM) sharing its views on the dissemination of information, mentoring clinicians and scientists, promoting patients' education, and commitment to maintaining high standards in the field of reproductive medicine. Dr. Georgeanna Jones (1970–71) and Dr. William Gibbons (2009–10) served as past presidents of ASRM. Dr. Howard was among the first to acknowledge the sensitive nature of ART and was a founder of the Ethics Committee. In parallel, several Jones Institute members have actively worked at the Society for Assisted Reproductive Technologies (SART), participating in efforts to maintain the highest standards in ART. In this regard, Drs. Robert Brzyski, Charles Coddington, and Jim Toner have been past presidents of SART, and Drs. Suheil Muasher and Sergio Oehninger have been members of the Executive Committee. Drs. Rosenwaks and Coddington were also President of the Society of Reproductive Endocrinology and Infertility (SREI) which is a governing body of the sub-specialty.

The Joneses

Getting to Know Dr. Georgeanna

We met Dr. Georgeanna in her teaching environment at the Jones Institute. There she was, a poised, elegant woman of boundless talent, mentoring a group of REI fellows and visitors from all over the world. She demanded strictness, discipline, and hard work from her students. But while we immediately recognized an image of authority, we started sensing something different, a true combination of a strong personality, impeccable ethics, and warmth, even sweetness on some occasions. Although she was deeply inquisitive, she introduced complex issues by asking simple questions: how can we apply the general physiological knowledge to the individual clinical situation? What experiment, either in an animal model or in the clinical scenario, can be designed to answer that question?

We remember vividly the first occasions we were privileged to see patients with her. When addressing her patients, Dr. Georgeanna exhibited a marvelous combination of empathy, reassurance, and optimism. She could be kind and gentle, and at the same time be quite firm in communicating her opinions and recommendations. Patients always responded to her ways, respected her, and loved her.

Other unforgettable moments took place daily in the Operating Room during the IVF cases. After egg harvesting Dr. Georgeanna would proudly carry the aspirated follicular fluid to the adjacent embryology lab where Lucinda and her team would find the egg. Nothing would interrupt her concentration and her excitement. Finding the eggs in a given patient (not many oocytes were recovered in those early days) was a daily celebration.

At that time Dr. Georgeanna wrote something that had a big impact on us. The argument arose over the view that the Catholic Church had an ethical objection to IVF if it is outside the bonds of conjugal love. In her reply to the Vatican in the autumn of 1987 she wrote: "Reproduction with family formation is surely one of the great pleasures and benefits resulting from the commitment made between two individuals joined in conjugal love . . . When our investigations indicate additional measures for correction of a defect, such as In Vitro Fertilization for the treatment of infertility, we should accept these findings as further evidence of God's will for us to be inquisitive and rational." This very well summarizes her view on Reproductive Medicine as an integral discipline. Her science could not be separated from her beliefs.

She was a humble but dedicated hostess of the IVF Journal Club gatherings at their home in Shirland Avenue, where all Jones faculty, scientists and embryologists, and external visitors from around the world discussed selected articles on a monthly basis. Foreign visitors and other trainees typically received a Jefferson Cup from Dr. Howard; that was a simple but touching way of them honoring their guests. Dr. Georgeanna was an exquisite combination of woman, wife, mother, and physician who broke through the gender barrier and became an inspiration to all. These gatherings fostered the sense of a team of which they were both so proud. Each person who presented and discussed papers at the journal club was given every consideration so that all ideas from many different perspectives were discussed and evaluated. No alcohol was served so that the focus of the discussion would not wander from the point of discussion at hand.

Dr. Howard's Vision and Legacy

We were all initially impressed by Dr. Howard's imposing, at the same time awe-inspiring figure of authority. However, Dr. Howard also emanated a true warmth and a certain sense of approachability that enriched his strong personality and ethics. Dr. Howard was a master of the art of oral communication, the pitch, tone, and rhythms of the spoken English language. A superb teacher and lecturer, he had a distinct ability to deliver ideas with impeccable clarity and elegance in that deep, firm, yet lively voice that never failed to fascinate his audiences and made him unforgettable.

Dr. Howard was always sensitive to addressing the challenging social, ethical, and religious questions raised by IVF (Crockin and Jones, 2009; Jones, 2013). And as important, he always foresaw the need to answer new emerging questions. It was in the last years that we witnessed his dedication to address these challenges with his fullest energy, particularly in three areas: (i) efforts toward eliminating multiple pregnancies after IVF (Kulkarni et al., 2013); (ii) understanding the efficiency of IVF (Jones et al., 2010); and (iii) supporting research for identification of the "best egg" to further improve IVF results. Many times in discussions in his later career, he was always trying to determine how to identify the best embryo even though it had been years since he was in clinic. These topics were his latest passion, and we are sure that once resolved, he would have moved on to the next one.

We always wondered in admiration about the roots of his self-motivation. What internal drive led him to persist with such determination? It appears that he simply felt a compelling need to get these answers; he was convinced that better results could be obtained. In this regard he was unstoppable. But if his self-motivation was remarkable, we found his inspirational leadership truly exceptional. His encouraging approach brought out the best in everyone. He was a natural born leader, deeply inquisitive, always in such delightful, occasionally humorous ways.

Like Dr. Georgeanna he was unselfish in sharing his knowledge, as unselfish as he and his Institute shared IVF with the rest of the world. Her journal review with the fellows was a wonderful time not only to give them deeper insight into the scientific methodology, but also into one's self as well. A few years ago, at the occasion of his 100th birthday, with the help of our REI colleague Silvina Bocca, MD, PhD, we created a painting in his honor seen today at the Jones Institute atrium, and called it "Seed of Life," a metaphor of Dr. Howard himself as he "exported" the seed of IVF for the benefit of patients in places throughout the world.

Dr. Howard was a one-of-a-kind teacher, mentor, and friend, and a main supporter at times of difficult decisions. Someone who at every turn inspired hope, ignited the imagination, and instilled love for untangling the complexities of the field, but also of the human condition itself. When confronted with difficult decisions we approached him looking for guidance, and he would never discourage us. Rather, he would say: "Think of this as an opportunity to improve the process."

Also at the time of his 100th birthday, Dr. Howard said to an audience: "Let me salute you who are far more important to the future than I (am)." And one more time citing his favored poet Robert Frost he said: "The woods are lovely, dark and deep / But I have promises to keep / And miles to go before I sleep / And miles to go before I sleep." And he concluded: "My miles are limited and I ask those that follow me to devote miles to filling the niche that I described."

Final Remarks

Eli Adashi, MD, eloquently described Dr. Howard's persona in an article published in *Fertility and Sterility* entitled: "Dr. Howard Jones: a giant in our midst" (Adashi, 2015): "Armed with unrequited curiosity, boundless energy, innate pragmatism, singular surgical skills, and a searing intellect, Dr. Jones did nothing less than transform an evolving discipline several times over. In the process, a life of unparalleled accomplishments unfolded during which the foundation of multiple present-day constructs has been laid."

A few of us share in the pride of being members of the extended Jones family, whether still practicing reproductive medicine at the Institute, or in different places of the country or rest of the world, and are driven to continue his legacy. As their trainees we have learnt to offer a friendly, compassionate, and caring environment where infertile couples can undergo diagnosis and treatment with cutting edge, state-of-the-art techniques, in the conviction that it should be done with concerns about safety, and with precise evaluation of new discoveries. While we are well aware of the challenges posed by academic medicine nowadays, we are certain that The Joneses vision and legacy of an Institute "Founded on Science and Dedicated to Life" will always remain a guiding light for generations to come.

References

Acosta AA, Swanson RJ, Ackerman SB, et al. *Human Spermatozoa in Assisted Reproduction*. 1990. Williams and Wilkins, Baltimore, USA.

Adashi EY. Howard Wilbur Jones, Jr., M.D.: a giant in our midst. *Fertil Steril* 2015;104:531–532.

Clark GF, Patankar MS, Hinsch KD, Oehninger S. New concepts in human sperm-zona pellucida interaction. *Hum Reprod* 1995;10:31–37.

Coddington CC, Franken DR, Burkman LJ, et al. Functional aspects of human sperm binding to the zona pellucida using the hemizona assay. *J Androl* 1991;12:1–8.

Crockin SL, Jones HW Jr. *Legal Conceptions: the Evolving Law and Policy of Assisted Reproductive Technologies.* 2009. The Johns Hopkins University Press, Baltimore, USA.

Gibbons WE, Gitlin SA, Lanzendorf SE, et al. Preimplantation genetic diagnosis for Tay–Sachs disease: successful pregnancy after pre-embryo biopsy and gene amplification by polymerase chain reaction. *Fertil Steril* 1995;63:723–728.

Goodman AL, Hodgen GD. The ovarian triad of the primate menstrual cycle. *Recent Prog Horm Res* 1983;39:1–73.

Hodgen GD. The dominant ovarian follicle. *Fertil Steril* 1982;38:281–300.

Jones HJ Jr, Oehninger S, Bocca S, Stadtmauer L, Mayer J. Reproductive efficiency of human oocytes fertilized in vitro. *Facts Views Vis Obgyn* 2010;2:169–171.

Jones HW Jr. The use of controlled ovarian hyperstimulation in clinical in vitro fertilization: the role of Georgeanna Jones. *Fertil Steril* 2008;90:e1–3.

Personhood Revisited – Reproductive Technology, Bioethics, Religion and the Law. 2013. Langdon Street Press, Minneapolis, USA.

In Vitro Fertilization Comes to America: Memoir of a MEDICAL BREAKTHROugh. 2014. Jamestowne Bookworks, Williamsburg, VA, USA.

Jones HW Jr, Acosta AA, Andrews MC, et al. Three years of in vitro fertilization at Norfolk. *Fertil Steril* 1984;42:826–834.

Jones HW Jr, Jones GS, Hodgen GD, Rosenwaks Z. *In Vitro Fertilization – Norfolk.* 1986. Williams and Wilkins, Baltimore, USA.

Kruger TF, Menkveld R, Stander FS, et al. Sperm morphologic features as a prognostic factor in in vitro fertilization. *Fertil Steril* 1986;46:1118–1123.

Kruger TF, Acosta AA, Simmons KF, et al. Predictive value of abnormal sperm morphology in in vitro fertilization. *Fertil Steril* 1988;49:112–117.

Kulkarni AD, Jamieson DJ, Jones HW Jr, et al. Fertility treatments and multiple births in the United States. *N Eng J Med* 2013;369:2218–2225.

Muasher SJ, Oehninger S, Simonetti S, et al. The value of basal and/or stimulated serum gonadotropin levels in prediction of stimulation response and in vitro fertilization outcome. *Fertil Steril* 1988;50:298–307.

Oehninger S, Kruger TF. *Male Infertility: Diagnosis and Treatment.* 2007. Informa UK Ltd, London, UK.

Oehninger S, Coddington CC, Scott R, et al. Hemizona assay: assessment of sperm dysfunction and prediction of in vitro fertilization outcome. *Fertil Steril* 1989;51:665–670.

Toner JP, Brzyski RG, Oehninger S, et al. Combined impact of the number of pre-ovulatory oocytes and cryopreservation on IVF outcome. *Hum Reprod* 1991a;6:284–289.

Toner JP, Hassiakos DK, Muasher SJ, Hsiu JG, Jones HW Jr. Endometrial receptivities after leuprolide suppression and gonadotropin stimulation: histology, steroid receptor concentrations, and implantation rates. *Ann N Y Acad Sci* 1991b;622:220–229.

Veeck LL. *Atlas of the Human Oocyte and Early Conceptus.* 1986. Williams and Wilkins, Baltimore, USA.

Yang H, Pan B. Citation classics in fertility and sterility, 1975–2004. *Fertil Steril* 2006;86:795–797.

The Development of In-Vitro Fertilization in North America After the Joneses
Moving the Field Forward After Elizabeth Carr

Matthew Connell and Alan H. DeCherney

Controlled Ovarian Stimulation

On December 28, 1981, Elizabeth Jordan Carr was born. She was the first baby born in the United States, and the fourteenth baby worldwide, using in-vitro fertilization (IVF). At this time, there were five IVF clinics: Drs. Howard and Georgeanna Jones at Eastern Virginia Medical School, Dr. Alan DeCherney at Yale, Dr. Martin Quigley at the University of Texas Health Science Center, Dr. Anne Wentz at Vanderbilt, and Dr. Richard Marrs at the University of Southern California (USC). There were five other ongoing pregnancies; four from the Jones Institute and one from USC (Thompson, 2016). IVF had truly arrived in the Unites States.

There is no doubt that the birth of Elizabeth Carr was an enormous moment in United States medical history; however, this was just the start. At the time, oocyte retrievals were done laparoscopically and the live birth per laparoscopic oocyte retrieval was 12% (Garcia et al., 1984). The Jones Institute was using stimulated cycles with low dose human menopausal gonadotropin (hMG), which contrasted with how IVF was being performed in other countries. Oocyte yield per laparoscopy and pregnancy rates were better with the use of hMG than natural cycle IVF. With this in mind, Dr. DeCherney and the group at Yale University (see Figure 8.1) initiated a high dose hMG protocol rather than low dose hMG use (Laufer et al., 1983). This protocol resulted in the higher oocyte yield per laparoscopy. Ovulation induction using high dose hMG for IVF was quickly adopted throughout the United States. This seminal work was the basis for stimulation protocols that are commonly used to today.

Controlled ovarian hyperstimulation (COH) provided more oocytes but it also provided powerful new insights into how the follicular phase was different in stimulated and natural cycles. Dr. DeCherney's group soon realized that patients given similar doses of hMG responded differently with variable levels of estradiol and numbers of follicles. These differences

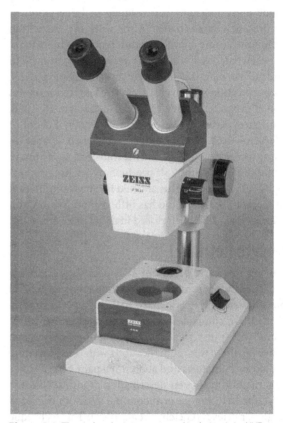

Figure 8.1 The authors' microscope used in their original IVF program. It is now in the Smithsonian Institute.

in the follicular phase were soon used as prognostic factors as patients tended to respond the same way in repeated cycles (Lyles et al., 1985; Pellicer et al., 1987). As patients were responding differently in the follicular phase, the term "poor responder" was used to describe patients with low estradiol levels and low numbers of follicles on ultrasound. While there was no single definition for poor responders, it was realized that they had a poor prognosis for live birth (Laufer et al., 1986). The patterns that emerged during COH allowed for the identification of predictors for success such as basal

FSH and estradiol levels and led to the development of menstrual cycle day 3 values of estradiol and FSH as markers of ovarian reserve (Scott et al., 1989; Smotrich et al., 1995). Testing ovarian reserve with estradiol and FSH is a practice that continues currently.

Medication

During the early years of IVF, hMG was used almost exclusively for COH. Early extraction techniques were crude and inefficient and resulted in large amounts of protein contaminants. Also, with the extraction techniques came significant differences in bioactivity between batches of hMG. This necessitated the need to add hCG to maintain the correct amount of bioactivity. As purification improved, there were less contaminates and ultimately urinary FSH was extracted. In 1989, Dr. Jeffrey Keen, at Washington University School of Medicine in St. Louis, Missouri, published a paper on using recombinant DNA and the transfection of human genes responsible for FSH production in Chinese hamster ovary cell lines. This allowed for mass production of recombinant FSH and has little contamination in it (Keene et al., 1989) (discussed in detail in Chapter 25).

Oocyte Retrieval

During this early period of IVF, oocytes were being retrieved by laparoscopy. This method required general anesthesia and was associated with postoperative pain. With these complications in mind, abdominal ultrasound with transvesical follicle aspiration was described; however, there were complications with this procedure including hematuria and abdominal pain. Shortly after this method had been described, a group in Chicago described a technique of abdominal ultrasound-guided vaginal retrieval (Gleicher et al., 1983). This technique did allow for the needle to be closer to the ovaries, but there was still a great distance between the needle and ultrasound probe. This soon changed with the advent of the vaginal ultrasound probe. Along with the IVF department at Yale, Dr. DeCherney designed a needle guide for the vaginal ultrasound probe, making follicular aspiration much easier. This technique quickly gained popularity as it had fewer complications and was better tolerated by patients. This method is universally practiced in modern day IVF.

Donor Oocytes

In 1983, John E. Buster's group at the UCLA Medical Center, described the first successful pregnancies after the donation of an oocyte *in vivo*. This was achieved by menstrual cycle synchronization between the donors and the recipients. The donors were inseminated on the day of the LH peak, and five days after the LH peak the donors underwent a uterine lavage where an embryo was recovered and then transferred to the recipients. Of the first 14 patients, embryos were recovered from five donors, and two of the five embryos were blastocysts that went on to become pregnancies (Buster et al., 1983). At the time, the group heralded this treatment for patients willing to accept a donor egg that had either surgically inaccessible ovaries, declined further surgery for oocyte retrieval, or had genetic reasons for needing a different chromosome complement (Buster et al., 1983). This method of oocyte donation was rather controversial and was superseded by in-vitro ovum donation and IVF. Zev Rosenwaks, Navot, and colleagues reported the first live birth from donated oocytes using IVF in the USA in 1986. The recipient was a 40-year-old patient with a history of multiple poor responses and poor fertilizations. The donor was given hMG and underwent retrieval of four oocytes which were fertilized with the husband's spermatozoa. Three oocytes fertilized and were transferred 43 h after oocyte retrieval. A healthy boy was born at term. The group advocated that donor oocytes could be used when surgery was contraindicated or when there had been multiple poor outcomes with traditional IVF (Rosenwaks et al., 1986). Since this time, egg donation has evolved and become a viable option for couples with age-related infertility, diminished ovarian reserve, or primary ovarian insufficiency. Good pregnancy and live birth rates have been achieved with vitrified eggs through a cryobank or the use of fresh donor oocytes.

Alternatives to Traditional IVF

As IVF techniques were being refined, others looked at alternatives and ways to expand treatment. In 1984, Ricardo Asch and his colleagues at the University of Texas described the first pregnancy using a laparoscopic approach to transfer gametes into the Fallopian tube (Asch et al., 1984). Gamete intra-Fallopian transfer (GIFT) sought to overcome failed pick up of the ovum by the fimbriae or failed sperm migration to the Fallopian tube. The group treated a 35-year-old woman with hMG followed by laparoscopic oocyte retrieval. These oocytes were loaded in a catheter with the prepared sperm. The catheter was placed in the Fallopian tube and the contents injected. The first GIFT attempt led to a successful twin pregnancy (Asch et al., 1984).

Later, this treatment was altered to zygote intra-Fallopian transfer; however, as IVF continued to improve, GIFT and ZIFT have fallen out of favor as a first line treatment modality.

Surrogacy

Human surrogacy became a reality in 1985. Utian and coworkers, in Cleveland, Ohio, at Mount Sinai Medical Center, described the first case in the *New England Journal of Medicine* (Utian et al., 1985). The patient was a 37-year-old woman who had a bilateral salpingectomy for tubo-ovarian abscesses and prior to IVF underwent a hysteropscopic myomectomy. She subsequently had a spontaneous uterine rupture at 28 weeks' gestation resulting in a cesarean hysterectomy and a fetal demise. The couple strongly preferred having a child with their own gametes. The couple had a 22-year-old friend that volunteered to carry the pregnancy. The group synchronized cycles utilizing oral contraceptive pills and the patient was started on clomiphene citrate and menotropins. On cycle day 10 the patient underwent laparoscopic oocyte retrieval followed by fertilization with the husband's spermatozoa. On the third day after retrieval one eight-cell embryo was transferred, resulting in a successful pregnancy (Utian et al., 1985). This breakthrough allowed couples to reproduce using their own genetic material. Surrogacy remains a viable option of treatment for patients, and its role has been expanded to patients suffering from uterine anomalies, multiple implantations failures, maternal medical conditions that preclude carrying a pregnancy, and to same sex male couples.

Male Infertility

Male factor infertility accounts for about 40% of the causes for the infertile couple (as of 2015). Over the years, clinicians have sought ways to overcome this. Around the world clinicians had made several strides. In Australia, sub-zonal injection of sperm brought new hope to couples with recurrent failed cycles and helped make way for intracytoplasmic sperm injection (ICSI). Microsurgical epidydimal sperm aspiration (MESA) and testicular sperm extraction (TESE) had been described. In the United States, several breakthroughs occurred to help overcome male factor infertility. Silber and colleagues at the University of California, Irvine, described MESA for men with congenital bilateral absence of vas deferens (CBAVD) in 1987 with the first live birth from this technique in 1988. The group described a series of 18 patients with CBAVD;

they were able to retrieve motile sperm from 17 of them and three pregnancies resulted from 10 transfers (Patrizio et al., 1988; Silber et al., 1987). A few years later a group at Boston University found that CBAVD was related to cystic fibrosis gene mutations and, in 1993, Silber et al. showed that this could be inherited (Patrizio et al., 1993). This work was important as it is now standard to assess for a CFTR gene mutation in cases of CBAVD and continues to give hope to those affected couples who would like to build families.

In 1996, another important genetic finding occurred in male infertility at the Howard Hughes Medical Institute in Cambridge, Massachusetts. Men with severe oligospermia or azoospermia were identified as having a deletion of the azoospermia factor (AZF) gene located on the long arm of the Y chromosome. AZFa, AZFb, and AZFc deletions were further categorized. Men with an AZFc deletion may have sperm found on MESA; however, this is transmissible to male offspring, who would likely be infertile as well (Reijo et al., 1996). Since this discovery, testing for these deletions has become a standard part of the evaluation of men with oligospermia. Another cause of azoospermia is Klinefelter's syndrome. In 1998, the group at Cornell successfully extracted sperm from a non-mosaic Klinefelter's patient that was used for ICSI and resulted in a live birth (Palermo et al., 1998). This practice is the mainstay therapy for Klinefelter's patients today.

Oncofertility

More than a decade ago it was well understood that the treatment of cancer in reproductive-age women was detrimental to their fertility. Fertility preservation for this reason was not a new idea but rather an uncoordinated effort to help women preserve their fertility. Many roadblocks existed, including reproductive endocrinologists understanding the need for emergency fertility preservation, and oncologists willing to let patients undergo these procedures prior to the initiation of treatment. Educational awareness began to change when Dr. Teresa Woodruff, in 2005, started the Oncofertility Consortium at Northwestern University. The mission was to serve as an authoritative voice for women diagnosed with conditions that involved fertility-threatening treatments. The Consortium's work has been centered on increasing patient awareness, helping communication between physicians of different specialties, and pursuing new options in therapy. Since 2005, many other institutions around the world have taken part in this important work. This groundbreaking advocacy led the American Society of Clinical Oncology and the American Society for Reproductive Medicine (ASRM) to both publish guidelines on fertility preservation in 2013 (Woodruff, 2015).

As a result of this effort, oncofertility has become part of fertility clinics' services around the world and oncologists are making fertility a priority after the diagnosis of a malignancy. This work has also been beneficial for patients with other diseases that have a detrimental influence on reproductive outcomes. This includes patients with rheumatologic diseases, hematologic conditions such as β-thalassemia, and certain metabolic disorders that all affect reproduction and gonadal function. Exploring options for fertility in these settings is paramount. Moving forward, options for fertility preservation in prepubescent children is being actively investigated and may include ovarian cryopreservation and development of primordial follicles into tertiary follicles in vitro for use later on in life (Woodruff, 2015).

Social Egg Freezing

The first pregnancy from a cryopreserved oocyte was in 1986 (Chen, 1986). However, it wasn't until 26 years later that the ASRM announced that oocyte cryopreservation would no longer be considered experimental. Shortly thereafter, ASRM and the Society for Assisted Reproductive Technology (SART) published a guideline regarding mature oocyte cryopreservation in 2013 Practice Committee of the American Society of Reproductive Medicine; Society for Assisted Reproduction (2013). This change was a result of the successes seen with vitrification of oocytes rather than the use of the slow-freeze method. With the use of vitrification, success rates approximate those of fresh oocytes used for IVF with intracytoplasmic sperm injection (ICSI). Initial analyses have been reassuring when comparing rates of congenital anomalies from vitrified oocytes with the general population from the United States (Noyes et al., 2009). The initial data are promising but more long term data need to be acquired.

Given the lack of long term data, ASRM was cautious and recommended against using egg freezing as a safeguard against age-related decline in fertility. However, oocyte cryopreservation has been heralded as a breakthrough for women's reproductive autonomy. A woman without a partner may freeze oocytes rather than using donor sperm to freeze embryos, allowing her to select her partner later in life. Couples that may not want embryos frozen may instead freeze oocytes.

This technology increasingly has been utilized since 2012. The media has given it increased attention as certain large corporations (i.e. Facebook and Apple) have offered to cover the cost of oocyte cryopreservation for their employees. This social egg freezing has been viewed by the public as "fertility insurance." There has been much ethical debate as to whether this social egg freezing is liberating for women or is pressuring women to further their career first (Rebar, 2016). Either way, this technology is currently being used and will likely continue to grow in the coming years.

Age and Fertility

In 1982 DeCherney and Berkowitz wrote an editorial in the *New England Journal of Medicine* defining the decrease in female fertility starting at approximately 35 years of age. This was based on the Federation CECOS study which included 2193 patients who underwent artificial insemination (donor) in France.

Laboratory Innovations
Culture Club

In the 1980s there had been years of work attempting to grow non-human embryos to the blastocyst stage. There were many laboratories attempting this work in different animals; however, there was no clear direction unifying this effort. At the time, this was hindering the treatment of infertility in humans with IVF. It was also understood that with the current poor environment, multiple embryos would need to be transferred to overcome the poor conditions and would increase the rates of multiple gestations. This work changed in 1984 when the National Institute of Child Health and Human Development (NIH) hired Dr. Richard Tasca to coordinate multiple investigators working on embryo development. This group became known as the Culture Club. Over the 14 years of its existence, there were multiple meetings to spearhead this research effort. The results were fantastic. The work resulted in over 240 publications. Dr. John Biggers created the KSOM media through a simplex optimization approach. Essentially, this allowed embryos to choose conditions that were favorable to the embryo. This base media is still used in labs around the world (Albertini and McGinnis, 2013).

Assisted Hatching

Around the world several advances in technology have helped improve IVF success rates. Groups in France and Australia worked to improve culture media to better mimic the human tubal and uterine environment. The breakthrough of ICSI helped couples with failed fertilization. In the United States, the early 1990s marked some significant breakthroughs. Jacques Cohen, an embryologist who worked with Steptoe and Edwards at Bourn Hall in the 1980s, pioneered many new techniques. In 1990, while at Emory University School of Medicine, he introduced a new concept to assist implantation. At the time, the ratio of live birth per embryo transferred was quite poor, and Cohen's group hypothesized that this was due to healthy embryos' inability to hatch from the zona pellucida and implant. With this in mind, they described piercing the zona pellucida with a microneedle. The embryo was considered pierced when the tip of the needle could be visualized in the perivitelline space (Cohen et al., 1990). This procedure became known as "assisted hatching." The result of this work was a doubling in the rate of implantation (Cohen et al.,1990). Over the years there has been debate as to what assisted hatching's contribution is to live birth rates; however, it has been shown to be helpful in some clinical scenarios and is a practice that is still carried out in many clinics today.

Testing for Aneuploidy and Diseases

Along with assisted hatching, Cohen, with Santiago Munné, James Grifo, and Zev Rosenwaks, described the first attempt at aneuploidy screening in 1995. At that time sex selection for embryos at risk of X-linked diseases was already being performed, and the group at Cornell took embryos that screened positive for a Y chromosome and performed fluorescence in-situ hybridization for chromosomes X, Y, 16, and 18 (Munne et al., 1995). This ground-breaking idea of preimplantation genetic screening (PGS) was meant to overcome the poor success rates of IVF by transferring euploid embryos only. While FISH has fallen out of favor for the better technique of PGS, this concept is still used today and with a growing number of IVF cycles utilizing PGS.

As the field continued evolve with the use of blastomere biopsy, Zev Rosenwaks' group expanded this technology for the diagnosis of genetic diseases. In 1999, a couple had undergone two induced abortions due to fetuses affected by sickle cell anemia. The group took the couple through IVF and on day 3 performed a blastomere biopsy. The blastomeres underwent analysis and unaffected embryos were transferred on day 4, with healthy twin girls born at term (Xu et al., 1999). Since this report, many other couples have utilized

this technology to avoid having offspring with lethal or life altering diseases. Currently, embryo biopsy has shifted to trophectoderm biopsy and is routinely used in practice.

Blastocyst Culture and Single Embryo Transfer

While work on embryos was being done to increase implantation rates, David Gardner and William Schoolcraft at the Colorado Center for Reproductive Medicine took on the challenge of growing embryos to the blastocyst stage in order to improve implantation rates and to promote single embryo transfers , thus reducing multiple gestations. To this point embryos were transferred at the cleavage stage as prior work on transferring blastocysts had not been successful. Gardner and Schoolcraft successfully showed that sequential serum free media could establish a reasonable blastocyst conversion rate, and that 90% of the patients received at least two blastocysts with a 70% pregnancy rate (Gardner et al., 1998). This landmark work pushed the field forward by improving implantation rates and decreasing the number of embryos transferred. Subsequently the group showed through a randomized trial that single embryo transfer (SET) could achieve reasonable pregnancy rates and dramatically decrease the twin rate (Gardner et al., 2004).

Donor Oocyte Cytoplasm

It was hypothesized that patients with poor outcomes in IVF may have deficiencies in the cytoplasm of their oocytes. To overcome this deficiency, cytoplasm from a donor oocyte would be transferred to the recipient oocyte. The first live birth from this technique was reported by Cohen in 1997. A 39-year-old patient had a history of four prior IVF cycles that failed due to poor embryo development. The patient was offered donor oocyte but declined as she desired genetically related children. The patient underwent COH with 20 oocytes of poor quality. Cytoplasm of seven donor oocytes was used for 14 of the patient's oocytes. After the cytoplasm was removed from the donor oocyte, confirmatory testing to assure the metaphase spindle was left intact was undertaken. Four embryos were transferred and a singleton pregnancy was established. Amniocentesis before the sixteenth week of gestation revealed nuclear DNA matching the parents and mitochondrial DNA homologous with maternal mitochondrial DNA.

A healthy girl was delivered at term (Cohen et al., 1997). This work continued until 2001. A total of 17 children were born from this technique in the United States. The FDA sent a cease and desist letter to clinics offering this service. As the long term effects of this technology were unknown, the federal government ruled this was experimental and without further studies was deemed unsafe.

Moral, Ethical, and Social Issues

Religion

Shortly after the birth of Elizabeth Carr, the Vatican published the *Dignitas Personae*. This document was instructions for respecting life. Within the document it is stated "the doctor is at the service of persons and of human procreation. He does not have the authority to dispose of them or to decide their fate." As an alternative, the Vatican offers that adoption should be a viable option for the treatment of infertile couples. The document continues by suggesting that IVF would seem to be helping create life but rather it imposes new threats against life by discarding embryos. Furthermore, the idea of preimplantation genetic diagnosis was considered shameful and reprehensible as it presumes the value of human life only within the context of normality and well-being. The Vatican states "thus opening the way to legitimizing infanticide and euthanasia as well." The Vatican continues to hold these views and principles.

Del-Zio vs. Vande Wiele

Interestingly, the first attempt at IVF was at New York's Columbia-Presbyterian Hospital. In 1973, Doris Del-Zio was 29 years old and suffering from tubal infertility. After multiple failed treatments, Dr. William Sweeney suggested IVF as a treatment, though at the time there hadn't been any success. Dr. Sweeney took Doris through ovulation induction and surgical aspiration of follicles. These follicles were taken to the laboratory of Dr. Landrum Shettles. The plan was to expose the oocytes to semen from her husband, and then grow the embryos for a few days and transfer them back. However, word spread of this plan and on the next day the chairman of the department of obstetrics and gynecology, Dr. Raymond Vande Wiele, removed the tube from the incubator, stopping cell division and ending the first attempt at IVF in the United States. The decision to end the experiment was based on the

premise that this was violating federal regulation and would hurt Columbia's grant funding for other work, and if the baby was abnormal it would expose the hospital to significant liability.

Outraged by the action of Dr. Vande Wiele, Dr. Shettles resigned from Columbia a month later and the Del-Zio family filed a lawsuit against Vande Weile and Columbia for intentional infliction of emotional distress. The couple was seeking $1.5 million dollars in damages. The trial took place in 1978 and on the seventh day of the trial Louise Brown was born which intensified the situation. The case concluded with the court finding Columbia at fault and awarded Mrs. Del-Zio $50,000 and Mr. Del-Zio $3. Ironically, five years later Dr. Vande Wiele became co-director of the first IVF clinic in New York City at Columbia.

The Case of Baby M

Surrogacy became a reality in 1985; however, in 1986 many countries in Europe outlawed surrogacy over the case involving Baby M. Mrs. Whitehead was a married woman with children of her own. She was asked by Elizabeth Stern if she would carry a child for her for $10,000, as Mrs. Stern had multiple sclerosis and was advised against becoming pregnant. Mrs. Whitehead underwent intrauterine insemination with William Stern's spermatozoa. As the pregnancy neared term the Whiteheads had a change of heart and did not feel that it was right to sell their child. They were also concerned about what they would tell their children. The birth occurred on March 27, 1986. The baby was given two names: Mrs. Whitehead named her Sarah and the Sterns named her Melissa. This case brought about the issue of third party parenting as the Whiteheads did not want to give up custody. New Jersey Judge Harvey Sorkow heard the case. It took a year of deliberation and the Sterns were awarded custody with the Whiteheads given rights for visitation. When Melissa Stern turned 18 she terminated parental rights with Mrs. Whitehead. This case went on to set the precedence for other controversial cases involving a third party (Sanger, 2007).

Cecil B. Jacobson vs. United States

In 1992, a federal court jury found Dr. Jacobson guilty on several counts of fraud and perjury. He was sentenced to five years in jail. The case stems from his medical practice in Fairfax County, Virginia. Over the years Dr. Jacobson had built a worldwide reputation for performing the first amniocentesis. Trouble began for Dr. Jacobson when a Washington DC investigative reporter broadcast reports of him giving patients hCG and telling the couples they were pregnant. It was later found that he had also been using his own semen to help couples achieve pregnancy and was telling couples the semen was from anonymous donors or medical students. He allegedly performed inseminations on 75 women without their knowledge. After genetic testing, 15 children were proven to be fathered by Dr. Jacobson. This case highlighted the importance of conducting the practice of reproductive medicine ethically, and the impropriety that can take place. While the United States does not regulate the use of donor semen at the national level, the United Kingdom adopted legislation the same year as this case to regulate donor insemination procedures.

The Ricardo Asch Affair

Dr. Ricardo Asch was the director of the infertility program at UC-Irvine. In 1994, it was discovered that he was utilizing patients' oocytes or embryos without their knowledge. These oocytes and embryos were being transferred for the use of other patients or being sold for research purposes. To further complicate matters, many fertility centers were unknowingly utilizing these stolen embryos for their patients. It has been reported that at least 15 live births occurred from this practice. Asch resigned and his two partners, Dr. Jose Balmaceda and Dr. Sergio Stone, were placed on administrative leave. Later, Drs. Asch and Balmaceda fled the country and Dr. Stone was found guilty for mail fraud and tax evasion (Fischer, 1999). This was the first reported theft of reproductive material. This case also highlighted the issues of research misconduct and misappropriation of funds in reproductive medicine. Research involving reproductive material should proceed forward only after proper ethical review and approval. To this day Dr. Asch lives in Argentina and has not been extradited to the United States.

Federal Regulation

In the United States, IVF has had some regulation, mostly regarding research with human embryos. In 1974, the National Research Act included protection of human subjects of biomedical research and ultimately encompassed embryos and thus prohibited human embryo research. In 1975 this decision was reversed by Casper Weinberger, the secretary of Health, Education, and Welfare. The new regulations allowed research

in the field of IVF if it was approved by the national Ethics Advisory Board. While this decision was made in 1975, the Ethics Advisory Board was not in place until 1978. Once assembled, the board unanimously recommended the federal funding of research in IVF. The 13-member panel (seven physicians, two lawyers, one businessman, one philosopher, one religious ethicist, and a member of a philanthropic organization) made this decision based on two points. First, the panel assumed IVF with embryo transfer is the next logical step in the treatment of infertility. Secondly, it felt that patients couldn't protect themselves from the risks of IVF if there wasn't research in the field.

Prior to the birth of Elizabeth Carr, the Joneses faced opposition in setting up the IVF center in Norfolk, Virginia. Hearings were held and several protests took place, but ultimately the Joneses were able to get approval in 1980. In 1985 Dr. Alan DeCherney chaired a meeting at the NIH to discuss forming a registry to be used for research, and in 1986 SART started voluntarily collecting data for research purposes, with the first report written in 1988 (Chang and DeCherney, 2003). The early 1990s saw an increase in unease with IVF clinics, as the costs were high, and success rates were misleading or overstated by a number of clinics. This spurred the Federal Trade Commission in 1992 to legally get involved for false advertising. This led Congress to pass the Fertility Clinic Success Rate and Certification Act which mandated that all clinics report their data yearly to the Centers for Disease Control and Prevention (CDC) (Thompson, 2016). Later that year, the CDC collaborated with SART to create a registry. Dr. DeCherney was president of ASRM at the time when the registry was being put in to place. The original intent was to have a registry that was not clinic specific, to avoid using it as an advertising tool; however, Dr. DeCherney let members vote and it was decided that the registry would be clinic specific. The first report of ART Success Rates was published by SART in 1995.

In 1993, Senator Edward Kennedy and Representative Henry Waxman enacted the National Institutes of Health Revitalization Act. Prior to this, funding for research with human embryos went through the Ethics Advisory Board and this act allowed the NIH to appoint a Human Embryo Research Panel to advise which areas were acceptable for federal funding. However, this oversight did not last long as the Dickey–Wicker Amendment was passed in 1995. This amendment restricted the use of federal funds for research that involved the creation, destruction, or injury of human embryos. To this day, this amendment remains as a legal obstacle for federal funding of human embryo research.

Mitochondrial Transfer

Mitochondrial disease can be devastating. PGD for mitochondrial disease is unreliable as different threshold amounts of abnormal mitochondria can present differently. In 2015, the United Kingdom approved mitochondrial transfer by allowing the Human Fertilisation and Embryology Authority to grant licences on a case-by-case basis. No regulatory authority exists in the United States and authorization would have to come from the FDA. The FDA asked the Institute of Medicine (IOM) to write a report addressing ethical, clinical, and policy issues of mitochondrial transfer. Dr. DeCherney sat on this committee, which met five times, for two days each time, over nine months in 2015. The IOM made several recommendations. First, clinical investigations should be limited to women at risk of transmitting the mitochondrial disease. Secondly, initial transfers should be done with male embryos only so that no further genetic information is passed on to other offspring. If research shows positive findings it may be expanded to female embryos. Thirdly, these initial investigations should be done at centers with expertise in these techniques. Finally, the committee further went on to say that if the FDA approves mitochondrial transfer, that societies should make strict guidelines to prevent clinics from using this technology for other purposes such as mitochondrial transfer in older patients (Falk et al., 2016; National Academies of Sciences, Engineering, and Medicine, 2016). Currently, the FDA has not yet approved mitochondrial transfer as a clinical tool in the United States, but this could happen in the future.

Conclusion

Since the birth of Elizabeth Carr, IVF in the United States has made extraordinary progress in helping couples to achieve their family planning goals. Many pioneering physicians and scientists have been involved in this work and to list all of them would be nearly impossible. These early years in the United States were exciting times and landmark papers were not uncommon. There were a few bumps in the road along the way as mentioned, but the practice of IVF has endured and flourished. The practice and science of IVF will continue to move forward and it will be exciting to see where it is at in the next 40 years.

References

Practice Committees of American society for Reproductive Medicine, Society for Assisted Reproductive Technology. Mature oocyte cryopreservation: a guideline. *Fertility and Sterility* 2013;99: 37–43.

Recommendations for practices utilizing gestational carriers: a committee opinion. *Fertility and Sterility* 2017;107: e3–e10.

Albertini DF, McGinnis LK. A catalyst for change in reproductive science: John D. Biggers as a mentor's mentor. *Journal of Assisted Reproduction and Genetics* 2013;30: 979–994.

Asch RH, Ellsworth LR, Balmaceda JP, Wong PC. Pregnancy after translaparoscopic gamete intrafallopian transfer. *Lancet* 1984;2: 1034–1035.

Buster JE, Bustillo M, Thorneycroft IH, et al. Non-surgical transfer of in vivo fertilised donated ova to five infertile women: report of two pregnancies. *Lancet* 1983;2: 223–224.

Chang WY, DeCherney AH. History of regulation of assisted reproductive technology (ART) in the USA: a work in progress. *Human Fertility* (Cambridge, England) 2003;6: 64–70.

Chen C. Pregnancy after human oocyte cryopreservation. *Lancet* 1986;1: 884–886.

Cohen J, Elsner C, Kort H, et al. Impairment of the hatching process following IVF in the human and improvement of implantation by assisting hatching using micromanipulation. *Human Reproduction* (Oxford, England) 1990;5: 7–13.

Cohen J, Scott R, Schimmel T, Levron J, Willadsen S. Birth of infant after transfer of anucleate donor oocyte cytoplasm into recipient eggs. *Lancet* 1997;350: 186–187.

DeCherney AH, Berkowitz TS. Female fecundity and age. *The New England Journal of Medicine* 1982; 306: 424–426.

Falk MJ, Decherney A, Kahn JP. Mitochondrial replacement techniques – implications for the clinical community. *The New England Journal of Medicine* 2016; 374: 1103–1106.

Fischer J. Misappropriation of human eggs and embryos and the tort of conversion: a relational view. *Loyola of Los Angeles Law Review* 1999; 2: 381–430.

Garcia J, Acosta A, Andrews MC, et al. In vitro fertilization in Norfolk, Virginia, 1980–1983. *Journal of In Vitro Fertilization and Embryo Transfer* 1984; 1: 24–28.

Gardner DK, Schoolcraft WB, Wagley L, et al. A prospective randomized trial of blastocyst culture and transfer in in-vitro fertilization. *Human Reproduction* (Oxford, England) 1998; 13: 3434–3440.

Gardner DK, Surrey E, Minjarez D, et al. Single blastocyst transfer: a prospective randomized trial. *Fertility and Sterility* 2004; 81: 551–555.

Gleicher N, Friberg J, Fullan N, et al. EGG retrieval for in vitro fertilisation by sonographically controlled vaginal culdocentesis. *Lancet* 1983; 2: 508–509.

Keene JL, Matzuk MM, Otani T, et al. Expression of biologically active human follitropin in Chinese hamster ovary cells. *The Journal of Biological Chemistry* 1989; 264: 4769–4775.

Laufer N, DeCherney AH, Haseltine FP, et al. The use of high-dose human menopausal gonadotropin in an in vitro fertilization program. *Fertility and Sterility* 1983; 40: 734–741.

Laufer N, DeCherney AH, Tarlatzis BC, Naftolin F. The association between preovulatory serum 17 beta-estradiol pattern and conception in human menopausal gonadotropin-human chorionic gonadotropin stimulation. *Fertility and Sterility* 1986; 46: 73–76.

Lyles R, Gibbons WE, Dodson MG, et al. Characterization and response of women undergoing repeat cycles of ovulation induction in an in vitro fertilization and embryo transfer program. *Fertility and Sterility* 1985; 44: 832–834.

Munne S, Sultan KM, Weier HU, et al. Assessment of numeric abnormalities of X, Y, 18, and 16 chromosomes in preimplantation human embryos before transfer. *American Journal of Obstetrics and Gynecology* 1995; 172: 1191–1199; discussion 1199–1201.

National Academies of Sciences, Engineering, and Medicine. *Mitochondrial Replacement Techniques: Ethical, Social, and Policy Considerations*, 2016. The National Academies Press, Washington, DC.

Noyes N, Porcu E, Borini A. Over 900 oocyte cryopreservation babies born with no apparent increase in congenital anomalies. *Reproductive Biomedicine Online* 2009; 18: 769–776.

Palermo GD, Schlegel PN, Sills ES, et al. Births after intracytoplasmic injection of sperm obtained by testicular extraction from men with nonmosaic Klinefelter's syndrome. *The New England Journal of Medicine* 1998; 338: 588–590.

Patrizio P, Silber S, Ord T, Balmaceda JP, Asch RH. Two births after microsurgical sperm aspiration in congenital absence of vas deferens. *Lancet* 1988; 2: 1364.

Patrizio P, Asch RH, Handelin B, Silber SJ. Aetiology of congenital absence of vas deferens: genetic study of three generations. *Human Reproduction* (Oxford, England) 1993; 8: 215–220.

Pellicer A, Lightman A, Diamond MP, et al. Outcome of in vitro fertilization in women with low response to ovarian stimulation. *Fertility and Sterility* 1987; 47: 812–815.

Rebar RW. Social and ethical implications of fertility preservation. *Fertility and Sterility* 2016; 105: 1449–1451.

Reijo R, Alagappan RK, Patrizio P, Page DC. Severe oligozoospermia resulting from deletions of azoospermia factor gene on Y chromosome. *Lancet* 1996; 347: 1290–1293.

Rosenwaks Z, Veeck LL, Liu HC. Pregnancy following transfer of in vitro fertilized donated oocytes. *Fertility and Sterility* 1986; 45: 417–420.

Sanger C. Developing markets in baby-making: in the matter of baby M. *Harvard Journal of Law and Gender* 2007; 30: 67–97.

Scott RT, Toner JP, Muasher SJ, et al. Follicle-stimulating hormone levels on cycle day 3 are predictive of in vitro fertilization outcome. *Fertility and Sterility* 1989; 51: 651–654.

Silber S, Ord T, Borrero C, Balmaceda J, Asch R. New treatment for infertility due to congenital absence of vas deferens. *Lancet* 1987; 2: 850–851.

Smotrich DB, Widra EA, Gindoff PR, et al. Prognostic value of day 3 estradiol on in vitro fertilization outcome. *Fertility and Sterility* 1995; 64: 1136–1140.

Thompson C. IVF global histories, USA: between Rock and a marketplace. *Reproductive Biomedicine & Society Online* 2016; 2: 128–135.

Utian WH, Sheean L, Goldfarb JM, Kiwi R. Successful pregnancy after in vitro fertilization and embryo transfer from an infertile woman to a surrogate. *The New England Journal of Medicine* 1985; 313: 1351–1352.

Woodruff TK. Oncofertility: a grand collaboration between reproductive medicine and oncology. *Reproduction* (Cambridge, England) 2015; 150: S1–10.

Xu K, Shi ZM, Veeck LL, Hughes MR, Rosenwaks Z. First unaffected pregnancy using preimplantation genetic diagnosis for sickle cell anemia. *Jama* 1999; 281: 1701–1706.

The Brussels Story and the Eureka Moment of Intracytoplasmic Sperm Injection

André Van Steirteghem

Introduction

Clinical IVF started at the University Hospital (UZ Brussel) of the Vrije Universiteit Brussel (VUB) in January 1983 under the guidance of Paul Devroey (the clinician) and André Van Steirteghem (reproductive biologist). The first IVF child was born in November 1983 and we are indebted to the Melbourne Monash University group where we attended the first IVF workshop in July 1982 and were allowed to stay as observers for several weeks after the workshop. On January 14, 1992, the first ICSI child was born.

In this chapter I will provide an historical overview on ICSI and attempt to answer the following questions: "Why did we start?," "What did we do?," "What did we find?," and "What does it mean?"

Why Did We Start?

After the birth of Louise Brown on July 25, 1978, IVF was gradually introduced in many countries and became a successful treatment for the alleviation of longstanding female-factor and idiopathic infertility. However, the hypothesis that bringing the male gametes closer to the oocytes would be an effective treatment in couples with reduced number of spermatozoa was not confirmed. A retrospective analysis of conventional IVF (cIVF) in tubal ($n = 480$) and male ($n = 175$) infertility indicated a lower fertilization rate, embryo transfer rate (89% versus 50%), and pregnancy rate (23% versus 13%) in male infertility (Tournaye et al., 1992). This finding implied that, for couples with a very low sperm count or azoospermia, it was necessary to resort to the use of artificial insemination with donor sperm (AID). As a consequence of this, several groups embarked on research aimed at assisting the fertilization process. Micromanipulation procedures were introduced. The two initial assisted fertilization procedures: zona drilling and partial zona dissection were not successful. Zona drilling involved making a hole in the zona pellucida of an oocyte, which was then incubated in a sperm suspension. Zona drilling worked well in mice but not in humans. Partial zona dissection was introduced afterwards. A mechanical slit was made in the oocytes, which were then incubated in a sperm suspension. Fertilization was obtained by this method but when it occurred there was a similar percentage of monospermic and polyspermic fertilization. Although some pregnancies and births occurred, inconsistent results meant that partial zona dissection was not widely applied in the clinic. Around the same time a few case reports were published on the next assisted fertilization procedure: subzonal insemination (SUZI), a micromanipulation technique involving the insertion of a few spermatozoa between the zona pellucida and the membrane of the oocyte.

What Did We Do?

In line with the policy of the Centre for Reproductive Medicine of VUB, new clinical application was preceded by experimental and translational research. Thanks to a grant from the Fund for Scientific Research Flanders, we investigated the following question: "Does the enhancement of the acrosome of mouse sperm (using chemical means or applying electroporation) result in fertilization and embryo development after a single 'treated' sperm was injected subzonally?" Our hypothesis proved to be correct: good fertilization and embryo development occurred, normal pups were born and they were able to reproduce (Palermo and Van Steirteghem, 1991). These experimental results led us to consider introduction of SUZI into the clinic for patients that had failed several cycles of conventional IVF. Ethical approval was asked for, and obtained from, the VUB Hospital Ethical Committee under the condition that all pregnancies and children born would be part of a thorough follow-up program. The patients were fully informed on the new procedure and agreed to the follow-up program, including a prenatal diagnosis by either chorionic villous sampling or amniocentesis. Clinical SUZI was started at VUB in 1990 and a

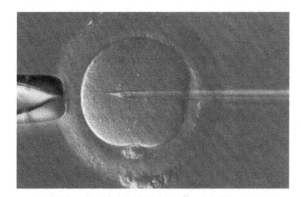

Figure 9.1 One of the first photographs of ICSI; this picture was shown by the late Anne McLaren at meetings.

number of pregnancies and births occurred after SUZI of a few spermatozoa, which had been treated prior to enhance the acrosome reaction (Palermo et al., 1992a). The technical procedure of SUZI is delicate and occasionally one of the sperm entered into the cytoplasm of the oocyte. In these cases of "failed SUZI" we observed normal fertilization as well as embryo development. These cases of "failed SUZI" were carefully observed for their development. In the event that only one such embryo was available it was transferred into the patient. We called this procedure intracytoplasmic sperm injection (ICSI). In April 1991 a patient became pregnant after replacing a single ICSI embryo and she delivered on January 14, 1992 – more than 25 years ago (Palermo et al., 1992b; Figure 9.1). After the initial ICSI observations we continued SUZI and also included ICSI on some oocytes in most cycles. It rapidly became very obvious that the results in terms of fertilization were much more consistent after ICSI than after SUZI, and we obtained ethical approval for ICSI under the same strict protocol regarding follow-up of any pregnancy. As of July 1992 the only assisted fertilization procedure practiced at VUB was ICSI (Van Steirteghem et al., 1993a, b). From late 1992 several live-video ICSI workshops were held at VUB, which helped a lot with the dissemination of ICSI worldwide. The VUB's openness to the world in showing ICSI was similar to the approach taken by the Melbourne groups for the introduction of conventional IVF.

What Did We Find?

ICSI proved to be a consistent treatment for the alleviation of infertility due to severe semen abnormalities, including cryptozoospermia. After the successes with

ejaculated spermatozoa we applied ICSI to epididymal or testicular spermatozoa in cases of azoospermia. Results of ICSI in cases of obstructive azoospermia using epididymal or testicular spermatozoa were similar to the results of ICSI with ejaculated sperm and the results of conventional IVF for female-factor or idiopathic infertility (Devroey et al., 1994; Silber et al., 1994; Tournaye et al., 1994). However, spermatozoa can be found in only half of the patients with non-obstructive azoospermia after testicular biopsy, even after extensive and prolonged searching. If no sperm can be found the sole alternative for these couples is the use of donor sperm (Vernaeve et al., 2006).

Around the time of the first ICSI successes, the first reports appeared of births after preimplantation genetic diagnosis – PGD, a very early form of prenatal diagnosis for couples at high risk of having a child with a genetic disease. PGD involves the removal of one (occasionally two) blastomere(s) from a developing embryo (usually at around the eight-cell stage). The use of ICSI as ART in these couples is indicated for two reasons: to avoid unexpected fertilization failures but also to avoid contamination with sperm DNA on cumulus cells adhering to the zona pellucida at the time of embryo biopsy.

At its inception, but even now, questions are asked about the risk to the offspring after cIVF but especially after ICSI, which is much more invasive than cIVF, bypasses a number of steps occurring in natural conception, and uses severely impaired sperm. The careful evaluation of pregnancies and children was always a condition of approval by the VUB Ethical Committee. Over the past 35 years (1982–2017) the number of ART children born in the VUB program is well over 26,000 and it is fair to summarize the outcome results as follows: there is a slight increase in fetal chromosomal abnormalities after ICSI, the congenital malformation rate is also slightly higher than after natural conception, but there is no difference between IVF and ICSI. Extensive register-based results on outcome, particularly from Scandinavian countries, support the single-center VUB results. In addition the outcome of well over 2500 PGD children at VUB is no different than the outcome after ICSI.

What Does It Mean?

Twenty-five years after the first ICSI birth it is fair to say that the successful introduction of ICSI has meant that the vast majority of cases with severe male-factor infertility, including some cases with azoospermia, can now have their wish for a child fulfilled. A number of groups have started to use ICSI for all patients, with the argument that unexpected fertilization failure can then be avoided. There are no data in the literature indicating that ICSI performs better than cIVF when semen parameters are normal or almost normal, except for PGD cases. The major drawback of ICSI is no different from other forms of ART: the multiple birth rate is still too high and avoiding this iatrogenic complication is the major challenge for all centers. The solution is available and simple – i.e. single embryo transfer, perhaps not for all age groups, but certainly for patients below 38 years of age in their first treatment cycles.

Acknowledgments

The author is indebted to his many colleagues who worked with him over the years at the Centre for Reproductive Medicine. Special thanks to my "partners in crime" Paul Devroey and Inge Liebaers and their many colleagues in the Fertility Clinic and the Centre for Medical Genetics.

References

Devroey P, Liu J, Nagy Z, et al. Normal fertilization of human oocytes after testicular sperm extraction and intracytoplasmic sperm injection. *Fertil Steril* 62, 639–641, 1994.

Palermo G, Van Steirteghem A. Enhancement of acrosome reaction and subzonal insemination of a single spermatozoon in mouse eggs. *Mol Reprod Dev* 30, 339–345, 1991.

Palermo G, Joris H, Devroey P, Van Steirteghem AC. Induction of acrosome reaction in human spermatozoa used for subzonal insemination. *Hum Reprod* 7, 248–254, 1992a.

Pregnancies after intracytoplasmic injection of single spermatozoon into an oocyte. *Lancet* 340, 17–18, 1992b.

Silber SJ, Nagy ZP, Liu J, et al. Conventional in-vitro fertilization versus intracytoplasmic sperm injection for patients requiring microsurgical sperm aspiration. *Hum Reprod* 9, 1705–1709, 1994.

Tournaye H, Devroey P, Camus M, et al. Comparison of in-vitro fertilization in male and tubal infertility: a 3 year survey. *Hum Reprod* 7, 218–222, 1992.

Tournaye H, Devroey P, Liu J, et al. Microsurgical epididymal sperm aspiration and intracytoplasmic sperm injection: a new effective approach to infertility as a result of congenital bilateral absence of the vas deferens. *Fertil Steril* 61, 1045–1051, 1994.

Van Steirteghem AC, Liu J, Joris H, et al. Higher success rate by intracytoplasmic sperm injection than by subzonal insemination. Report of a second series of 300 consecutive treatment cycles. *Hum Reprod* 8, 1055–1060, 1993a.

Van Steirteghem AC, Nagy Z, Joris H, et al. High fertilization and implantation rates after intracytoplasmic sperm injection. *Hum Reprod* 8, 1061–1066, 1993b.

Vernaeve V, Verheyen G, Goossens A, et al. How successful is repeat testicular sperm extraction in patients with azoospermia? *Hum Reprod* 21, 1551–1554, 2006.

The Development of In-Vitro Fertilization in Austria

Wilfried Feichtinger

This chapter is based on an article by Peter Kemeter, originally published in 2007 in German that appeared in the *Journal für Fertilität und Reproduktion*, KUP Verlag, A-3003 Gablitz, Austria, with kind permission of the publisher and author.

At 4.25 pm on August 5, 1982, Austria's first IVF baby, a baby from an egg fertilized outside the body, was born at the Second Vienna University Women's Hospital (Second VUWH). The healthy boy weighed 3.65 kg, was 52 cm in height and was named Zlatan by his parents Jovanka and Dragan Jovanovic. It was sensational news in Austria, and made a big splash across the media.

As leader of the team of doctors, I would like to tell the story of how this pregnancy and birth were achieved, and also about the early days of IVF as I experienced them. I spent the first 13 years of my work in IVF at three different locations, working with Peter Kemeter, and therefore long stretches of this story are also an account of our collaboration.

Preliminary Studies at the Second VUWH

At the Second VUWH, reproductive medicine had been one of the main focuses of the previous director, Hugo Husslein, since the 1970s . The catalyst was one research project in particular, supported by the Ford Foundation. First Peter introduced radioimmunoassay (RIA) to the laboratory in the autumn of 1973, then a new method to precisely determine the hormone levels in blood. Then he organized gynecological operations so that they could be carried out in the ovulation phase of the cycle, to obtain material for examination. Over time he became very familiar with endocrinology and reproduction, and the results of his studies led to several interesting works, which also led to Florian Friedrich, Gerhard Breitenecker, and Peter Kemeter being invited to Detroit and Miami to present their studies.

I Begin Training to Become a Specialist and Start Doing Science

I joined the team in September 1977 to start my training as a specialist. I was regularly assigned to the hormone and sterility clinic operated by Florian Friedrich and Peter Kemeter as head of medicine. Peter described me then as "charming, with a devil-may-care attitude, jovial and always in the mood for a joke," which obviously was popular with staff and patients. I could also speak Russian because my mother was Russian, which helped me talk to patients in their native Slavic languages, mostly with people from Yugoslavia. Unlike most trainees, I was also interested in research. By 1980 I was carrying out studies myself, after planning them with the others. It was said that I proved to have a considerable talent for organization, and great determination.

The First IVF Trials

In early 1979, when I heard that Steptoe and Edwards were going to present their method of IVF, which they had used in the birth of the world's first IVF baby, I was very excited and eager to attend, and decided to fly to London on my own initiative and without an invitation, to learn the methods of these pioneers and perhaps meet them in person (Figure 10.1). The knowledge gained in London enabled us to make concrete progress in IVF. We began to plan diagnostic laparoscopies to be carried out as soon as possible before ovulation. Peter already knew this timing from the Ford project described above, as well as extracting oocytes from mature follicles using suction. An incubator was set up in the laboratory according to specifications from Steptoe and Edwards for the cultivation of oocytes. The acting head of the clinic, Alfred Kratochwil, worked on the program as a pioneer of follicle imaging using ultrasound. Peter selected patients with unexplained problems from the sterility

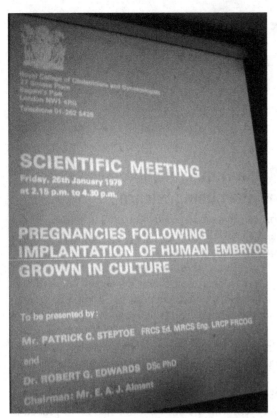

Figure 10.1 Photo taken by the author at the ensigns of the historic scientific meeting, January 1979, in London.

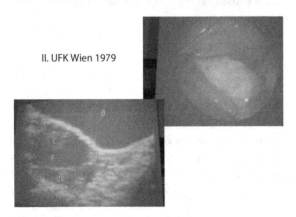

Figure 10.2 Comparison of a follicle as seen on ultrasound and later during laparoscopy (c = cumulus oophorus), Second University Clinic of OBGYN Vienna.

at night as the operating staff were not prepared to work so late for our scientific studies. The laparoscopies were done by the operating team, and Peter or I joined them for the extraction of the oocytes and for examining them.

The incubator was in the laboratory, a considerable distance from the OR, and the conditions for maturation were still very uncontrolled. In hindsight, it is easy to see why this process produced such limited success, because the timing was right in just 33% of cases, and we were also only able to find the oocyte in 25% of cases – although this was in unstimulated cycles (Feichtinger et al., 1981).

The Project Grows

On October 31, 1979, Herbert Janisch came from the First VUWH, preceded by a reputation as an exceptional surgeon, to take over our clinic. He brought Stefan Szalay with him, the most senior doctor and his right-hand man. Janisch gave him the task of developing a successful IVF program, with a focus on sterility, without being aware that we were already working on this.

unit for the program, who gave consent, and collected urine samples after the tenth day of their cycles for determining LH levels. When an increase in LH was detected and a Graafian follicle could be seen using ultrasound, the laparoscopy was scheduled for 26–32 h later (Figure 10.2). Of course, we avoided working

At a meeting of the senior doctors, Janisch explained his plans to entrust Stefan Szalay with IVF. I told him that we already had an IVF programme, what preliminary work Peter and I had already done, and what results we had had. Using a microscope, I showed Janisch an oocyte we had just found. He seemed surprised, because it was the first time he heard about this project. I told him the reasons we suspected were behind our low rate of success, and how improvements could be made, which we thought could be done by extending the project and providing better coordination. I suggested a team be formed, consisting of Stefan, Peter and myself, because it seemed urgent to me to collect oocytes round the clock, which meant also at night. Janisch immediately agreed, all he asked was that his consent for every case should be obtained beforehand.

After the program became the responsibility of the boss, a lot of things became easier for us. For example, anesthetists, operation room nurses, and the other members of the team could no longer refuse to work in the night because it was "just for research."

An external telephone was finally installed in Kemeter's laboratory. This was Laboratory A16, a special clinic for people who wanted to have a baby and for hormone disorders. It was quite different to the main work of the clinic, and the working environment was much more pleasant and personal than in the rest of the building. Laboratory A16 developed into the center of the IVF program, because it was here that patients and their partners were recruited for the program, their files were kept here, and they were also cared for here, both before and after the IVF.

The Long and Difficult Journey to Success

The program continued, following a procedure where the selected patients were introduced to the head of medicine; then, after he gave his consent, they were enrolled in what was called "The Follicle Program." Most were suspected of tubal damage, with otherwise normal test results. Then began cycle monitoring, a few days before ovulation was expected to begin; the patient took three urine samples for testing for LH using HI-Gonavis. As soon as an increase was detected, the patient was admitted to hospital and, once or twice daily, follicle measurement was carried out via ultrasound. The laparoscopy was then carried out using follicular puncture, between 26 h and 32 h after the first clear increase of LH in the urine, usually by Stefan and myself, sometimes also by Adolf Beck. The incubator was installed in a room right next to the OR. I now took over the major part of oocyte cultivation. Insemination of the oocytes with the prepared semen of the husband was done by whichever one of us three had the night shift, often in the evening or during the night.

In July 1980, Peter and I visited the 10th World Fertility Congress in Madrid. I reported our experiences with ultrasound measurement of ovarian follicles in the follicle program, and afterwards got talking to the British pioneer Bob Edwards. He already knew my name from my earlier work, and now I had the chance to tell him that we had also started an IVF program.

Our program's results had improved after the reorganization that took place under Janisch, because our timing in the first half of 1980 was 60% accurate, while it was 92% accurate in the second half of the year. The number of oocytes being found during the same period increased from 32% to 54%. It was only with cell division that we were still waiting for good results. We had not often managed to bring them further than the pronuclear stage.

Disappointed, we sought help from the second most successful center in the world, run by Alex Lopata in Melbourne, Australia. Stefan and I were able to spend two weeks at Lopata's center (Figure 10.3) learning about their methods, and when we returned in October 1980, we changed the culture medium according to his specifications. Cell division soon happened, and in one of six cases even a short-lived pregnancy, a biochemical pregnancy (Feichtinger et al., 1982). I still remember very well how we invited all the staff to a celebration at a nearby bar after the first regular cell division, to celebrate our success.

I collected all the data from the ongoing program and, as soon as we had a number of cases, I wrote a paper, even if there wasn't yet any real success, with the motto "publish or perish" in mind. I credited the others involved as co-authors, with the head of medicine listed last, before presenting it to him.

With his agreement – which he almost always gave – I sent it to the selected journal for publication. Janisch was naturally very interested in having his clinic's successes published. IVF was generating much more interest back then than it does today and so all my papers were accepted (Feichtinger et al., 1982).

Peter came back from holiday in the summer of 1981, and I told him that I had received an invitation

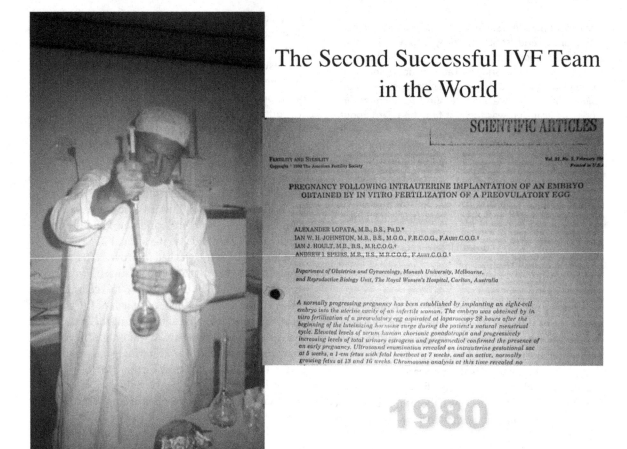

The Second Successful IVF Team in the World

SCIENTIFIC ARTICLES

PREGNANCY FOLLOWING INTRAUTERINE IMPLANTATION OF AN EMBRYO OBTAINED BY IN VITRO FERTILIZATION OF A PREOVULATORY EGG

1980

Figure 10.3 Our great teacher Alex Lopata.

from Bob Edwards and Patrick Steptoe for the two of us to take part in the First Bourn Hall Meeting. Edwards and Steptoe had set up their IVF clinic at Bourn Hall near Cambridge, after the birth of Louise Brown, the first IVF child in the world. The intention of this meeting was for every IVF center that had already had success to be able to share their experience. We were already able to report one pregnancy, even if it had not lasted long, which made us the sixth most successful center in the world and so we were invited too.

Peter was delighted, but too soon. Stefan had already gone to the head of medicine and made the case that he should be one of the people to go to the meeting. After all, he had been brought from the 1st VUWH for IVF. Janisch decided that Peter would have to stay home and keep things running while Stefan went in his stead to Bourn Hall. Janisch immediately sent a

letter to Edwards where he thanked him for the invitation and explained that Stefan would be attending instead of Peter. Bob Edwards reacted in astonishment ("How could Janisch, somebody he didn't even know, take it on himself to send somebody unknown in the world of reproduction instead of somebody with Peter's international reputation?") but he didn't answer the letter because he was told that Peter was going to go along with what Janisch wanted, to avoid tension within the team.

We learned something important from this meeting, something presented by the second most successful center in Australia, headed by Alan Trounson at Monash University. He reported considerably better success when the woman's ovaries were stimulated before the IVF with clomiphene, and they didn't wait for a spontaneous increase in LH, but triggered ovulation with an injection of HCG. We adopted this strategy and the yield of oocytes immediately increased along with fertilization, and, as mentioned at the start, the first pregnancy came in November 1981. Two more pregnancies were achieved in the same month (Feichtinger et al., 1982).

The IVF Treatment of the Jovanovices

The woman who would go on to be the mother of the first IVF baby in Austria was Jovanka Jovanovic (Figure 10.4), a 26-year-old administrative assistant

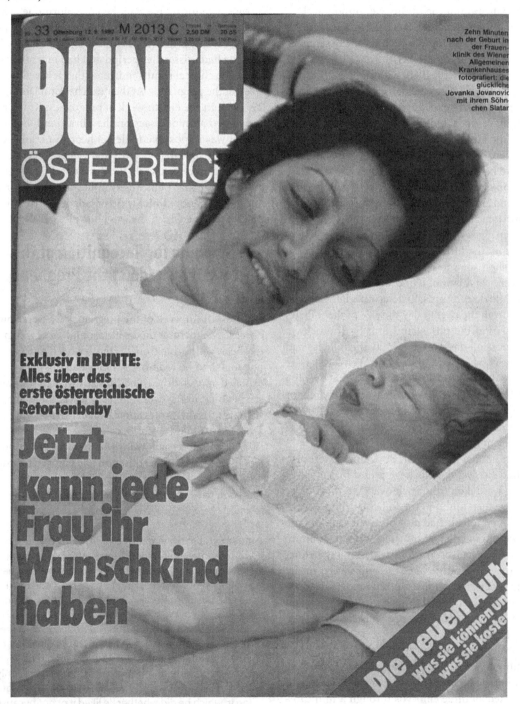

Figure 10.4 Cover page of the popular Austrian magazine "BUNTE" with Jovanka Jovanovic and our first "testube-baby" Zlatan.

at a construction company. On February 19, 1980, she was transferred from the health service clinic in Andreasgasse to our hormone and sterilization clinic, because of six years of sterility. Peter took her medical history and carried out the first gynecological examination. On palpation of the uterus, he found a lack of mobility and immediately suspected blockages in the region of the Fallopian tubes, which led me to send her for a hysterosalpingogram (HSG).

She came on June 10, 1980, with the results of the HSG, which showed blockage of both Fallopian tubes. After the results were explained to her, she said, "The house we have been building in Yugoslavia is finished, and my husband said that now we should soon have children. I think he should get a divorce." It was explained to her that a laparoscopy, for a more precise investigation of the Fallopian tubes, was advisable and that we could also attempt IVF, if she agreed. She gave her permission, and the boss also gave the green light. She was then given Clomiphene tablets, which were to be taken from the fifth to the ninth day of her cycle. Before this she made another visit on the third day of her cycle for cervical dilation. Blood was taken every day, from the tenth day onwards, to determine her estrogen levels, and from the twelfth day the size of the follicles was measured at the ultrasound unit by Kratochwil. On the fourteenth day, November 20, the follicles had attained the correct size and the oestrogen levels were right, so we decided to trigger ovulation that evening using HCG. The patient was admitted and prepared for laparoscopy and extraction of the oocytes exactly 36 h later. Stefan carried out this procedure in the operating room on the morning of October 22, 1981.

Other team members, Peter, Beck, and I, were also there. After incising the blockage found by the HSG, one oocyte was taken from each ovary. In total, three oocytes were then found in the follicular fluid, meaning one hidden follicle had also been sucked out. The oocytes were immediately transferred to the culture medium, which had been fumigated the day before, brought to a temperature of 37 °C and placed in the incubator. Then two drops (approximately 180,000 spermatozoon) were added to each oocyte, which had been also been prepared the previous day from the sperm of the husband.

The next morning we saw that all three oocytes had been fertilized. A day later they had divided to produce one group of eight cells and two groups of four cells. I now injected all three embryos through a thin catheter into the uterus, while the patient stayed still on her elbows and knees. Then she had to lie on her stomach for another 4 h, before being able to go home the next day.

On the eighth day after the IVF, Peter removed the stitches, and from the tenth day blood was taken to determine hormone levels. On the tenth day there was already a gentle increase in the HCG hormone, which indicated that a pregnancy had occurred. At the next check, on December 16, 1981, Mrs. Jovanovic told us that she had missed her period and had morning sickness. The clinical results indicated that it was the sixth week of the pregnancy. At the next check on December 29, 1981, in the eighth week of pregnancy, Kratochwil found two amniotic sacs on the ultrasound, but back then it was impossible to detect heart function. After some light spotting we gave her a depot injection of progestogens once a week. I was present at this examination and at that point referred her to me personally at the pregnancy clinic, which made her virtually my private patient, which she was quite pleased about.

The Struggle for Recognition of the Success Overshadows the Pregnancy and Birth

Until the ninth week of the pregnancy we were able to observe two foetuses on the ultrasound, each with positive heart action, but from the tenth week there was only one foetus to be found. The other had obviously been expelled or reabsorbed. I had already written the manuscript about our success and sent it, via the manager's secretary, to the professional journal *Geburtshilfe und Frauenheilkunde* (Feichtinger et al., 1982) under the title "Pregnancies with twins after oocyte extraction via laparoscopy, in vitro fertilisation and embryo transfer."

There was still time to change the title, but interest was soon to be directed more at the order of authors.

After a visit to the women's clinic in Munich, I met Prof. Holzmann, an editor for the journal "Geburtshilfe und Frauenheilkunde," and I discovered that Janisch had recently sent a letter asking to have his name moved to first position. He also asked if the other authors knew about it. We hadn't heard a thing about it, and we wrote a letter to the publisher telling them that all the authors had agreed that the original list of authors, with me in the first position, should be kept. We put this letter in front of Janisch, which was only lacking his signature, and asked him to join us in signing it, which he did whether he liked it or not because

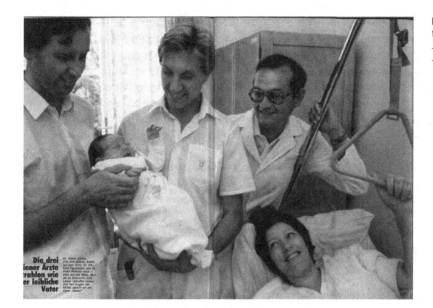

Figure 10.5 The happy successful team from left to right: S. Szalay, Baby Zlatan Jovanovic, W. Feichtinger, P. Kemeter, and Jovanka Jovanovic after the birth.

otherwise we would have prevented publication with a restraining order. Instead of leaving it at that, for good measure I said to the boss, "...by the way, I won't do the specialist exam that you introduced to our clinic, because it's illegal."

Of course, the atmosphere among the IVF team instantly became very bad. I contacted the medical council and other disciplinary bodies, and I went on the offensive in the media. Janisch took revenge, for example by giving me duties that took me away from IVF. Because of the media interest we were expecting, I suggested to Stefan and Peter that we contact a lawyer friend of his and sign an exclusive contract with a magazine called "Die Bunte" in our name, to give us more influence on how the media reported events. Together, we presented this suggestion to Janisch, who agreed to it.

In the mean time, Mrs. Jovanovic's pregnancy was proceeding without complications. The boss was kept informed about the progress of the pregnancy and examined her himself in the thirty-eighth week. He ordered that five days before the predicted date of birth a placental function test was to be carried out; and if this exhibited defective function, a Cesarean section should be done.

This proved unnecessary, and contractions started spontaneously on August 5, 1982. Expulsion was delayed

and Janisch ordered forceps to be used to aid delivery, which I did without complication (Figure 10.5).

The next birth from our first series of successful IVF procedures also excited a lot of curiosity in the media, because it was the birth of Austria's first IVF twins, and the first on the continent. The patient had chosen Peter as her obstetrician and so it was he who carried out the Cesarean section that was necessary because of an abnormal presentation, assisted by myself and Stefan. Two healthy young girls were brought into the world at Rudolfinerhaus on November 10, 1982. The father was enormously proud, he wrote a long report and sent it to a number of newspapers, who then wrote articles.

Peter Kemeter's Exit from the Second VUWH and the Founding of the First IVF Outpatient Clinic

In view of the difficult situation at the clinic, Peter came to the decision to leave, in order to set up an IVF unit at the private clinic he had already founded in 1979. He was sure that the many stages of IVF treatment would be easier to organize and coordinate at a smaller unit rather than a large clinic. He therefore resigned on December 31, 1982, and had suggested to me that I should practise IVF with him during the time he was not on other duties. I agreed and we wasted no time in founding the joint venture "Extra-corporale

Fertilisierung" at 76 Hadikgasse in Penzing on November 25, 1982 (Figure 10.6). A bathroom served us as IVF laboratory (Figure 10.7), and Peter's private office later became our operating room (Figure 10.8).

Naturally we did not have an operating room to perform laporoscopies, so we had to look for one. We found one at the Rudolfinerhaus private hospital, but this was located in the 19th district, which was relatively far away. We had to transport the oocytes in a battery powered transport incubator. I persuaded

the reliable doctor's assistant Christa Hochfellner (Figure 10.9) to leave Laboratory A16 and join us, which she did. She was now a receptionist and doctor's assistant and soon learned to measure follicles using ultrasound without supervision, when neither of us had time. Our new system worked and we were soon able to treat couples and bring them the joy of pregnancy (Feichtinger et al., 1983).

I immediately began to talk to the media and publicize our work, which meant more and more patients

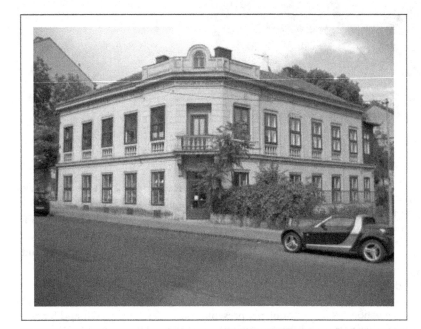

Figure 10.6 Peter's house, Hadikgasse 76 in Vienna: the first outpatient IVF clinic in the world.

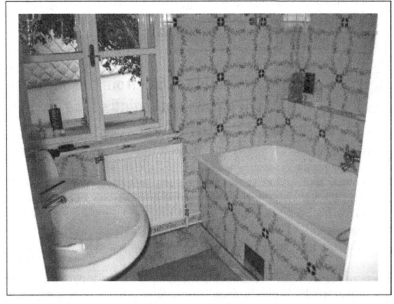

Figure 10.7 The incubator was placed on this bath-tub.

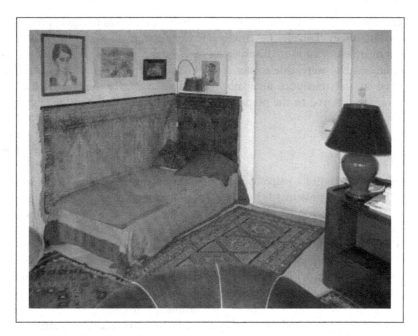

Figure 10.8 On this couch we did our first ultrasound-guided egg retrievals.

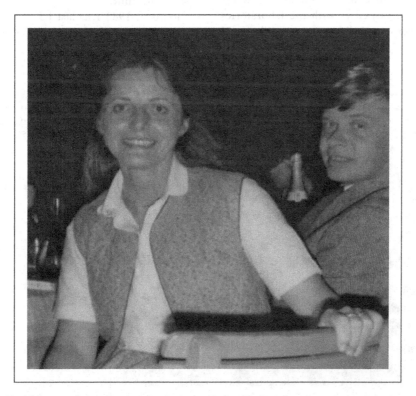

Figure 10.9 Christa Hochfellner, our first embryologist and assistant. (Gerhard Breitenecker, pioneer in Austria having started radioimmuno-assays and genetics, chief of the lab of the university clinic, is seen in the back of the picture.)

and their partners came to us. We had a much more familiar relationship with them than at the clinic, and we also made the treatment a lot more transparent for them; for example, they were able to watch as the oocytes arrived in the transport incubator (Figure 10.10), and were transferred to the prepared Petri dishes using a pipette.

Who Dares, Wins

All this wasn't enough for me, and I had already sent a flyer in October 1981 for a congress in 1983 at the Hofburg in Vienna, which now had to be organized. With the aid of a company called Med Congress, I immediately got to work. And now the difference between us and the clinic became very clear. All communication was speedy and direct, with no bureaucracy in the way and without conflict between peoples' different interests.

The schedule for each day was as follows: in the morning there were consultations with patients, where we presented the treatment plans for those who came to us in the IVF program. Christa used the plan to coordinate the appointments with the patients and their partners, as well as with the laboratories and the Rudolfinerhaus. I didn't arrive until after 4

pm, because I was needed at the clinic until then, or I went directly to Rudolfinerhaus to do laparoscopies and extract oocytes. Peter usually came too because what we were striving for was that both of us would be able to master the entire treatment and continue to hone our skills. Then the oocytes were brought in the transport incubator by car to us in Hadikgasse. Sometimes the partner of the patient brought them, if we had things to do elsewhere. Once we were visited by the biologist Tatjana Kniewald from the team at the Erlanger Women's Clinic who were responsible for Germany's first IVF child. She observed the laparoscopy, and it turned out that there was no space left in the transport incubator for a test tube with follicular fluid. She quickly slipped the test tube between her breasts, to keep it at body temperature. It turned out later that it was the follicle from this precise test tube that Tatjana so conscientiously incubated that produced the child.

I made sure that our outpatients' IVF treatment was covered by the media, and soon reports appeared in Austrian and foreign media about "two Viennese doctors who do IVF as outpatients" which was a first in the world at the time.

In April 1983 I at last left the Second VUWH, because I was on borrowed time there, and because

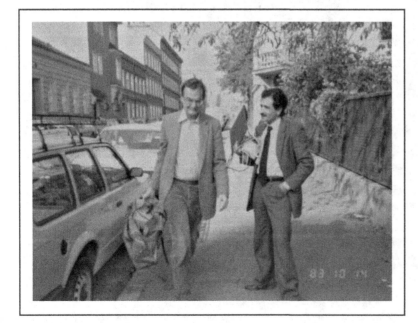

Figure 10.10 Peter Kemeter arrives from the private hospital with oocytes in a transport incubator at our outpatient clinic, and meets the husband of the patient.

Janisch had put other members of staff on the IVF program. Stefan Szalay had already left the clinic, to become the senior consultant at the hospital in Klagenfurt. He soon also started an IVF clinic in nearby Krumpendorf.

The First World Congress on IVF, Among Other Things

The congress took place between June 22 and 24, 1983, and was a great success. It was attended, not by the 200 participants we expected, but by 360, and the scientific program was extremely interesting. At the end there was a round-table discussion, where it was the "ethical questions" in particular that were discussed. We published the most important contributions in a book. One of my clearest memories is of the seminar at Rudolfinerhaus. We had prepared ten couples who wanted children. They agreed to take part in exchange for not having to pay for their treatment.

In the morning the 80 participants were given a demonstration of hormonal stimulation of the ovaries, monitoring follicle maturation via ultrasound, triggering ovulation with HCG and timing of oocyte extraction. At the end, all the participants went through to the OR to observe the laparoscopy, or went to the second auditorium in order to – in a first for us – observe as Lars Hamberger from Göteborg extracted the oocytes from the ovaries using suction through a long needle, inserted through the abdominal wall and the entire bladder. The others watched in the second auditorium with translation from German into English, French and Italian by Dr. Angelo Conti, from Switzerland, because there wasn't enough room for everyone in the first.

After eating lunch together at a traditional tavern, located just behind Rudolfinerhaus, things continued with a demonstration of oocyte cultivation, semen preparation, and insemination. And of course we also demonstrated the last step of the treatment, the transfer of the embryo.

Between 4 pm and 5 pm, a general discussion took place in the auditorium, which was always lively, open, friendly, and humorous – most of the participants had by then become friends. At the end of the day most people made their way back to the tavern, where contacts were made and experiences were shared long into the night. Even today I sometimes talk to former participants at international congresses, who assure me

that they are still successfully using most of what they learned from us.

Simplification of the Method

We were in Hadikgasse for two years in total, where we worked on the IVF method, not to improve it, but to simplify it. Among other things, we followed a suggestion from our German colleague Dr. Maas, to use transparent plastic Petri dishes instead of test tubes for oocyte cultivation (Feichtinger & Kemeter 1983), because they fit under a microscope and the oocytes did not need to be moved using a pipette to be examined. We now performed the transfer speedily on the day after the puncture, and not two days later. Finally we also decided to perform the puncture through the stomach wall and the entire bladder using ultrasound. This spared the patients an operation under general anesthetic, and the entire treatment was now possible at our institute as an outpatient procedure. But our interest in the science underlying our technique was as strong as ever. Prompted by a conversation with Alan Trounson, we were able to do a study that showed for the first time that fertilization of the oocyte and maturation of the embryos was also possible in pure serum. Unfortunately, the rate of division was worse than with a synthetic culture medium, which meant this method did not find a practical application.

Enough Space at Last for All Our Activities

The lack of space in our institute was becoming ever more of a frustration, especially because of the increase in patients, so we searched for something bigger. We rented a large villa in Hietzing (Figure 10.11) not far from us, in Trauttmannsdorfgasse, and we founded a partnership named the Institute of Reproductive Endocrinology and In Vitro Fertilisation on December 29, 1984. After some alterations and new furniture, our work became a pleasure. We were also able to take on more staff, a nurse, and an additional doctor's assistant.

The following five years were also a very productive time. Many articles about our clinic appeared in newspapers and magazines, and this brought us patients from Germany, Holland, Norway, Italy, Switzerland, and many other countries. For example, I gave an

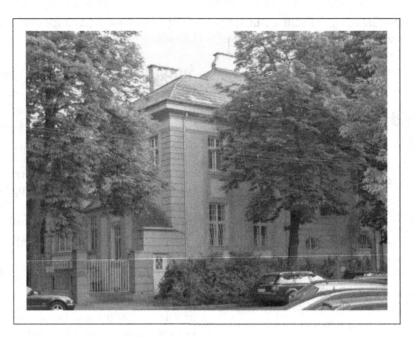

Figure 10.11 Our second outpatient IVF clinic in Trauttmansdorffgasse 3A, Vienna.

interview to a Dutch magazine, and soon after a sudden influx of patients came from Holland for treatment, because there wasn't a really successful IVF center there at that time.

There were also many developments in our method. To improve our success rate, we increased hormone stimulation of the ovaries, which also meant that more embryos were left over. We didn't want to throw them away, and so we had to freeze them. This led us to work on various methods of cryoconservation.

Our ultrasound equipment was produced by a company called Kretztechnik, from Zipf in Upper Austria. The company provided us with a newly developed vaginal scanner, which allowed us to see the genital organs of the woman better than an abdominal scanner. They soon after also gave us a needle guide that could be mounted on the left or right side of the scanner, allowing us to perform follicular aspiration through the vault of the vagina using ultrasound (Figure 10.12). We were able to achieve normal pregnancies with oocytes extracted using this transvaginal technique (Feichtinger & Kemeter, 1986; Kemeter & Feichtinger, 1986).

We were also able to improve and simplify the stimulation of the ovaries. A modification of the fixed protocol presented by Frydmann et al. at the congress at the Hofburg in 1983 proved very useful. We

did a study based on experience gained at the Second VUWH about female androgen metabolism, which revealed that giving additional prednisolone via lowering androgens and of the LH, improves the quality of the oocytes and the pregnancy rate. This stimulation protocol would later become known as the "Kemeter–Feichtinger protocol."

For women who no longer had any oocytes or had lost them, or because of a hereditary condition, we ran an oocyte donation program that was soon successful and produced the first child from donated oocytes on the continent (Feichtinger & Kemeter, 1985).

The next novelty for Austria was the birth of a child from an embryo that had been frozen and stored, after being unfrozen and inserted into the uterus.

We also, for the first time, managed to terminate a tubal pregnancy through infiltration with methotrexate through the vagina (Feichtinger & Kemeter, 1987).

Because Peter and I did the IVF work in the laboratory ourselves, we sometimes got in each other's way because we both always wanted to be first to see if the oocytes were fertilized and how the embryo developed from there. We therefore soon decided to divide up all our work relating to IVF treatment by the week. This meant each of us had every other week free for other activities, for example doing scientific work. This system worked exceptionally well right up until the end.

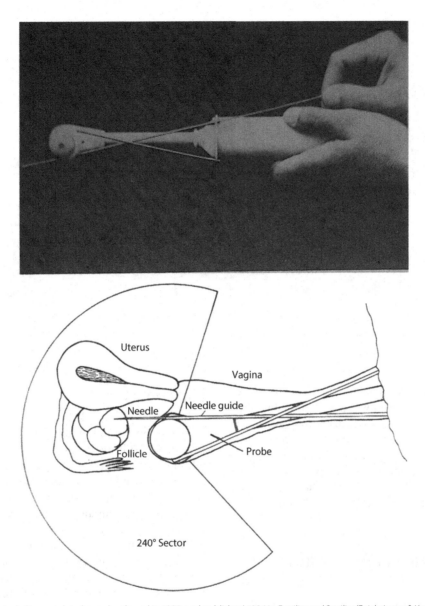

Figure 10.12 Vaginal ultrasound probe as developed in 1985, and published 1986 in *Fertility and Sterility* (Feichtinger & Kemeter, 1986).

Our Institute Becomes an Internationally Famous Teaching Center

Our publications meant that we were very often visited by colleagues from other IVF centers, for instance from Israel, Syria, Egypt, Germany, Switzerland, France, Greece, and China. There was a constant coming and going; sometimes we had guests from different centers at the same time (Figure 10.13).

In 1986 I organized the next international congress at the Hofburg. This time a colleague from South Africa did hands-on training with mice in the cellar, though it wasn't as popular as in 1983.

Our Habilitation Studies

During this period I submitted my thesis, which is a postdoctoral university degree that provides the qualifications necessary to be a lecturer. It was very arduous for very understandable reasons. This qualification

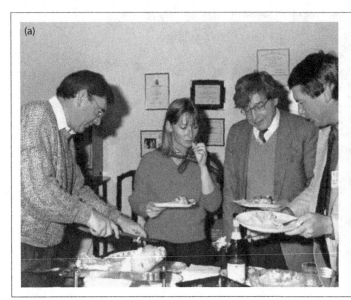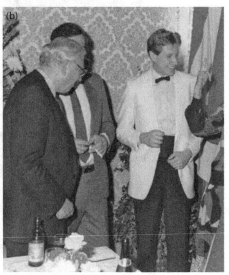

Figure 10.13 From left to right: (a) Ian Johnston (Australia), Yvonne duPlessis (Australia), Robert Edwards (England), John Mc Bain (Australia), (b) Patrick Steptoe (on the left) Wilfried Feichtinger (on the right).

is difficult for people who are not enrolled at university, and in my case there was the additional problem that I had left the university under a cloud and in particular had made enemies of the management of the two women's clinics. I therefore asked for a new panel and arranged references from international pioneers in IVF, so that it all worked out in the second round in October 1986. Peter did not gain the qualification until 1990.

Celebration of our Twenty-fifth Anniversary

This anniversary was a natural opportunity for us three – Peter, Stefan, and I – who had long since gone our separate ways, to celebrate with the birthday boy, Zlatan, and his mother, Jovanka. Unfortunately, his father, Dragan, could not take part because he had died two years previously. At a round table organized by a newspaper, the *Kronenzeitung*, we thought about his life and heard about the life of the Jovanovic family over the intervening 25 years. Zlatan has become a healthy, contented young man and is sure to find his way – reason enough for us to congratulate him (Figure 10.14).

Final Notes

I often like to think back to the early days of IVF, and I am happy and proud to have been able to be part of it, and that I still am. It was an interesting, productive, adventurous, energetic, and, sometimes, difficult time for me. Peter and I were a good team in the early days, when it was all about little else than IVF; I was more the organizer and communicator with the outside world, while he was more the one who was responsible for the daily work with patients; he was more for endocrinology, I more for technical issues; he more for consultations with patients, I more for the simplification of processes, etc. – in a nutshell, there were advantages for both of us. Peter's interests then went wider than IVF and were very different to my interests, so it was better for both of us to go our separate ways.

All in all, my reward for all the work, conflict, and problems has always been the wonderful feeling that comes when I can help others. But it was always more or less a team effort, because without the collaboration and help of others, none of it would have been possible. That's why I would like to conclude by thanking everyone very much, both the people mentioned above and those not mentioned, who have stood by my side during my life and helped me – this success is also theirs.

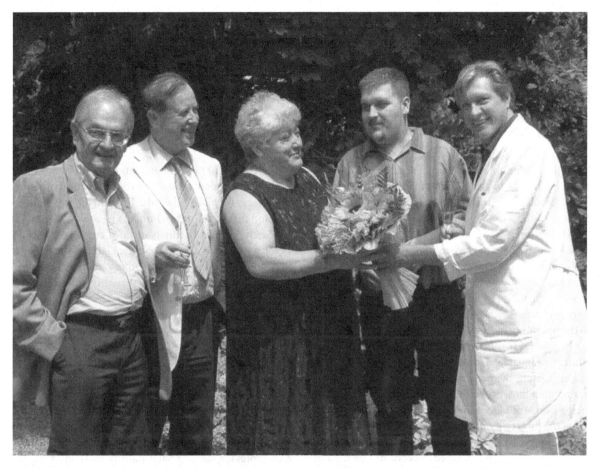

Figure 10.14 From the left to the right: Peter Kemeter, Stefan Szalay, Jovanka and Zlatan Jovanovic at Zlatan's 25th birthday in 2007.

References

Feichtinger, W., Kemeter, P. A simplified technique for fertilization and culture of human preimplantation embryos in vitro. *Acta. Eur. Fertil.* 1983;14: 125–128.

Pregnancy after total ovariectomy achieved by ovum donation. *Lancet.* 1985; 2: 722–723.

Transvaginal sector scan sonography for needle guided transvaginal follicle aspiration and other applications in gynecologic routine and research. *Fertil. Steril.* 1986;45: 722–725.

Feichtinger, W., Kemeter, P. Conservative treatment of ectopic pregnancy by transvaginal aspiration under sonographic control and methotrexate injection. *Lancet* 1987;1: 381–382.

Feichtinger, W., Szalay, S., Beck, A., Kemeter, P., Janisch, H. Results of laparoscopic recovery of preovulatory human oocytes from non-stimulated ovaries in an ongoing in vitro fertilization program. *Fertil. Steril.* 1981;36: 707–711.

Feichtinger, W., Szalay, S., Kemeter, P., et al. 1982. The preovulatory follicle and oocyte. In: Edwards RG (ed.) *Human Conception In Vitro.* Academic Press, London, pp. 73–83.

Feichtinger, W., Kemeter, P., Szalay, S., Beck, A., Janisch, H. Could aspiration of the Graafian follicle cause luteal phase deficiency? *Fertil. Steril.* 1982; 37: 205–208.

Feichtinger, W., Szalay, S., Kemeter, P., Beck, A., Janisch, H. Zwillingsschwangerschaft nach laparoskopischer Eizellgewinnung, In-vitro-Fertilisierung und Embryotransfer. *Geburtshilfe Frauenheilkd.* 1982; 42: 197–199.

Feichtinger, W., Kemeter, P., Szalay, S. The Vienna program of in vitro fertilization and embryo-transfer – a successful clinical treatment. *Eur. J. Obstet. Gynecol. Reprod. Biol.* 1983;15: 63–70.

Kemeter, P., Feichtinger, W. News and views: Trans-vaginal oocyte retrieval: an update. *Hum. Reprod.* 1986;1: 278.

The Development of In-Vitro Fertilization in France

René F. Frydman

In the 1970s, the aim for a young French gynecologist-obstetrician was to develop microsurgery techniques for tubal disease. This occurrence was very frequent because of the social evolution of French society after the explosion of May 1968. As a consequence of the sexual revolution, the spread of sexually transmitted infections became more common and, as a direct consequence, salpingitis and obstruction of the Fallopian tubes occurred. Fertility care was limited to tubal microsurgery, which often required three or four hours in the operating room with dismal pregnancy rates.

In 1976, *The Lancet* reported the first human clinical pregnancy from in-vitro fertilization (IVF). Unfortunately, the pregnancy was extra-uterine but it invigorated the world of human reproduction and created a future of potential. I decided at this moment to focus my career on reproductive medicine.

In France, Dr. Jean Cohen, who met Bob Edwards in 1975 in Tokyo, also decided to work in this field of medicine. In 1978, Edwards accepted Cohen's invitation to speak to the French Fertility Society about in-vitro fertilization. At this time, I was working under Professor Emile Papiernick in Clamart, who was investigating the relationship between egg quality and pathological perinatal outcomes, such as growth restriction (small for dates). One of the eminent biologists of Professor Papiernick's team, Ondine Bomsell, kindly introduced me to Bob Edwards. Edwards was very enthusiastic and supported the development of an in-vitro fertilization program in France.

I focused my attention initially to laparoscopic oocyte retrieval. As a surgeon, it was relatively easy (at that time!) to propose to all patients undergoing diagnostic laparoscopy to schedule the surgery on the assumed day of ovulation. If a preovulatory follicle was visualized, I attempted aspiration and sent the follicular fluid to Ondine Bomsell, who was working in a laboratory within the same hospital. She would try to locate and characterize the morphology of the oocyte.

In 1961, Charles Thibaud, an eminent biologist in France, succeeded in the in-vitro fertilization of rabbit oocytes, as had Bob Edwards. Thibaud did not want to develop this technique in humans.

Many French scientists did not support a human IVF program. Professor Beaulieu claimed the need to first do IVF in the monkey. Others, such as Professor Lejeune, argued that human sexuality should not be separated from reproduction.

After the birth of Louise Brown in 1978, two French teams were determined to establish an IVF program. Jacqueline Mandelbaun, a gynecologist, and Michele Plachot, a biologist cytogeneticist and a member of Professor De Grouchy's team at Necker Hospital in central Paris, developed an IVF center. At that time, no maternity care was established at Necker. They sought two clinicians who would agree to develop this program: Jean Cohen in hospital de Sevres (south of Paris) and Professor Jacques Salat Baroux in Tenon hospital (north of Paris). After a few months of the physicians working at different practices, they decided to split into two completely separate entities (lab and operating room) in each hospital (Sevres and Tenon).

In Clamart, Ondine Bomsell resigned to join the IVF program. I recruited Jacques Testart, an animal biologist on Professor Thibaut's team, to join our team under the auspice of Professor Emile Papiernick.

In 1980, John Leeton came to London for an IVF conference. At this time, the first Australian baby had been born. I travelled across the English Channel to listen to him, and at the end of the conference, I asked Leeton if he would join Jaques Testart and me to help us upgrade our program.

I told him that we had a grant for the travel and stay, but, in fact, his invitation letter gave us the possibility to obtain a grant for our Australian journey. We obtained experimental oocytes, which were to be fertilized, in a neonatal incubator, which was created by Jaques Testart and would serve as our first IVF laboratory (now visible in the permanent exhibition of the

Musée de l'Homme in Paris). We were interested in observing how the other successful team operated.

We stayed for two weeks in Melbourne with Ian Johnson, Carl Wood, John Leeton, Alex Lopata, and Alan Trounson. When we returned to France, we began our first embryo transfers. A few months later, we obtained our first biochemical pregnancy. At the same time, Jean Cohen's group had not achieved fertilization. In order to identify the cause of this, we decided to do the fertilization in the Clamart laboratory from an oocyte collected by Cohen in hospital of Sevres. Two days later, I brought the developed embryo from Clamart in a catheter and Jean Cohen completed the embryo transfer. The embryo implanted but a miscarriage occurred two weeks later.

After this collaboration, the activity in Clamart increased and led to the birth of Amandine, the first test tube baby born in France on February 23, 1982.

In September 1981, Bob Edwards invited an estimated twenty scientists who were pioneers in this field to Bourn Hall to share their experiences in IVF.

The birth of Amandine in February 1982 and Alexia some months later (Jean Cohen's team) began an ideological battle between pro- and con-IVF in our country. As a result, the French national ethics committee was created in 1984 and three bioethics laws were voted on (in 1994, 2004, 2011). Presently, the ethics debate still exists and is very dynamic. Many restrictions have been placed on the practice of IVF in France compared to many countries. For instance, five years passed between the theoretical authorization of PGD in 1994 and the final agreement in 1999.

In France, our team reported the first birth after a frozen-thawed embryo transfer in 1986, after PGD

in 2000, after in-vitro maturation in 2003, and after oocyte freezing in 2011.

We lost six years between the scientific Japanese publication about vitrification (2005) and the legal authorization of its use (2011) in France. Many restrictions continue to exist in France even at the time of writing, in 2017.

- No possibility of treatment for single women or homosexual couples.
- No possibility for anonymous gamete donation.
- The majority of oocyte donations are done outside of the country because of the non-optimal organization of the oocyte donation program.
- Post-mortem sperm extraction is forbidden.
- No possibilities for a young woman to preserve her fertility by oocyte collection/freezing.
- No PGS is allowed, even if pregnant women can make a genetic assessment of the fetus at three months of gestation (although the meaning of this remains unclear).

Testart and I organized one of the first international meetings of IVF in 1983 in Cargese (Corsica) where more than 200 participated. Jean Cohen and Bob Edwards made the first proposition of a European Society with its own *Journal*. Now the ESRHE meetings attract thousands of scientists and clinicians! The development of the medical and social aspects of infertility was set up in Europe and everywhere else in the world. Forty years is a short period from a historical point of view, a similar time that was necessary for the Hebrews to find the Promised Land!

The Development of In-Vitro Fertilization in Italy

Luca Gianaroli, Serena Sgargi, Maria Cristina Magli, and Anna Pia Ferraretti

The Pioneers

In the 1960s, some clinics in Italy started to deal with fertility problems. In 1965, a young clinician named Guido Ragni, owing to his interest in gynecological endocrinology, was assigned to the often neglected Infertility Unit of the Clinica Mangiagalli in Milan (Northern Italy), which at the time mainly provided consultations. After 13 years spent managing the Unit almost by himself, he asked the director of the hospital to start IVF treatments, spurred by the positive outcomes coming from the United Kingdom. The refusal was categorical, for religious reasons: such treatments could not be acceptable for a practicing Catholic.

Wishing to proceed in this direction, Dr. Ragni completed a brief internship in the USA under the supervision of the Joneses. He then moved to a different hospital in Milan, directed by Professor Piegiorgio Crosignani, who was more open-minded than his previous boss towards these treatments. Gynecologist-biologist Anna Mattei, who had learnt laboratory techniques from Professor David Baird in Edinburgh, soon joined him. The first procedures were performed in a single room, Dr. Ragni's office, which was used as a consultation room and as a lab. The ultraviolet (UV) laminar flow cabinet could be good for tanning (but not for the eyes) if one fell asleep under it while studying for long hours at night! Since an operating theater was not available for these procedures, Dr. Ragni and his colleagues had to use ultrasound-guided oocyte retrieval, and the equipment was built by a blacksmith based upon the instructions of Dr. Ragni himself and of his colleague Dr. Giancarlo Lombroso Finzi. Their first baby was born in 1985 to a 28-year-old patient suffering from tubal infertility. In 1990 the Unit was finally transferred to more suitable facilities, which allowed a constant increase in the number of procedures performed and provided high-quality treatments in a public setting.

Also back in the 1960s, Sicilian gynecologist Ettore Cittadini was completing his residency at the Infertility Unit of the Hôpital Broca in Paris, directed by Professor Raoul Palmer. There, he was given the task to train a new visiting gynecologist from the UK, Patrick Steptoe, who soon became familiar with laparoscopic oocyte retrieval (Cittadini et al., 1984). At the beginning of the 1980s, Professor Cittadini moved to Melbourne, to work with Carl Wood, who at that point routinely performed these techniques, in spite of religious opposition to his work. Alongside clinical activities, experimental research on stimulation protocols and embryo cryopreservation were performed. While in Melbourne, Professor Cittadini personally ordered all the necessary equipment to start clinical and laboratory activities in Palermo in 1982. After several unsuccessful attempts, Eleonora Zaccheddu was born on May 18, 1984, to a couple who had been trying to have children for more than eight years. The baby was named Eleonora after Eleonora Cefalù, the scientist who performed all the laboratory procedures related to her conception. At first, Eleonora was denied baptism due to the way in which she had been conceived. The authorization was only given weeks later (Cittadini, 2012).

Vincenzo Abate was a young physician when he left Naples, his hometown, in the early 1950s to continue his studies at Columbia University, in the United States. After working for some time at a clinic in Harlem, he was transferred to the New York Polyclinic, where Professor Kupperman, a luminary in endocrinology, suggested he visit Dr. Tjler's laboratory in Los Angeles, where one of the first sperm banks had been established. This laboratory had been visited also by Edwards and Steptoe, Louise Brown's "fathers." From there he moved to Australia, where he was present at the birth of the first Australian IVF baby, and he then returned to Italy. In spite of his international experience, he had to complete his Italian specialization in Obstetrics and Gynecology in Pisa before being able to start his own IVF clinic in Naples. His collaboration with Australian professionals, instead of Italian ones, raised hostility towards this initiative, but in spite of that Dr. Abate and his team welcomed the first Italian IVF baby, Alessandra, in 1983. In later years, he had to face a legal controversy concerning the "paternity" of GIFT, but he continued to work hard in this field, supported by the positive results achieved over the years.

In Bologna, in the late 1970s, two young clinicians who had just graduated, Luca Gianaroli and Anna Pia Ferraretti, were becoming increasingly interested in infertility treatment. In order to learn more about these experimental techniques, Dr. Ferraretti was sent by Professor Carlo Flamigni to Virginia, while Dr. Gianaroli obtained a publicly-funded grant which enabled him to get an internship in Melbourne.

In Australia, Dr. Gianaroli worked closely with Alan Trounson, who had started to apply IVF techniques successfully used experimentally on animals to human patients, and he learnt more about fertilization procedures, working both on veterinary and clinical procedures. At the same time, in Norfolk, Virginia, Dr. Ferraretti grasped the secrets of gynecological endocrinology from Georgeanna and Howard Jones, being part of the team responsible for the birth of the first American IVF baby in 1981.

When they came back, they joined forces and skills to set up the first University IVF Clinic in Bologna. The number of patients was constantly increasing, while funds for the functioning of the Unit were hard to get, so Dr. Gianaroli and Dr. Ferraretti decided also to start a private IVF clinic. In spite of the first year of unsuccessful attempts, in 1985 a couple of twins and a singleton were born from patients treated at the public hospital and at the private practice. A few months later, a baby girl was born following oocyte donation, an innovative technique learnt in Australia. She was the first Italian baby born thanks to this procedure, and she herself recently gave birth to a perfectly healthy boy.

The team of the Bologna IVF unit was enriched by other professionals, but difficulties in obtaining the equipment and technologies required forced Dr. Gianaroli and Dr. Ferraretti to leave the hospital and to opt for careers in private practice. At the beginning of the 1990s, when the first ICSI babies were being conceived, Maria Cristina Magli, a biologist with a completely different professional experience, joined the team and started her career in embryology.

In spite of their different backgrounds, stories and personalities, Italian IVF pioneers also have several things in common. Firstly, all of them accepted having

to move abroad, even to the other side of the world, to learn and discover these new techniques, of which they saw the huge potential. Moreover, they all agree on the fact that, alongside initial mistrust and hostility, the main difficulties in the early days were due to surgical risks and to the impossibility of planning oocyte retrieval times. All of them remember rushing to the operating theater in the middle of the night, sleeping at the hospital or leaving restaurants in a hurry to adapt to the physiological rhythms of patients and cells. All this happened in an era when mobile phones did not yet exist. In addition, in spite of surgical skills, oocyte retrievals and GIFT were risky and invasive procedures that often led to abdominal bleeding due to technical limitations, including the lack of laparoscopic cameras.

Significant improvement in later years derived from the personalization of stimulation protocols, allowing more accurate planning of procedures, from ultrasound-guided oocyte aspiration, which reduced surgical risks, from embryo cryopreservation and vitrification, and from the continuous development of new techniques and equipment in the clinical and laboratory settings.

The pioneers' gratitude also goes to those patients who entrusted them their biggest hopes and wishes, at a time when these techniques were experimental and extremely invasive. Their stubbornness, determination, and firm belief in science and in the skills of clinicians and scientists, allowed professionals to achieve those results that led to the acknowledgement of Assisted Reproduction as a potential treatment for infertility also in Italy.

The Late 1980s and the 1990s

The increasingly positive results obtained by the Italian pioneers and by their apprentices contributed to the diffusion of ART in Italy, making it one of the leading countries for these techniques. For example, Antonio Fasolino from Salerno, in Southern Italy, joined the initial group of pioneers and decided to apply his laparoscopic skills to IVF. In order to learn these techniques, he got in touch with Dr. Gianaroli and Dr. Ferraretti in Bologna and he joined them for some time for a specific training. After that, he established a satellite Center of Bologna headquarters in his hometown. While the surgical techniques applied to IVF were well established in Salerno, laboratory techniques were still experimental and the training of biologists was no "piece of cake."

After some unsuccessful attempts, a pregnancy finally came to term, leading to the birth of twins following donor GIFT.

Until 2004, there was no specific IVF legislation in Italy and all techniques available at that time were routinely performed in the country with positive outcomes for an increasing number of indications. Some centers were leading pioneers in terms of scientific research and development of new techniques and couples came to Italy from abroad to undergo specific treatments, turning the country into a popular destination for so-called "Reproductive Tourism."

In fact, after an initial period during which Italian clinicians and embryologists were starting to put into practice what they had learnt abroad, pregnancies were obtained shortly after positive results had been achieved by means of innovative procedures first published worldwide (Figure 12.1). International collaborations also allowed new techniques to develop that were initially considered experimental, but that are now routinely used by clinics worldwide.

In the early 1990s, a young Spanish student working in the USA, Santiago Munné, was searching for a lab that would allow him to work on his theory related to the possibility of analyzing chromosomes collected from embryos to predict their genetic status. Dr. Munné was hosted in Bologna (where he first started to appreciate Italian wines!) to generate those experiments that constitute the initial steps of Preimplantation Genetic Screening (Gianaroli et al., 1997 a, b). This collaboration is still ongoing and it led to achievements of the utmost relevance in this field (Munné et al., 2012).

In the same period, following the request of a Catholic patient who was not in favor of embryo freezing, there was a need to develop a safe and effective technique to cryopreserve oocytes instead. A Russian PhD student with a background in submarine engineering was sent to Bologna by Alan Trounson to work closely with local professionals on this issue. In 1999, the first live birth following oocyte vitrification was published in *Human Reproduction*, and this technique has now become a standard procedure all over the world (Kuleshova et al., 1999).

The Year 2000 Onwards

Things, however, dramatically started to change in 2003, when the center-right Government led by Silvio Berlusconi submitted to the Parliament a draft law concerning Medically Assisted Reproduction (MAR), supposedly with the aim of regulating a field that, until then, had only been subject to professional guidelines and good practice principles issued by the Italian Medical Council. The draft immediately appeared controversial, resulting in a violent political and social clash between those in favor of it and those who opposed the restrictions it imposed. In fact, the proposed law implied several limitations, most of which were unsubstantiated by any medical or scientific evidence. These limitations were:

- a ban on gamete and embryo donation,
- an obligation to generate a maximum of three embryos, to be transferred simultaneously, regardless of the patient's specific characteristics,

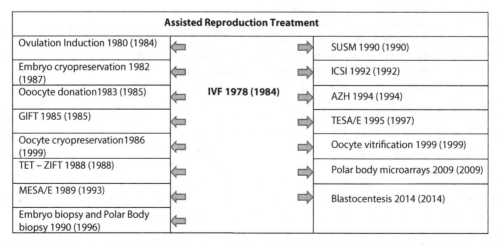

Assisted Reproduction Treatment

Ovulation Induction 1980 (1984)		SUSM 1990 (1990)
Embryo cryopreservation 1982 (1987)		ICSI 1992 (1992)
Ooocyte donation1983 (1985)	IVF 1978 (1984)	AZH 1994 (1994)
GIFT 1985 (1985)		TESA/E 1995 (1997)
Oocyte cryopreservation1986 (1999)		Oocyte vitrification 1999 (1999)
TET – ZIFT 1988 (1988)		Polar body microarrays 2009 (2009)
MESA/E 1989 (1993)		Blastocentesis 2014 (2014)
Embryo biopsy and Polar Body biopsy 1990 (1996)		

Figure 12.1 The year next to the technique indicates the date of the first pregnancy reported in the literature. The year in brackets indicates the date of the first pregnancy reported by S.I.S.Me.R.'s staff members.

- impossibility to assess the genetic status of gametes and embryos,
- a ban on embryo cryopreservation, except under specific conditions causing a risk to the health of the mother,
- a ban on surrogacy,
- a ban on scientific research on embryos.

Moreover, severe punishments, ranging from hefty fines to imprisonment, for those clinics and those professionals who acted against these provisions were established. Professionals who had been successfully working in the field of MAR for years, immediately rose against this draft, to uphold the principle of good medical practice, followed shortly after by patients' associations, political parties, and other entities and organizations opposing this proposal.

On the other hand, supporters of the bill and religious institutions claimed that the above-mentioned limitations only aimed at disciplining what they defined as "reproductive anarchy" and at protecting the conceptus throughout all phases of its development, albeit to the detriment of prospective parents' best interests in terms of physical and psychological well-being.

In spite of the escalating conflict, Parliament approved this draft law, which became effective in February 2004 under the notorious name of Law 40 (Benagiano and Gianaroli, 2004). From one day to another, clinicians and embryologists had to radically change their way of working, and patients who had gone through long procedures and waiting lists to undergo specific treatments, especially those implying gamete donation, were suddenly excluded from the therapies they needed.

A national referendum was immediately announced in an attempt to abolish the newly-established law. However, due to a vehement strategy conducted by supporters of the law, and aiming at giving a negative connotation to this kind of treatment, in 2005 the referendum failed to reach the required quorum and the law remained in place as it was.

It was difficult being IVF professionals in those days. Those who publicly opposed the new law were denigrated in newspapers and other mass media by supporters of its provisions and their professionalism was constantly called into question. This, though, did not stop the majority of them, and in spite of failing at this first referendum, patients and professionals did not give up and they turned to the courts to re-affirm their rights. After a first verdict of a regional court, which basically supported the provisions of Law 40,

verdicts from local and other regional courts followed, this time supporting the interests of patients.

Legal battles, however, lasted many years, during which thousands of patients every year were forced to go abroad to get access to those medical procedures that were prohibited in Italy, facing all risks and economical burdens related to this choice. This was a choice that not all couples had, though. Involuntary childlessness due to the prohibitions imposed by the law and to the impossibility to afford treatments abroad is difficult to estimate, but its impact was certainly dramatic for every single couple that had to face it.

IVF professionals also went through tough times. They were compelled by law to work against the principles of good medical practice and they had to face misinformation and mistrust. Frustration at the impossibility of providing patients with the best treatment options available was also a significant psychological burden.

Embryologists wanting to keep their skills in gamete and embryo cryopreservation, Preimplantation Genetic Diagnosis (PGD, now PGT), and gamete and embryo donation were sent by the most forward-thinking centers to countries where these techniques were allowed, to maintain their training and keep up with advancements in these fields.

The only positive effect of Law 40/2004, was the forced improvement of oocyte cryopreservation techniques, mostly thanks to the work of Eleonora Porcu. These techniques were later applied to oocyte donation and fertility preservation (Porcu and Venturoli, 2006). A few years later, however, the increasing number of verdicts against Law 40/2004, which reached the unbelievably high number of more than 30, resulted in the intervention of the Constitutional Court, and hope started to rise again.

In 2009, the Constitutional Court ruled that the obligation to generate a maximum of three embryos to be transferred simultaneously and the ban on cryopreservation were unconstitutional. *De facto*, this verdict restored the prevalence of medical expertise in the definition of the most appropriate treatment depending on each couple's specific characteristics. It also gave the possibility to generate more embryos and to cryopreserve them if necessary, so that PGD techniques became feasible again, although only in the case of infertile couples (Ruling 151/2009) (Benagiano and Gianaroli, 2010).

The Constitutional Court was besought again in 2014, following more rulings from local and regional courts regarding gamete donation. In April 2014, the Constitutional Court ruled that the ban on gamete donation was unconstitutional based on the fact that it infringed upon the rights of couples and individuals to start a family, to get access to the best medical treatment available for their specific pathology, and to self-determination. Considering that the inability to conceive is an acknowledged pathology, the ban also led to a discrimination among infertile patients based on their cause of infertility, which was obviously very unfortunate and inappropriate (Ruling 162/2014) (Benagiano et al., 2014).

Even so, the ruling of the Constitutional Court did not magically solve the issues related to gamete donation. In fact, in the aftermath of it, the debate shifted on how to regulate these treatments and on the potential need to abrogate Law 40/2004 and to replace it with a new one taking into account the pronouncements of the court. The process, however, turned out to be quite difficult due to conflicting points of view regarding reimbursement for donors, anonymity, and other practicalities. The Ministry of Health issued guidelines for the provision of gamete donation treatments, the most problematic of which was the prohibition to reimburse donors in any way. This greatly contributes to the shortage of donors (especially women), which makes it difficult to face the increasing demand for this kind of treatment.

In the wake of positive results achieved in previous legal actions (including one in front of the European Court of Human Rights), the Constitutional Court was consulted a year later regarding the legitimacy of the ban on PGT for fertile couples who were carriers of, or suffering from, genetic diseases. This was an extremely delicate issue, as it had many personal and emotional implications, especially for those couples who had lost children or whose children were suffering terribly due to pathologies whose transmission could have been prevented thanks to these techniques. Once again, the Constitutional Court ruled in favor of applicants twice (rulings 96/2015 and 229/2015), thus inflicting the finishing blow to the original version of Law 40/2004.

Full legitimacy of PGT as an integral part of Assisted Reproduction Treatments for specific indications was reaffirmed by a ruling of the Court of Appeal of Milan, which also condemned a public hospital to provide it to patients at another center at its own expense, in case it failed to provide it directly. This means that, if required, PGD should be available through the national healthcare service, raising a variety of issues, mostly related to the costs of these procedures.

Current Issues and Future Perspectives

At present, MAR in Italy is regulated by the residual provisions of a dismantled Law 40/2004. Although at present almost all techniques are legal and feasible in the country, the decade of bans between 2004 and 2014 caused irreparable damage to personal and social awareness towards infertility, its causes, its prevention, and its treatment, which is especially reflected by the difficulties in finding potential donors and in discussing these issues openly.

Some political parties attempted to propose new draft laws on this subject, but opposing views on it made it impossible to find, if not a consensus, a vast majority. Drafts were then kept on stand-by in order not to jeopardize the fragile political balance that has characterized Italy in the last decades.

Nowadays, there are several pending issues regarding assisted reproduction in Italy. In a country with an extremely low birth rate and an ageing population, provision of these treatments, along with a range of related policies in support of young people and families, should be a priority. However, this does not seem to be the case, as availability of these treatments is still below the cutoff recommended by international standards (1500 cycles per million inhabitants). Moreover, if analyzed critically, the cumulative number of cycles per million inhabitants will show major disparities in availability among different Italian regions, causing people to move to get access to treatments.

Reimbursement policies also vary among regions, and so does the provision of treatments through the national healthcare service.

Low awareness of fertility issues does not allow effective prevention of some of the causes (especially those related to lifestyle factors) and it makes it difficult to sensitize young people to gamete donation. This is made even harder by the lack of reimbursement for those who decide to become donors.

Another aspect not to be underestimated is the management of surplus embryos that, according to current regulations, must be cryopreserved without time limit. This is a huge cost for centers and a waste of a precious resource of genetic material that could be used fruitfully for scientific and clinical research. The Italian paradox in this field is that stem cells from embryos cryopreserved in Italy cannot be donated by their owners for scientific research projects, but it is possible to purchase embryonic stem cells from abroad at very high costs.

In addition, the law that recently acknowledged same-sex couples now raises the issue of their potential access to assisted reproduction within their family project. It is likely that the debate on this matter will be particularly heated and that politicians will not be eager to face it at a time of political instability.

Finally, the influence of wide areas of society on popular perception of IVF techniques should not be underestimated. Prejudice and misconceptions are still very common in spite of the efforts of professionals, and most time they are fostered on purpose for personal and political interests. Attention on these issues should be kept high in order to avoid attempts to restore some of the bans of Law 40/2004, which took so much effort to be dismantled.

The Italian pioneers are now getting old and most of them retired from their clinical activities after training younger professionals who gradually took their place, some of them with passion and skills learnt from direct experience in the early days of IVF and from the hardships of the struggle against Law 40/2004.

It is interesting to notice that, in spite of the troubled history of IVF in Italy in the past 20 years, most Italian professionals were able to keep high-quality standards of treatment and to contribute to cutting-edge studies from the clinical and laboratory point of view. It is significant that blastocentesis, the latest innovation in PGT (Gianaroli et al., 2014 a; Magli et al., 2016) was recently developed in a country where it was prohibited from 2004 to 2009, to the detriment of hundreds of patients (Gianaroli et al., 2014b).

In the struggle to keep Italy connected to other European countries with more advanced legislation, a vital role was played by ESHRE and by Italian professionals involved in its activities. In particular, Dr. Gianaroli's chairmanship between 2009 and 2011 helped Italy to start the process of re-alignment of Italian policies and results to European data following the abolition of the main restrictions of Law 40/2004 in 2009. Involvement in European multicenter trials also helped professionals to keep in touch with current practices and to preserve scientific credibility at an international level.

Although there is a strong evidence of the negative effects of Law 40/2004 on treatment outcomes and clinical and laboratory procedures, powerful lobbies (especially religious ones), are still trying to impose similar restrictions in other European countries. Malta's current legislation is basically a clone of the Italian law, forcing patients to move abroad to seek appropriate treatments, while the attempt of introducing similar provision in national legislation in Poland and Lithuania was stopped thanks to the strong opposition of professionals, patients, citizens, and of the leading scientific society in Europe, ESHRE.

A Glance Towards the Future

Although the events that characterize its history are many and its pace of development is very fast, medically assisted reproduction is still a relatively "young" area of medicine and biology.

A vital role in the future evolution of this field will be played by scientific research aiming at improving results and at increasing safety and effectiveness. Italian clinicians and scientists should be able to learn from their past and to keep pace with innovations. They should also co-operate with political and legislative institutions to assist them in the elaboration and implementation of legislations complying with international scientific standards, principles of good medical practice, and technological advancements.

Finally they should commit to scientific research as . . ."Where scientific research is performed, more babies are born."

Acknowledgments

The authors would like to thank:
- Vincenzo Abate, Ettore Cittadini, Antonio Fasolino, and Guido Ragni for sharing their memories of the early days of IVF in Italy with them during the writing of this chapter,
- Piergiorgio Crosignani, for linking the Italian scientific community to the European Society of Human Reproduction and Embryology for many years,
- Giuseppe Benagiano, for denouncing in scientific papers the despicable influence of religious lobbies on political decisions in Italy.

References

Benagiano G., Gianaroli L. The new Italian IVF legislation. *Reprod Biomed Online* 2004, 9:117–125.

The Consitutional Court modifies Italian legislation on assisted reproduction technology. *Reprod Biomed Online* 2010;20:261–266.

Benagiano G, Filippi V, Sgargi S, Gianaroli L. Italian Constitutional Court removes the prohibition on gamete donation in Italy. *Reprod Biomed Online.* 2014;29:662–664.

Cittadini E. *Nata a Palermo. Storia della Fecondazione in vitro in Italia.* 2012, Cofese Edizioni, Palermo.

Cittadini E, Geraci D, Cefalù E, et al. *Il tempo del Sogno. Storia della Fecondazione in vitro.* 1984, Sellerio Editore, Palermo.

Gianaroli L, Magli MC, Munné S, et al. Will preimplantation genetic diagnosis assist patients with a poor prognosis to achieve pregnancy? *Hum Reprod* 1997a;12:1762–1767.

Gianaroli L, Magli MC, Ferraretti AP, et al. Preimplantation genetic diagnosis increases the implantation rate in human in vitro fertilization by avoiding the transfer of chromosomally abnormal embryos. *Fertil Steril* 1997b, 68:1128–1131.

Gianaroli L, Magli MC, Pomante A, et al. Blastocentesis: a source of DNA for preimplantation genetic testing. Results from a pilot study. *Fertil Steril* 2014a;102:1692–1699.

Gianaroli L, Crivello A, Stanghellini I, et al. Reiterative changes in the Italian regulation on IVF: the effect on PGD patients' reproductive decisions. *Reprod Biomed Online* 2014b, 28:125–32.

Kuleshova L, Gianaroli L, Magli MC, Ferraretti AP, Trounson AO. Birth following vitrification of a small number of human oocytes. *Hum Reprod* 1999; 14: 3077–3079.

Magli MC, Pomante A, Cafueri G, et al. Preimplantation genetic testing: polar bodies, blastomeres, trophectoderm cells or blastocoelic fluid? *Fertil Steril* 2016;105:676–683.e5.

Munné S, Held KR, Magli MC, et al. Intra-age, inter-center and inter-cycle diffrences in chromosome abnormalities in oocytes. *Fertil Steril* 2012;97:935–942.

Porcu E, Venturoli S. Progress with oocyte cryopreservation. *Curr Opin Obstet Gynecol.* 2006;18:273–279.

Ruling 151/2009 of the Italian Constitutional Court. Gazzetta Ufficiale della Repubblica Italiana 13/05/2009 n. 19.

Ruling 162/2014 of the Italian Constitutional Court. Gazzetta Ufficiale della Repubblica Italiana 18/06/2014 n. 26.

Ruling 96/2015 of the Italian Constitutional Court. Gazzetta Ufficiale della Repubblica Italiana 10/06/2015 n. 23.

Ruling 229/2015 of the Italian Constitutional Court. Gazzetta Ufficiale della Repubblica Italiana 18/11/2015 n. 46.

Ruling of the Court of Appeals of Milan. www.biodirotto.org/index.php/item/900-pma-dgp-milano.

The Development of In-Vitro Fertilization in Scandinavia

Lars Hamberger, Torbjörn Hillensjö, and Matts Wikland

Introduction

Although Sweden is a small country, in the 1960s and 1970s there were certain pioneers in endocrinology and infertility who laid the foundation for what was to come later in the area of in-vitro fertilization (IVF). At the Karolinska Institute in Stockholm, Egon Diczfalusy founded and chaired a reproductive endocrinology laboratory, which became internationally well-known. In particular the group developed sensitive and specific radioimmunoassays for steroid hormones, and simplified the techniques for use in clinical routines. Another endocrinologist, Leif Wide from Uppsala, studied the various isoforms of circulating follicle stimulating hormone (FSH) and discovered their different glycosylation patterns and the circulating half-lives of the hormone. Also from Uppsala came Carl Gemzell, who, in collaboration with Paul Roos, applied human pituitary gonadotrophins for ovulation induction in anovulatory patients. In Gothenburg the gynecological microsurgeon Kurt Swolin developed reconstructive tubal surgery and operative laparoscopy with great success. Thus, by the end of the 1970s, there were a few medical options for infertile patients in the case of tubal factor or anovulatory infertility. However, these few centers were not sufficient to help the large numbers of infertile couples.

Fertility Research in Gothenburg

Two groups at the University of Gothenburg, the Department of Physiology, and Obstetrics and Gynecology, were well equipped to enter the field of assisted reproduction. At the Department of Physiology, Professor Kurt Ahrén led a group of young scientists who were involved in basic research on ovarian function in experimental animals. The group collaborated with well-known international research groups, including Hans Lindner's group at the Weizmann Institute in Israel, John Marsh and William LeMaire at the University of Miami, and with Cornelia

Channing at the University of Maryland in Baltimore. These collaborations included studies of the ovulatory process, oocyte and cumulus maturation, regulation of follicle steroid production, and corpus luteum function. After graduating in physiology several young scientists moved to the Department of Obstetrics and Gynecology, headed by Professor Nils Wiquist, to get the requisite clinical training in order to specialize in obstetrics and gynecology. The clinic had a well-equipped research laboratory, enabling the study of human ovarian cells obtained at elective surgery. Thus, it was possible for these young doctors to continue basic research on human material. Also in this laboratory, muscle physiology was studied using strips obtained from the uterus or oviduct. All these projects on ovarian physiology were basic studies, not really aiming at enhancing fertility but at developing newer forms of contraception. This was often presented as the long-term goal in applications for research grants. Maybe this fact could explain why it took one year after the birth of Louise Brown in 1978 before the group in Gothenburg started a common project to enter the IVF field in order to alleviate infertility.

The IVF Team in Gothenburg

The original IVF team in Gothenburg consisted of the following people (Figure 13.1): Lars Hamberger MD PhD, who presented his thesis in physiology on rat ovarian granulosa and theca cells in 1970 and who later became a clinician while continuing research in reproductive biology; Lars Nilsson MD PhD, who had presented his thesis in physiology on rat preovulatory follicles in 1974 and who later, as a gynecologist, developed an interest in reproductive endocrinology; Per Olof Janson MD PhD, who presented his thesis in physiology of ovarian blood flow in 1975 and who was a well-established clinician with a particular interest in reproductive endocrinology and surgery; Matts Wikland MD PhD, who completed his PhD thesis

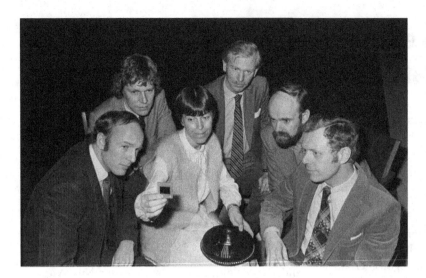

Figure 13.1 The IVF team in Gothenburg 1982. To the left is Lars Nilsson and to the right of him Torbjörn Hillensjö then Lars Hamberger, Matts Wikland, and Per Olof Janson. In the middle is Anita Sjögren (photo: Alf Wihede).

1983 on uterine contractility and was a well-qualified gynecologist who introduced ultrasound for monitoring the cycle and for retrieving eggs; Torbjörn Hillensjö MD PhD, who presented his thesis in physiology on preovulatory follicular function in the rat in 1975, and after postdoctoral work in the laboratory of Cornelia Channing continued his experimental research and joined the group in 1979, and several years later he completed his training in obstetrics and gynecology; and Anita Sjögren, an experienced laboratory technician, who started her career in physiology where, among other things, she was an expert on various microtechniques, and some years after joining the group she presented a Master's thesis on the effect of prolactin on human granulosa cells in cultures. Last but not least, a very important addition to the team was nurse Karin Hammarberg (Figure 13.2), who had the challenging job of building up the clinical routines and procedures and organizing the waiting list. She became the first clinical co-ordinator of the IVF program at Sahlgrenska University Hospital. Karin later moved to Australia where she became an important person within the IVF community and also wrote a PhD thesis with the focus on psychosocial aspects of infertility and infertility treatment.

Initial Trials of IVF in Gothenburg

The initial steps in establishing IVF were taken in 1979, one year after the birth of Louise Brown. In the local newspaper, there was an article in which Lars

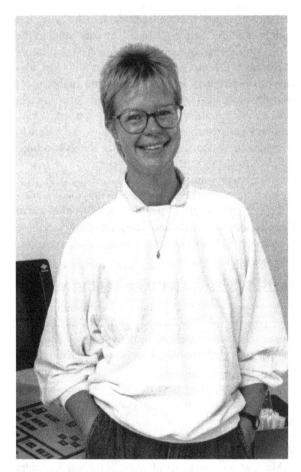

Figure 13.2 Karin Hammarberg, the first nurse-coordinator at the IVF team in Gothenburg (photo: Per Landén).

Hamberger and Nils Wiquist were interviewed and asked about the possibility of establishing the IVF method in Gothenburg. The optimistic answer was that they believed an IVF baby would be born within two years. This did not seem realistic, while at the same time it put pressure on the group. The initial trials to fertilize human eggs were in patients scheduled for sterilization in the late follicular phase. Most were mini-laparotomy procedures, which gave good access to the largest follicle. Apart from isolating the egg, different cell types were isolated and used for cell culture in different research projects. Follicular fluid was recovered and frozen for later steroid analysis. Initially there was a very poor recovery of oocytes, most probably due to bad timing of the cycle or patient factors. Later, recovery improved after administration of hCG to the patients. However, most oocytes were immature, or degenerated and failed to fertilize. We realized that there was a long way to go, and our resources for the project were poor.

Time-lapse Photography

In 1979 Lars Hamberger was contacted by the photographer Lennart Nilsson who had read about the possibility of seeing and photographing human eggs outside the body, where they developed for up to five days before the eggs were transferred to the uterus. He wanted to document the fertilization and early development, not only by using still pictures but also by using time-lapse techniques. In this way, utilizing our laboratory and the team in Gothenburg, he started to make a film of the early development of the human embryo. One problem was that the bright light that had to be used during the filming had a potentially negative effect on the egg. The photographer Carlo Löfman managed to get a West German spy camera that could take pictures in low light. The laboratory where the camera was located was heated to 37 °C to obtain optimal development of the embryos.

Lennart Nilsson and the team from Swedish Television arrived, bringing their equipment to the laboratory. They brought an excellent incubator, and they rebuilt the laboratory to contain "a lab within the lab" to ensure temperature control. For time-lapse photography Lennart Nilsson did not approve of inverted microscopes, since he considered the optics at the time inferior to the conventional microscope. The egg and the sperm were placed in culture medium under oil in a quartz dish, giving good optical conditions. The lenses of the microscope were covered with quartz cylinders and the lens was slowly and cautiously lowered into the oil. Based on some reports from hamster eggs it was thought that visible light could damage the oocyte during prolonged observation, thus the special low light camera was used. Most of the time it was quite difficult to localize the egg with the 100-fold magnification lens. Usually the filming would start on Friday afternoon, since the operations were scheduled on Friday mornings. Lennart Nilsson would take a flight from Stockholm and arrive in Gothenburg around lunchtime. More than once no egg was recovered and he had to return to Stockholm. When an egg was recovered, it was mixed with donor sperm from the andrology laboratory and now and then one or two pronuclei resulted, but cleavage often failed. Lennart would spend the whole weekend in the heated lab before he gave up. Through Lennart Nilsson we gained access to an important manuscript written by Pierre Soupart. In this unpublished manuscript there were many details about important practical steps (note that in 1979 there were hardly any publications about the procedures of human IVF). Among many things, he recommended Hams F10 medium rather than medium 199 for culturing of embryos, which we had used. We also adopted his method of sperm preparation and capacitation. After these changes, our results were more predictable but still we could not record regular cleavage. Because of a moratorium on this type of research in the United States, Pierre Soupart could not get research grants and continue his important studies, but he consulted with other physicians on the technique and also tried to help Lennart Nilsson in his endeavor. Unfortunately, Dr. Soupart died of lung cancer in 1981, only 58 years old.

Although fertilization and cleavage were recorded regularly, initially it was difficult to get good results using time-lapse. Finally, this was achieved and everyone was very happy and proud.

International Fertility Congress Berlin

In the spring of 1981 there was an international congress in Berlin, and Lars Hamberger was able to get permission to show the film by Lennart Nilsson separately from the scientific program, since the deadline for abstracts had passed. The film was shown during the lunch break and it created great interest in the audience. Among others, Bob Edwards was very positive. At this congress, another Swedish IVF group also appeared. It was a group from Malmö General Hospital who reported data on their research project on IVF, which had started in 1978–79 (Wramsby et al., 1981). The leader of the team was Professor Stig Kullander,

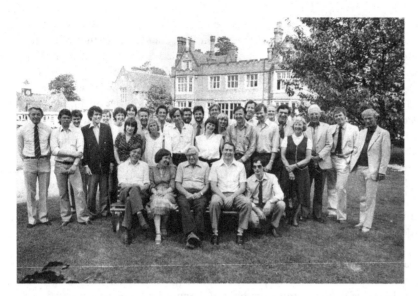

Figure 13.3 Attendees at the Bourn Hall meeting in 1981. It was a long time before the photographer, Lennart Nilsson, was pleased with how people looked, and had taken this picture. Finally he shouted "look successful" (photo: Lennart Nilsson).

and the others in the team included senior gynecologist Percy Liedholm and two young gynecologists, Per Sundström and Håkan Wramsby. We were quite surprised and impressed by their progress in the field and it became evident that we had strong competition within our own country. Dr. Per Sundström collaborated with Professor Ove Nilsson in Uppsala, using scanning electron microscopy to document events related to fertilization and cleavage of the human egg. Dr. Håkan Wramsby was involved in studies of the chromosomes in the oocyte, and collaborated with Professor Yanagimachi in Hawaii. Academically the work from the Malmö group resulted in two PhD theses and in 1983 their work resulted in the second IVF child born in Sweden.

Experience from the Bourn Hall Meeting

In the autumn of 1981 a meeting was arranged by Bob Edwards and Patrick Steptoe at Bourn Hall in Cambridge. Around 30 doctors and scientists were invited from all over the world (Figure 13.3). Our team was invited, probably due to the time-lapse film, which had been shown at the Berlin meeting. Lars Hamberger, Lennart Nilsson, and Torbjörn Hillensjö participated. The meeting was quite informal and each group presented their procedures relating to patient monitoring, egg retrieval, sperm preparation, culture procedures, embryo transfer, and luteal support. Each topic was discussed in detail. We were also invited to see the lab and shown various procedures by Jane Purdy, who was the embryologist. One topic, which was discussed at

length, was the pros and cons of the natural and stimulated cycle. Edwards and Steptoe had long argued for the natural cycle and close monitoring of the LH surge. From the mid to late follicular phase, urinary LH was measured every 4 h and laparoscopy undertaken 30 h after the start of the LH surge. The patients were staying at Bourn Hall and laparoscopies were scheduled irrespective of the time of the day. Some groups had experience of stimulated cycles, chlomiphene citrate (Lopata, Wood, Trounson), or hMG (Georgiana and Howard Jones). With regards to culture medium, Earle´s simple medium supplied with heat-inactivated patient serum was advocated. With regards to luteal support Howard and Georgeanna Jones strongly recommended progesterone whereas others used hCG. The meeting was in fact a practical workshop and all participants appeared to be very pleased to be part of it. In 1981 the IVF world was small, and everyone benefited from an open atmosphere.

After returning from the Bourn Hall meeting, several changes were made to our IVF program. We learned that the quality of the water used for medium preparation was extremely important, and that conventional double-distilled laboratory water was not sufficient. We therefore started to use Analar water, which was obtained in big bottles and shipped from England. We made our own Earle´s medium, since no commercial products were available. To increase environmental stability in the incubator, we began to place the culture dishes in a desiccator within the incubator. It was gassed with a mixture of 5% CO_2 in air. We became increasingly concerned about keeping the humidity high since we did not cover the medium with oil. Another procedure that we changed was to let the oocytes pre-incubate longer, for 5–6 h before the sperm was added, in accordance with the recommendations made by Alan Trounson. All these changes, together with improved patient monitoring, led gradually to better results in terms of fertilization and cleavage, and embryo fragmentation declined.

How Ultrasound Became an Important Tool for Clinical IVF

Clinical IVF started in Sweden at the time when ultrasound imaging in obstetrics and gynecology was developing rapidly and becoming used more often in daily clinical work. In 1978, Hackelöer and Robinson published a study where, for the first time, it was shown that ultrasound imaging of follicular size could be used for the prediction of oocyte maturation (Hackelöer and Robinson, 1978). At that time, radiologists had already been using ultrasound for guided puncture of cysts in the kidney, as well as for percutaneous biopsy of abdominal tumors, for some years, a technique described by the Danish ultrasound pioneer and urological surgeon Dr. Hans Henrik Holm (Holm et al., 1972). At the university clinic of Obstetrics and Gynecology in Gothenburg, ultrasound in both obstetrics and gynecology by tradition had been an important diagnostic tool. There were two people in particular who started the use of ultrasound in obstetrics and gynecology in Gothenburg and they were Dr. Jan Lundberg and Dr. Klas-Henry Hökegård. Their tradition in using diagnostic ultrasound made the IVF teams in Gothenburg curious about the use of ultrasound imagining as a tool for clinical IVF.

There were two obvious clinical parts of the IVF cycle where ultrasound imaging could be useful – they were monitoring of follicular maturation and the oocyte pick-up procedure. Monitoring of oocyte maturation for clinical purposes in both stimulated and natural cycles was initially done by measuring hormones such as estrogens, progesterone and luteinizing hormone (LH) in the urine and later in blood. At that time, the hormone assays were time-consuming and not very accurate. Thus, using ultrasound for imaging follicles and their daily growth had practical advantages over the tedious work of collecting urine 24 h a day to analyze hormones.

The Gothenburg IVF team in 1980, initiated by Dr. Lars Nilsson and Dr. Matts Wikland, started to explore the use of ultrasound imagining of follicular size as a method for predicting oocyte maturation and for

oocyte pick-up in IVF cycles (Wikland et al., 1983). To learn the technique of scanning ovaries with follicles we visited Dr. Bernhard-Joachim Hackelöer in Marburg, Germany, where he was active at the time. In those days, only abdominal ultrasound was available for scanning ovaries. Furthermore, owing to the position of the ovaries deep in the lower pelvis they could only be clearly visualized by ultrasound when the patient had a full bladder, a technique often uncomfortable for the patient. Sitting in the waiting-room with a full bladder not knowing exactly when the examination was to be performed was unpleasant.

Monitoring the IVF Cycle

IVF was initially performed in natural cycles. However, there were difficulties collecting the oocyte at the right time; either it was too early and the oocyte was not mature or ovulation had occured. For such reasons the stimulated cycle became more frequently used, since it also meant that several mature oocytes could be retrieved. Thus, the ovarian response to hormonal stimulation had to be monitored, since we needed to know how far we could go and when the oocytes were mature (Klopper et al., 1974). As mentioned above, in the early days of IVF the available tool for monitoring was measuring ovarian hormones such as oestrogens and LH in the urine or blood. It was time-consuming and not so accurate. For this reason, in Gothenburg we decided early on to utilize ultrasound imaging of follicular growth as a tool for monitoring the stimulated IVF cycle, since the method gave immediate information about the ovarian response. The method was first evaluated in the natural cycle, but it was soon realized that it was in stimulated cycles where it could be really useful. It was Dr. Pekka Ylöstalo, coming from the Finnish IVF team in Helsinki including Professor Markku Seppälä and Dr. Aarne Koskimies, who tried early on to evaluate the value of measuring follicular growth by ultrasound in cycles stimulated by clomiphene and gonadotrophins (Ylöstalo et al., 1981). In our group in Gothenburg we made an early decision to monitor the stimulated cycles by ultrasound. We also based the oocyte pick-up time in the majority of IVF cycles on the size of the largest follicles, as measured by ultrasound (Nilsson et al., 1985). Ultrasound scanning of follicular size as a method for monitoring oocyte maturation and prediction of the time for human chorionic gonadotrophin (hCG) and oocyte pick-up has today become the main method for monitoring ovarian response in stimulated IVF cycles irrespective of the protocol used (Wittmaack et al., 1994).

115

Oocyte Pick-up

In the beginning of the IVF era, oocyte pick-up was performed laparoscopically, a technique that had to be performed under general anesthesia. It was time-consuming and involved a certain risk to the patient. If the oocyte pick-up was to be performed as an outpatient procedure, there was a need for simplifying it. Since mature follicles are large (15–25mm in diameter) and cystic structures that can be imaged by ultrasound, the Danish group and we thought it must be possible to puncture them with the guidance of ultrasound. With the experience of the ultrasound-guided percutaneous puncture technique described above by Dr. Holm in Denmark it was not surprising that the IVF team in Copenhagen at Rigshospitalet with Dr. Suzan Lenz, Dr. Jörgen Glenn Lauritsen, and Dr. Svend Lindenberg, who at that time worked in the lab, would be amongst the pioneers to demonstrate successful oocyte collection under the guidance of abdominal real-time ultrasound (Lenz et al., 1981).

Parallel with the Danish group, our IVF team in Gothenburg also started to explore the technique for ultrasound-guided follicle aspiration to be used in IVF cycles (Hamberger et al., 1982). In this early work, we learnt much from a radiologist, Dr. Mats Asztély, who worked at the Department of Radiology in our hospital and who was a pioneer in carrying out ultrasound-guided percutaneous puncture of cysts in the kidney. The technique we initially utilized was abdominal scanning by a linear array real-time transducer, percutaneous puncturing through a full urinary bladder under general anesthesia, but later it was carried out under local anesthesia (Figure 13.4) (Wikland et al., 1983). It was not as technically demanding as a laparoscopy, but owing to the pain that some patients experienced when it was performed under local anesthesia, it was preferable to perform the procedure under general anesthesia. As such, the advantages of this procedure in comparison to laparoscopy were not appreciated. Because of this, our IVF team in Gothenburg started to explore the possibilities of performing ultrasound scanning via the vagina or vaginal sonography. The vaginal route made it possible to get close to the ovaries with an empty urinary bladder. Furthermore, since it was possible to avoid puncturing the urinary bladder, the procedure could be performed under local anesthesia.

In 1983, our group started to work on vaginal ultrasound scanning. At that time, we used small abdominal mechanical sector transducers, which were possible to use in the vagina. However, in those days

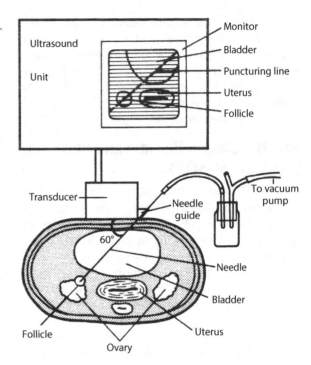

Figure 13.4 Principals of abdominal ultrasonically-guided follicle puncture.

the abdominal transducers available were not ideal for vaginal scanning and particularly not for transvaginal puncture.

The Importance of Collaborating with the Industry

In the early days of clinical IVF, it was not possible to buy equipment like needles, tubes, collection tubes for oocytes, and needle guides for the ultrasound transducer from companies specializing in IVF equipment. In those days, no such companies existed. In Gothenburg we approached a small Swedish company specializing in manufacturing medical instruments and had them manufacture the equipment we needed for the oocyte pick-up procedure. Later, this company, Swemed Lab International, and another Swedish, Gothenburg-based company, Vitrolife, originally specializing in producing culture media, focused all their efforts on manufacturing products for IVF, many of which were designed by our group.

Owing to our experience of the excellent quality of images of ovaries via vaginal scanning, and the fact that in those days we only had abdominal transducers not designed for vaginal scanning, we had to find an ultrasound company that could help us to manufacture a transducer that was designed for vaginal scanning.

In 1984, we started a collaboration with the Danish ultrasound company, Brüel and Kjaer. They had previously developed a mechanical ultrasound probe for cranial scanning during neurosurgical procedures, but it never became used widely. After we contacted them and described what we needed for vaginal scanning, they realized that by modifying a transducer originally meant for neurosurgical procedures, it could be used as a vaginal transducer. With this new transducer, the ovaries and follicles could easily be scanned and oocyte aspiration performed (Figure 13.5) as an outpatient procedure under local anesthesia by using a modified paracervical block (Wikland et al., 1985). It did not take long before other manufacturers of diagnostic ultrasound understood the potential of vaginal sonography for gynecological diagnostic and interventional procedures and consequently started to design and manufacture vaginal probes. In our opinion, clinical IVF was probably the starting point for vaginal sonography, which subsequently has become such an important tool in both diagnostic and interventional gynecological ultrasound examinations.

It did not take long for other IVF groups to realize the potential of this new technique. Another Scandinavian group that also started to utilize the technique for oocyte pick-up very early was the Norwegian IVF team in Trondheim with and Dr. Jarl A Kahn, Professor Kåre Molne, and the embryologist Arne Sunde. Another European group that began early to practice vaginal sonography was the IVF team in Austria (Feichtinger and Kemeter, 1986).

Transvaginal ultrasound-guided oocyte retrieval (TVOR) has since become the gold standard for oocyte aspiration in ART. Even though there has been no large prospective controlled randomized trial comparing laparoscopic-guided and transvaginal-guided oocyte retrieval, the latter has become the method of choice. The reason for this is probably that TVOR is a simple and safe method that, in the majority of patients, results in the recovery of many oocytes, enough to guarantee a good chance of achieving pregnancy.

The technique has, over the years, been improved in many ways. The ultrasound equipment has become more sophisticated, resulting in extremely refined images as compared to results from equipment used in the early days. This has meant a lot for the safety and ease of use of the technique.

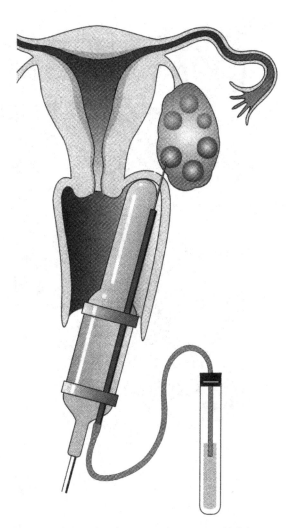

Figure 13.5 Principles of transvaginal scanning and follicle aspiration.

Scandinavian Collaboration

An open atmosphere prevailed between the Scandinavian IVF groups, and clinics were very willing to support other clinics. It was a win–win situation rather than competition. Meetings were arranged in the Nordic countries, the first one in Helsingör, Denmark, in 1981, and the second one in Geilo, Norway, in 1983. The first Scandinavian IVF child was born in Gothenburg, Sweden, in September 1982. The Geilo meeting therefore received considerable interest from the media and was covered by TV news. The meeting held in April 1983 (Figure 13.6) was arranged by the IVF team in Trondheim, Norway, and was a great success. The town of Geilo is known for excellent down-hill

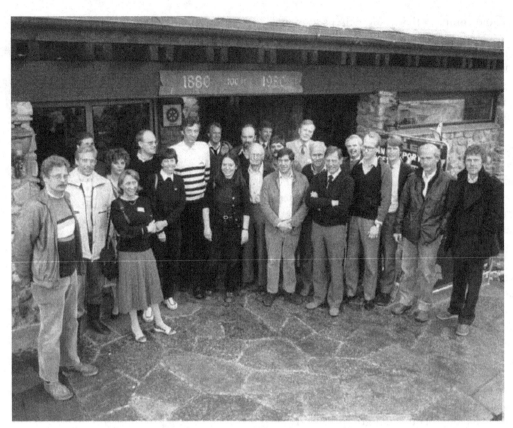

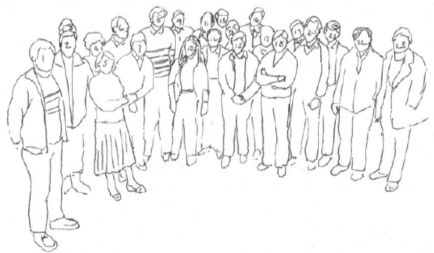

1 Per Lundmo	2 Germond Unsgird	3	4	5 Anne Halverson	6 Hakan Wramsby	7 Anita Sjogren
8 Per Sundstrom	9 Leif Hagglund	10 Ritza Storeng	11 Matts Wikland	12 J Jensen	13 J. Glen Lauritsen	14 Arne Sunde
15 Jarl Kahn	16 Anders Berg	17 Kare Molne	18 Petter Fylling	19 Berni Kjessler	20 Svend Lindenberg	21 Johan Hazekamp
22 Lars Hamberger	23 Torbjorn Hillensjo					

Figure 13.6 Group photograph of the attendees of the Nordic IVF meeting in 1983 in Geilo, Norway. Numbered key.

Table 13.1 Summary of the birth of the first IVF child in the different Scandinavian countries

Country	Year of birth	IVF team
Sweden	1982	Gothenburg
Denmark	1983	Rigshospitalet Copenhagen
Norway	1984	Trondheim
Finland	1984	Helsinki

skiing and the meeting consisted of workshops held in the morning and evening, while the afternoon was reserved for skiing. Not only gynecologists and scientists participated in the meeting, but also embryologists, laboratory technicians, and nurses. From this time onwards, Scandinavian IVF meetings have been held every 18 months in one of the Nordic countries. With time, these meetings have grown in size to several hundred participants. Not only have they stimulated scientific research and communication, but they also have aided education, training, and networking in this new field.

Pioneering Groups in Scandinavian IVF

As previously mentioned, the first IVF child in Sweden was born in September 1982 (Gothenburg group) and the second was born in 1983 (Malmö group). In Denmark, the first IVF child was born in 1983 (Rigshospitalet Copenhagen). In Norway, the first IVF child was born in 1984 (Trondheim group) and the same year the first IVF child in Finland was born (Helsinki group). A summary is shown in Table 13.1.

References

Feichtinger W, Kemeter P. Transvaginal sector scan sonography for needle guided transvaginal follicle aspiration and other applications in gynecologic routine and research. *Fertil Steril* 1986;45:722–725.

Hackelöer BJ, Robinson HP. Ultrasound examination of the growing ovarian follicle and of the corpus luteum during the normal physiology of menstrual cycle. *Geburtshilfe Frauenheilkd* 1978;38:163–168.

Hamberger, L, Wikland M, Nilsson L. Methods for aspiration of human oocytes by various techniques. *Acta Med Rom* 1982;20:370–379.

Holm HH, Kristensen JK, Rasmussen SN, Northeved A, Barlebo H. Ultrasound as a guide in percutaneous puncture technique. *Ultrasonics* 1972;10:83–86.

Klopper A, Aiman J, Besser M. Ovarian steroidogenesis resulting from treatment with menopausal gonadotropin. *Eur J ObstetGynecol Reprod Biol* 1974;4:25–30.

Lenz S, Lauritsen JG, Kjellow M. Collection of human oocytes for in vitro fertilization by ultrasonically guided puncture. *Lancet* 1981;1:1163–1164.

Nilsson L, Wikland M, Hamberger L, et al. Simplification of the method of in vitro fertilization: sonographic measurements of follicular diameter as the sole index of follicular maturity. *J In Vitro Fert Embryo Transf* 1985;2:17–22.

Wikland M, Nilsson L, Hansson R, Hamberger L, Janson PO. Collection of human oocytes by the use of sonography. *Fertil Steril* 1983;39:603–608.

Wikland M, Enk L, Hamberger L. Transvesical and transvaginal approaches for the aspiration of follicles by use of ultrasound. *Ann N Y Acad Sci* 1985;442:182–194.

Wittmaack FM, Kreger DO, Blasco L, et al. Effect of follicular size on oocyte retrieval, fertilization, cleavage, and embryo quality in in vitro fertilization cycles: a 6-year data collection. *Fertil Steril* 1994;62:1205–1210.

Wramsby H, Kullander S, Liedholm P, et al. The success rate of in vitro fertilization of human oocytes in relation to the concentration of different hormones in follicular fluid and plasma. *Fertil Steril* 1981;36:448–454.

Ylöstalo P, Lindgren P, Nillius SJ. Ultrasonic measurement of ovarian follicles, ovarian and uterine size during induction of ovulation with human gonadotrophins. *Acta Endocrinol* 1981;98:592–598.

The Development of In-Vitro Fertilization in Spain

Antonio Pellicer

The story of in-vitro fertilization (IVF) and assisted reproduction technology (ART) in Spain has been marked by the existence of two different assisted reproduction laws, enacted in 1988 and 2006. Both have had a significant impact on our practice, but both have turned out to be quite permissive laws and have allowed medical advances to be made over the years. As a result, international registries have consistently shown Spain as a country with acceptable ART outcomes compared to our neighbors, and as a European leader in the oocyte donation field (Calhaz-Jorge et al., 2016). Moreover, and in parallel, research and development have always been a driving force in some centers, such as the Instituto Valenciano de Infertilidad (IVI). IVI has become one of the world's leading groups in creating a culture of science in Spain, which has been an incentive to others and has made Spain a significant country in the production of scientific work in ART.

The Beginning

The first efforts made to be able to reproduce what was already a reality in the UK, the USA, Austria, France, or Germany addressed the creation of teams of clinicians and embryologists in Barcelona. Some well-known physicians, who were already established in the private sector in that city, combined efforts in a multidisciplinary group with the goal of accomplishing the first IVF pregnancy in Spain. However, it was the group from the Dexeus Institute, formed by Dr. Pedro Barri and young embryologists Gloria Calderón and Anna Veiga, who deserved the merit of having accomplished the first term pregnancy back in 1984. They also published the first term pregnancy after the replacement of frozen-thawed embryos (Barri et al., 1984; Veiga et al., 1987).

In parallel, public hospitals reacted to the challenge of offering similar standards to their patients. Spain is a country with full universal health coverage to all citizens, and ART was soon included in the list of pathologies to be treated in public hospitals. However, it was a difficult time because public health providers' interest was not concentrated on ART; rather infertility was considered a scarcity and not a disease. Nevertheless, the Hospital de Cruces in Bilbao and the Hospital Clinic in Valencia were both successful in establishing full pregnancies in 1985 after some failed attempts (Pellicer et al., 1984).

As a result of my personal frustration with the public system and future prospects, it soon became clear to me that the only way to contribute to modern ART would be to create an Institution which, while maintaining the principles and spirit of the University (teaching and research), would also be able to handle patients with the highest standards of quality and clinical outcomes. This is why and how IVI was born in 1990 as the result of public authorities' lack of care with ART.

Professor Robert G. Edwards in Spain

Bob Edwards was very close to both the University of Valencia and IVI. In the late 1980s and the early 1990s he attended several meetings that we organized in Valencia. These conferences were the perfect place where the initial ESHRE steps were decided since we had many relevant people as guests and speakers in those meetings, who later became chairmen of ESHRE, with Bob being the driving force for them all and for the future of ESHRE.

Bob was awarded the Gold Metal of the Instituto Universitario Dexeus in 1985. In 1992, long before he was recognized and received the Nobel Prize of Medicine and Physiology, he became Doctor Honoris Causa by the University of Valencia. In his speech to the teaching community, he pointed out the difficulties he had encountered until that time to fully develop IVF as a standard infertility treatment. He told the audience not only about the scientific challenges, but also about the social conflicts that his work generated, especially in the UK.

In 2002, when we opened the new facilities in Valencia, Bob was our guest (Figure 14.1). I still remember that in those days he was interested in the

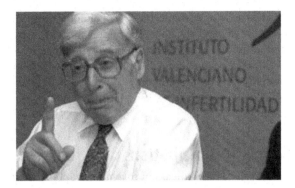

Figure 14.1 Professor Robert G. Edwards in Valencia in 2002.

non-invasive diagnosis of embryo viability, a topic that still remains unsolved today, but to which we have dedicated many hours of research, and I wish we could share with him our findings (Tejera et al., 2016). He was always very supportive and friendly.

I certainly cannot say how many times Bob Edwards was invited to visit Spain to attend meetings. All I can say is that he was always so enthusiastic, and he transmitted to the young fellows his curiosity for, and interest in, gaining knowledge in the field. He was certainly very important for the further development of ART in Spain until his age no longer allowed him to travel.

Regulations

Spain has passed two fundamental Laws in Assisted Reproduction. The first was published in November 1988 and a review law was published in 2006. Both regulations were quite permissive because they allowed and prohibited a series of techniques that, in the end, have modified our daily practice and determined the development of ART in Spain.

Some specifics of our law as regards potential users is the free access to ART of any individual, regardless of his/her age (>18 years), civil status, or sexual orientation. Oocyte donation is also allowed with the particularity of anonymity and compensation to donors. Patients can freeze their oocytes for non-medical reasons, and preimplantation genetic diagnosis (PGD) is allowed, although the approval of the Comisión Nacional de Reproducción Humana Asistida (CNRHA) is required in some uncommon cases.

The CNRHA was created in 1997 as a consultant commission that depended on the Spanish Ministry of Health. Among its many functions, the CNRHA should review PGD applications, the research protocols that involve embryos, as well as the activities surrounding oocyte donation, such as compensation or advertisement. The CNRHA should also establish the accreditation and follow-up requisites for the different techniques employed in ART centers.

In Spain, the maximum number of embryos allowed to be replaced in the uterus is three, but today there is a tendency towards reaching 100% single embryo transfer. It will take some time, but we will get there.

Research is allowed with embryos donated for this purpose or with embryonic stem cells, but requires a written project that has to be positively approved by the corresponding regulatory authorities, and each embryo used must have traceability in order to make clear what its final destination has been. It is completely forbidden to create human embryos for the sole purpose of research. Surrogacy and gender selection are specifically forbidden in Spanish law.

Oocyte Donation in Spain

From the very beginning, Spain has taken a very realistic approach to oocyte donation. It was authorized in the law published in 1988 with some characteristics that made the technique truly available not only for Spaniards, but also for foreigners. First, oocyte donation was anonymous. A registry should be created to control all donations in the country, which is still not finished 30 years later. This is a problem because we do not want to help some women possibly becoming oocyte donation "professionals." In any event, a few years ago the CNRHA postulated that a woman should be stimulated up to six times in her reproductive life. Thus overstimulation of donors should not happen. Moreover, the occurrence of ovarian hyperstimulation is specifically punished in Spanish law, showing another example of donor's protection against potential abuse.

Second, there is the matter of compensation to donors for the discomfort caused and working hours lost, which is controversial. The amount of money was carefully calculated back in 1988 and has basically not increased since then. It was established at around €900, and the CNRHA takes care that this policy is followed among groups. This has been a matter of controversy because in some neighboring countries, such as France and Italy, oocyte donation is allowed, but not compensated at all. Others, however, have adopted the Spanish system and compensate women for such generous effort. This is the case in the UK, Belgium, Portugal, Greece, and others.

As a result, some countries, including Spain, have become the final destination of couples searching for oocyte donation. This started to become known as medical tourism, but is actually a phenomenon that shows the global functioning of today's medical care. Information is available on the Internet and patients seek their chances elsewhere if their own country is unable to provide help. Oocyte and sperm donations were probably the first techniques to completely open the doors of ART anywhere in the world, but were followed by other treatments, such as surrogacy and gender selection.

Spain was right in compensating donors and making donations anonymous. The UK, for example, where compensation is also allowed, has very few donors because of non-anonymous programs. Patients who decide to undergo oocyte donation feel quite comfortable with anonymity. Although lack of a full description of their donors may be worrying, they trust the medical team, and the fact that nobody will request information about those donated eggs in the future is quite reassuring for them.

Not favoring an oocyte donation policy based on compensation to donors and anonymity is, in my modest opinion, a mistake for several reasons. Oocyte donation is absolutely necessary for many women because of the age at which they decide to have children. There is no other realistic choice and the technique has proved extraordinarily efficient in achieving term pregnancies (Garrido et al., 2012).

Whether or not oocyte donation should be forbidden can be discussed, but the position of some countries in allowing egg donation, but prohibiting compensation to donors, is cynical because, in the end, there are no active donors in these countries and patients need to travel abroad. Moreover, what is even worse is the position of other European countries where compensation is not allowed, but the import of gametes according to European Union (EU) directives is common practice. Thus the women who are stimulated are not their citizens, while women receive treatment for egg donations in their own country with foreign oocytes. To my understanding, a common and permissive regulation should be made valid in EU territory.

Another reason why I believe that oocyte donation has been of paramount importance in ART is because it is scientifically sound. Oocyte donation has allowed us to separate the relevance of the embryo and endometrium in successful implantation. By using this technique and designing smart clinical trials, we have learned, for example, the role of endometriosis in infertility (Diaz et al., 2000), the importance of having uterine fibroids (Horcajadas et al., 2008), adenomyosis (Martinez-Conejero et al., 2011), or the effects of chemotherapy and radiotherapy on subsequent pregnancies (Muñoz et al., 2015), just to mention a few examples.

Scientific Contributions

As a result of the clinical improvements supported by permissive laws and investments in research and development, over the years Spain has been an important contributor to the scientific literature. In fact, bibliometric manuscripts have described Spain as one of the hubs of reproductive medicine (Aleixandre-Benavent et al., 2015) and I have been recognized as author number 8 in the world with the largest number of citations (Gransalke, 2015). A series of landmark manuscripts were published, some of which have really changed clinical practice. IVI became one of the few private institutions which, despite providing outstanding medical care, also invested in research and development as a pillar of its own growth, a strange, albeit successful, phenomenon in a world where science seems to be restricted to universities.

For example, we were the first to establish co-culture systems of human embryos with cells of maternal origin (Simón et al., 1999). The technique proved better at obtaining good quality embryos than commercial media. However, the widespread diffusion of co-culture was not achieved mainly because of the complicated preparation process.

After ICSI was published by Palermo et al. (1992), we were concerned about how to develop a successful way of preserving valuable sperm in patients with severe male factor infertility. We described a technique that has since been employed as a reference for many years and communicated the first pregnancies (Romero et al., 1996; Gil-Salom et al., 1996).

The most comprehensive studies to the pathophysiology of ovarian hyperstimulation syndrome (OHSS) were also published in Spain. Balasch et al. (1996) described the syndrome in the early days when women were actually subjected to high risks because the mechanisms that underlay OHSS were completely unknown and proposed approaches to treatment. We studied in detail the role of VEGF and dopamine agonists in OHSS development and management (Gomez et al., 2006; Alvarez et al., 2007). Moreover, we introduced the use of dopamine agonists as an accepted treatment of an already established OHSS (Busso et al., 2010).

Another important contribution to the world of ART also came from IVI. Cobo et al. (2010) published a randomized clinical trial that compared the use of fresh and vitrified human oocytes in oocyte donation, and showed no inferiority of egg vitrification. This manuscript changed practice; indeed today many programs and oocyte banks use oocyte vitrification regularly. It also opened the doors to oocyte freezing for oncological and non-oncological reasons. For the former it proved to be a great treatment alternative together with ovarian tissue freezing (Domingo et al., 2012). The latter is a concept that is still being developed, but is one of extraordinary social relevance (Cobo et al., 2016).

In as much as a closer look at the endometrium as a necessary partner in human implantation was a concept that was also further developed in the IVI Foundation Labs under Carlos Simon's direction, we were able to develop a customized test to check for the window of implantation after defining the relevant genes to implantation in humans (Diaz-Gimeno et al., 2011). The endometrial receptivity assay (ERA) is a commercially available test that is widely employed today.

References

Aleixandre-Benavent R, Simon C, Fauser BC. Trends in clinical reproductive medicine research: 10 years of growth. *Fertil Steril* 2015; 104: 131–137.

Alvarez C, Martí-Bonmatí L, Novella-Maestre E, et al. Dopamine agonist cabergoline reduces hemoconcentration and ascites in hyperstimulated women undergoing assisted reproduction. *J Clin Endocrinol Metab* 2007; 92: 2931–2937.

Balasch J, Fábregues F, Arroyo V, et al. Treatment of severe ovarian hyperstimulation syndrome by a conservative medical approach. *Acta Obstet Gynecol Scand* 1996; 75: 662–667.

Barri PN, Veiga A, Calderón G, et al. Primeros resultados del programa FIV del Instituto Dexeus. *Prog Obstet Ginecol* 1984; 27: 27–32.

Busso C, Fernández M, García-Velasco JA, et al. The non-ergot derived dopamine agonist quinagolide in prevention of early ovarian hyperstimulation syndrome in IVF patients: a randomized, double-blind, placebo-controlled trial. *Hum Reprod* 2010; 25: 995–1004.

Calhaz-Jorge C, de Geyter C, Kupka MS, et al. Assisted reproductive technology in Europe, 2012: results generated from European registers by ESHRE. *Hum Reprod* 2016; 31: 1638–1652.

Cobo A, Meseguer M, Remohí J, Pellicer A. Use of cryo-banked oocytes in an ovum donation programme: a prospective, randomized, controlled, clinical trial. *Hum Reprod* 2010; 25: 2239–2246.

Cobo A, García-Velasco JA, Coello A, et al. Oocytes vitrification as an efficient option for elective fertility preservation. *Fertil Steril* 2016; 105(3): 755–764. e8.

Díaz I, Navarro J, Blasco L, et al. Impact of stages III–VI of endometriosis on recipients of sibling oocytes: matched case-control study. *Fertil Steril* 2000; 74: 31–34.

Diaz-Gimeno P, Horcajadas JA, Martínez-Conejero JA, et al. A genomic diagnostic tool for human endometrial receptivity based on the transcriptomic signature. *Fertil Steril* 2011; 95: 50–60.

Domingo J, Guillén V, Ayllón A, et al. Ovarian response to controlled ovarian hyperstimulation in cancer patients is diminished even before oncological treatment. *Fertil Steril* 2012; 97: 930–934.

Garrido N, Bellver J, Remohí J, Alamá P, Pellicer A. Cumulative newborn rates increase with the total number of transferred embryos according to an analysis of 15792 ovum donation cycles. *Fertil Steril* 2012; 98: 341–346.

Gil-Salom M, Romero J, Mínguez Y, et al. Pregnancies after intracytoplasmic sperm injection with cryopreserved testicular spermatozoa. *Hum Reprod* 1996; 11: 1309–1313.

Gómez R, González-Izquierdo M, Zimmermann RC, et al. Low-dose dopamine agonist administration blocks vascular endothelial growth factor (VEGF)-mediated vascular hyperpermeability without altering VEGF receptor 2-dependent luteal angiogenesis in a rat ovarian hyperstimulated model. *Endocrinology* 2006; 147: 5400–5411.

Gransalke K. Reproductive Biomedicine, Publication Analysis 2007–2013. *Lab Times* 2015; 4: 32–34.

Horcajadas JA, Goyri E, Higón MA, et al. Endometrial receptivity and implantation are not affected by the presence of uterine intramural leiomyomas: a clinical and functional genomics analysis. *J Clin Endocrinol Metab* 2008; 93: 3490–3498.

Martínez-Conejero JA, Morgan M, Montesinos M, et al. Adenomyosis does not affect implantation, but is associated with miscarriage in patients undergoing oocyte donation. *Fertil Steril* 2011; 96: 943–950.

Muñoz E, Fernandez I, Martinez M, et al. Oocyte donation outcome after oncological treatment in cancer survivors. *Fertil Steril* 2015; 103: 205–213.

Palermo G, Joris H, Devroey P, Van Steirteghem AC. Pregnancies after intracytoplasmic injection of single spermatozoon into an oocyte. *Lancet* 1992; 340: 17–18.

Pellicer A, Pérez-Gil M, Tortajada M, Bonilla-Musoles F. Fertilización "in vitro", transferencia embrionaria y gestación gemelar anembrionada. *Rev Esp Obst y Gin* 1984; 43: 569–574.

Romero J, Remohí J, Mínguez Y, et al. Fertilization after intracytoplasmic sperm injection with cryopreserved testicular sperm. *Fertil Steril* 1996; 65: 877–879.

Simón C, Mercader A, García-Velasco JA, et al. Co-Culture of human embryos with autologous human endometrial epithelial cells in patients with implantation failure. *J Clin Endocrinol Metab* 1999; 84: 2638–2646.

Tejera A, Castelló D, De los Santos JM, et al. Combination of metabolism measurement and a time-lapse sytem provides an embryo selection method based on oxygen uptake and chronology of cytokinesis timing. *Fertil Steril* 2016; 106: 119–126.

Veiga A, Calderón G, Barri PN, Coroleu B. Pregnancy after the replacement of a frozen-thawed embryo with < 50% intact blastomeres. *Hum Reprod* 1987; 2: 321–323.

The Development of In-Vitro Fertilization in Greece, Germany, and The Netherlands

Basil C. Tarlatzis, Klaus Diedrich, and Bart Fauser

The Beginning of IVF in Greece

Children were always very important for the Greek family. When I started my residency training in obstetrics and gynecology in 1977, treatment of infertility was part of the gynecological practice, albeit with the methods available, which were mainly tubal microsurgery (laparoscopic surgery was just starting), ovulation induction with clomiphene citrate, and donor insemination. Everything changed on July 25, 1978, when Steptoe and Edwards announced the birth of Louise Brown. Later that year, October 2–6, 1978, attending the Fifth ESCO Congress in Venice and listening to Patrick Steptoe, also on behalf of Robert Edwards, giving the Main Lecture on "Pregnancies following in vitro fertilization techniques in the human" (Figure 15.1), I knew that this was what I wanted to do. Thus, started my long and exciting journey in the "brave new world" of assisted reproduction.

The amazing progress and rapid spread of in-vitro fertilization around the globe prompted several gynecologists from Greece to try to learn the scientific and technical details of IVF, in order to be able to apply it locally. Some tried immediately to get access to Steptoe and Edwards, but the two pioneers did not feel ready to share information at this early stage on what they considered still preliminary and experimental. Hence, colleagues sought training options in the IVF Centers that were opening up in different countries: some, like me, in the United States, and others in Australia or in Europe, particularly the United Kingdom.

In the early 1980s, when IVF was not available in Greece, infertile couples tried to get IVF treatment abroad. Hence, in 1981, a couple from Athens who were treated by Steptoe in Bourn Hall became pregnant. A boy was delivered in early 1982 by the mother's gynecologist K. Kolias and P. Steptoe himself at "MITERA" private maternity clinic. This represents the first IVF baby delivered in Greece but not the first conceived by IVF performed in Greece, since the procedure was done in the UK.

The first attempts to set up properly organized IVF Centers in Greece started in the mid 1980s. That was the time that I also came back from the USA, after training and working for three years (1982–1985) in the IVF Program of Yale University, with Alan DeCherney, Neri Laufer, and several other distinguished colleagues. The Yale Program (Figure 15.2) was one of the first in the USA, after Norfolk, and was extremely active both clinically and in research (Laufer et al., 1984; Tarlatzis et al., 1984a). These were exciting times, since everything in the IVF procedure, both in the clinical and the embryology laboratory aspects, was *terra incognita* and had to be developed from scratch, based on previous animal work that Neri and I had previously done (Laufer et al., 1983; Tarlatzis et al., 1984b).

In the summer of 1985, with this experience in my bags, I decided to return to Greece in order to establish the first IVF Center in Thessaloniki and probably (one of the first) in the country. To that aim, I joined forces with two prominent gynecologists: Professor John Bontis, who had trained with Lord Robert Winston at Hammersmith Hospital, London, UK, in tubal microsurgery and laparoscopy, and Professor Serge Mantalenakis, who had done basic research on embryo implantation with Gregory Pincus in the Wooster Foundation, Massachusetts, USA (Figure 15.3). The team also included the gynecologist specializing in ultrasonography Dr. Makis Lagos, the biologist Thomai Sanopoulou, BA, MSc,, for the laboratory and the midwife Betty Gavriilidou as coordinator.

At that time, Greece did not have any legislation or regulation concerning the organization of an IVF unit. Hence, since oocyte pick-up was still done by laparoscopy under general anesthesia, we decided that it would be safer for the patients to place the IVF Center inside the private General Clinic "Geniki Kliniki," which also had an Obstetrics & Gynecology Section and an ICU. The first few months were devoted to designing and rearranging the rooms, ordering the necessary instruments and equipment, and identifying the providers of

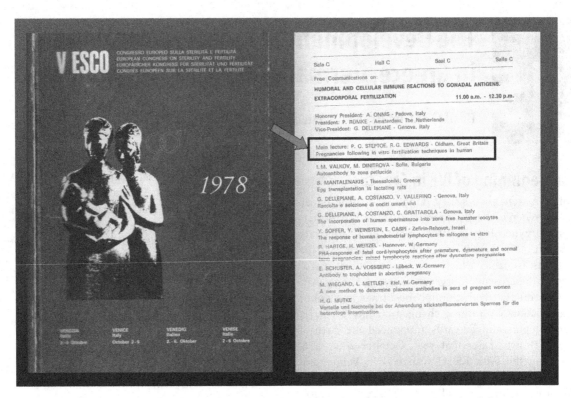

Figure 15.1 The Main Lecture by Patrick C. Steptoe and Robert G. Edwards in the Fifth ESCO Congress in Venice (1978), describing "Pregnancies following in vitro fertilization techniques in the human."

the disposables. Obviously, we faced many challenges. As there were no ready-made culture media, we had to prepare them in-house. Similarly, there were very few disposables and even less were available in Greece; thus, we had to find out what existed in our market and, for the rest, either import them directly or construct them locally. I remember vividly pulling pipettes for oocyte denudation over the Bunsen burner myself, and I still have a few glass pieces in one of my fingers from a failed attempt. The end result was quite satisfactory: the laboratory was next to the operating theater, communicating directly with it, while all the equipment was state of the art (for 1985, of course!).

At the same time, we began patient consultations for the clinical activities that started towards the end of 1985. Initially, I was also doing the laboratory part, as in Yale, and, concomitantly, I was training our biologist, who did not have any previous experience in clinical embryology. After some biochemical pregnancies and early miscarriages, at the end of October 1986, we had a positive βHCG test of what was going to be our first viable pregnancy (Tarlatzis et al., 1988). Shortly thereafter, a second pregnancy was obtained by Dr.

Spyros Sarris. Dr. Sarris, a well-known gynecologist, who was trained in tubal microsurgery and infertility in University College London, UK, organized his IVF Center in 1986 within "LITO" private maternity clinic in Athens. His pregnancy was confirmed by a positive pregnancy test on November 19, 1986. These first two pregnancies were announced in a Special Symposium organized by the Hellenic Society of Fertility and Sterility on November 22, 1986 in Athens and were covered by the press (Figures 15.4 and 15.5). Our pregnancy developed uneventfully and on July 8, 1987, a baby boy (I.Y.) was delivered with cesarean section performed in "GENIKI KLINIKI" of Thessaloniki, by J. Bontis, S. Lagos, and myself (Figure 15.6). This is the first baby conceived by IVF and delivered in Greece (Figure 15.7). The second baby was delivered by Dr. Sarris at the end of July 1987, in Athens.

At approximately the same period, a third pregnancy was reported in Athens by Drs. Yovich and Massouras (Yovich et al., 1987). Dr. Massouras, a very successful gynecologist in Athens, trained in laparoscopy with Patrick Steptoe in the UK and developed close professional but also personal relations with

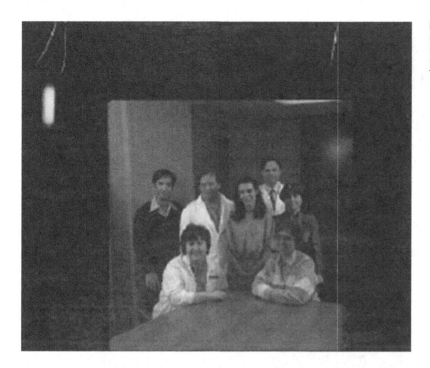

Figure 15.2 The Yale IVF Team (1984). From left to right: D. Sweeney and Mary Lake Polan (seated), Neri Laufer, Alan H. DeCherney, Joyce Masters, Basil C. Tarlatzis, and Fanny Nero.

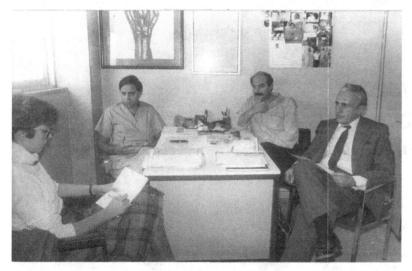

Figure 15.3 The IVF Team in "GENIKI KLINIKI" of Thessaloniki (1985). From left to right: a medical journalist, Basil C. Tarlatzis, John Bontis, and Serge Mantalenakis.

him. After the birth of Louise Brown, he immediately got interested in IVF; in that context, he tried to promote in Greece the first book of R. G. Edwards and P. C. Steptoe, *A Matter of Life*, immediately after its publication. I still remember Harris Massouras visiting our Hospital "Hippokrateion" in Thessaloniki, around 1980, and making a passionate presentation of the book and the very basics of IVF, in an auditorium packed with gynecologists, endocrinologists, trainees like me, medical students, and midwives. Based

on his relationship with Steptoe, he tried to establish a collaboration with him and Edwards, in order to set up an IVF Center in Athens together. Unfortunately, his efforts did not materialize but he did manage to collaborate in 1986 with Dr. John Yovich and PIVET Infertility Management Service and thus obtain his first pregnancy, which was also delivered in the summer of 1987.

After this slow start, IVF grew very rapidly, with IVF Centers appearing in every part of Greece, from

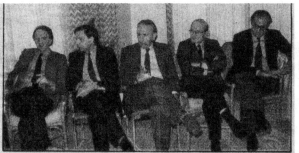

Figure 15.4 Press Conference of the Hellenic Society of Fertility and Sterility concerning the first IVF babies in Greece. From left to right: S. Sarris, B. C. Tarlatzis, S. Mantalenakis, J. Danezis and Th. Mantzavinos (Eleftherotypia, November 22, 1986).

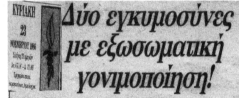

Figure 15.5 Newspaper headline announcing the first two IVF pregnancies in Greece (Eleftherotypia, November 23, 1986).

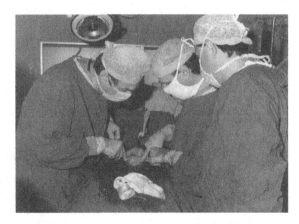

Figure 15.6 Delivery by cesarian section of the first IVF baby in Greece by (from left to right) J. Bontis, M. Lagos, and B. C. Tarlatzis (July 8, 1987).

north to south and east to west. At the peak of this activity, approximately 55 IVF Centers were operating, of which 46 were in the private sector and nine in the public (eight in University Hospitals and one in a Public Hospital). However, the economic crisis that started in 2009 significantly affected the IVF activity, since patients had to pay totally out of their own pocket for the clinical and laboratory application of the different procedures. That led to a great reduction of the cycles done, by approximately 35–40% all around the country, forcing several units either to close or to merge with others. Hence, according to the data of the National Authority for Medically Assisted Reproduction, in 2017, 44 units from both the private and public sectors

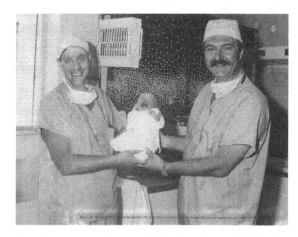

Figure 15.7 Basil C. Tarlatzis and John Bontis holding the first IVF baby born in Greece, immediately after delivery (July 8,1987).

have applied so far for a license, which has been granted to 43 of them (www.eaiya.gov.gr).

As in many other countries, the legal regulation of IVF followed its clinical application. In 1986, in the aforementioned Symposium and Press Conference, the Hellenic Society of Fertility and Sterility had proposed to the Ministry of Health to start, in collaboration with the scientific societies, the process to regulate and license the IVF Centers. The first Advisory Committee was established in 1991, followed by another one in 1996, and made proposals to the Ministry covering all aspects of IVF application. I was part of both Committees, as well as of the third one established in 2002, which, based on these proposals, but also on the international experience, prepared the actual law regulating the whole field of medically assisted reproduction (MAR). This law was accepted by the Greek Parliament in 2005 (law 3305/2005) and, together with law 3089/2002 from the Ministry of Justice, which amended our Family Law in order to include the new forms of families created by MAR, constituted the basis for the application of Assisted Reproductive Technologies (ART) in Greece. According to law 3305/2005, the National Authority for Medically Assisted Reproduction was established – I was appointed Deputy Chairman of the first one – in order to promote the implementation of the law, the licensing of the MAR Units and the oversight of their activities. Our legal framework, with the significant contribution of the previous and current Authority, has done an excellent service to infertile couples and to society, since it is liberal, practically allowing and regulating all assisted reproduction technologies in Greece.

The History of IVF in Germany

Together with Professors Krebs and van der Ven, I started an IVF Program in 1979 with animal experiments (rabbits). We retrieved oocytes by flushing the tubes and fertilized them with spermatozoa from the rabbit uterine cavity. After a while, we could fertilize the oocytes, culture the embryos and transfer them into the uterine cavity: we could achieve pregnancies. In 1981, I travelled to visit Professor Lopata in Melbourne and learnt IVF in the human, which was well established in the Royal Women's Hospital. After my return from Melbourne, we started to treat patients in October 1981 and after 12 trials we achieved the first pregnancy and delivery in 1983, which was the second successful IVF attempt in Germany (Diedrich et al., 1982). The first child was born in Erlangen University with Professor Trotnow in 1982 (Trotnow et al., 1981). Our IVF Program Professor Krebs and his Group, Professors Lehmann, Diedrich, van der Ven, and the biologist Dr. Al-Hasani, was well established and up until 1985 we achieved 32 pregnancies. At that time, we – Professors Krebs, Diedrich, van der Ven and Dr. Al-Hasani – worked at the University of Bonn. Hence, in 1985, we organized the first ESHRE Congress in Bonn with 700 participants and we were very proud to have this opportunity (Figure 15.8).

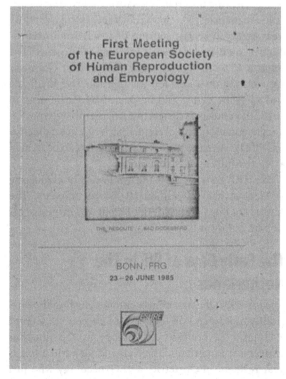

Figure 15.8 The Bonn ESHRE Meeting 1985.

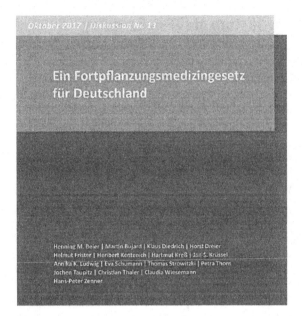

Figure 15.9 The proposed new Law in Reproductive Medicine, Germany, 2017.

In 1990 the Embryo Protection Law came into effect in Germany. It was very strict and we were allowed to fertilize only up to three oocytes and we had to transfer every embryo. Freezing of embryos was not allowed. By transferring three embryos we achieved many multiple pregnancies, which was not a successful infertility treatment. Currently, a group of specialists in reproductive medicine, lawyers, ethicists, and geneticists (Figure 15.9) in reproductive medicine in Germany are working on a new law for reproductive medicine and we hope that it will be passed by Parliament in 2018, allowing us to do elective single embryo transfer, oocyte donation, and preimplantation genetic diagnosis (PGD). Then the patients in Germany can be treated as successfully as outside Germany.

ESHRE grew very fast and our last Annual Meeting in Geneva had more than 10,000 participants. The "father" of this very fast development was Professor Sir Robert G. Edwards from Cambridge.

The Early Days of IVF in The Netherlands

In early 1977, the first conversation regarding the possibility of human IVF took place between Dr. Gerard Zeilmaker (a professor of biology at the Erasmus University, Rotterdam, The Netherlands) and a third-year resident in Obstetrics and Gynecology who just

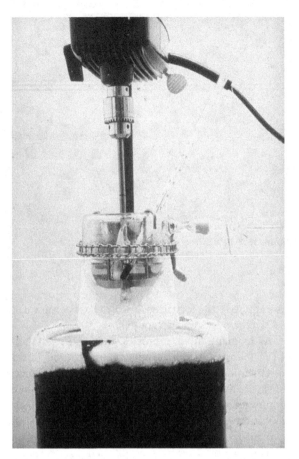

Figure 15.10 Early-day cryopreservation equipment used in Rotterdam, The Netherlands.

arrived in Rotterdam, Dr. Bert Alberda. Previously, Dr. Zeilmaker had successfully developed IVF in the mouse model and had unsuccessfully approached other University Infertility Centers in The Netherlands aiming for a collaboration to develop human IVF.

Initial attempts in Rotterdam focused on generating oocytes from women undergoing tubal surgery or laparoscopy. Such procedures were planned on cycle day 15 following ovarian stimulation using clomiphene citrate and hCG. This approach turned out to be successful in approximately 50% of women and, in 1978, fertilization of a human oocyte was achieved for the first time in the laboratory of Professor Zeilmaker. At that time, it was not yet allowed to transfer the embryo, and therefore all embryos obtained were cryopreserved at the eight-cell stage (Figure 15.10). During the early years, donor sperm was used to generate embryos.

After three years of struggling with the head of the Department, Board of Directors, and the local

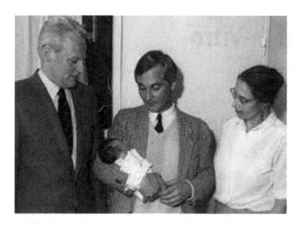

Figure 15.11 Birth of the first IVF baby in The Netherlands in 1983. From left to right: Professor Zeilmaker, Dr. Alberda, and Dr. van Gent.

institutional Ethics Review Board, approval to transfer human embryos was finally obtained in late 1981. Initially two IVF cycles (including oocyte retrieval by laparoscopy) were performed per month and only privately insured patients were allowed to be treated. A first biochemical pregnancy following IVF was achieved in May 1982. This was followed by an ongoing pregnancy in August that year, which resulted in the birth of the first IVF baby (Stefanie Li) in The Netherlands on May 15, 1983 (Figure 15.11). For reasons of privacy, it was decided at the time to not report this birth in the international literature.

Initially, oocyte collection was performed during diagnostic laparoscopy (also including tubal perfusion with a blue dye) for the work up of infertility. The transfer of fresh embryos following such a procedure was not considered realistic, and therefore all embryos were frozen as routine procedure. The first ongoing pregnancies following the transfer of intact frozen-thawed embryos were reported in 1984 (Zeilmaker et al., 1984). Subsequent studies by the laboratory team also focused on extended embryo culture (van Os et al., 1989).

Over the years, the volume of couples undergoing IVF in Rotterdam increased to 50 annually. This was still not considered enough by Dr. Zeilmaker, and he developed the concept of a so-called transport IVF program, where patients underwent counselling, ovarian stimulation, and oocyte collection in another regional hospital, followed by transportation of the oocytes to the University Hospital by the patients themselves. Subsequently, in-vitro fertilization of oocytes and the embryo transfer was performed at the Erasmus University in Rotterdam (Jansen et al., 1986). This developed into a large transport IVF program, which still exists today throughout The Netherlands. A relatively small number of IVF laboratories (all running many hundreds and sometimes thousands of IVF cycles annually), all collaborate with several hospitals performing the clinical IVF procedures.

References

Diedrich K, Lehmann F, Krebs D. In-vitro fertilization of human eggs and embryo transfer. *Geburtshilfe Frauenheilkd* 1982; 42:530–532.

Jansen CA, van Beek JJ, Verhoeff A, Alberda AT, Zeilmaker GM. In vitro fertilization and embryo transfer with transport of oocytes. *Lancet* 1986; March 22: 676.

Laufer N, Pratt BM, DeCherney AH, et al. The in vivo and in vitro effects of clomiphene citrate on ovulation, fertilization, and development of cultured mouse oocytes. *American Journal of Obstetrics and Gynecology* 1983; 147:633–639.

Laufer N, DeCherney AH, Haseltine FP, et al. Human in vitro fertilization employing individualized ovulation induction by human menopausal gonadotropins. *Journal of In Vitro Fertilization Embryo Transfer* 1984; 1:56–62.

Tarlatzis BC, Laufer N, DeCherney AH. The use of ovarian ultrasonography in monitoring ovulation induction. *Journal of In Vitro Fertilization Embryo Transfer* 1984a; 1:226–232.

Tarlatzis BC, Sanyal MK, Biggers WJ, Naftolin F. Continuous culture of the postimplantation rat conceptus. *Biology of Reproduction* 1984b; 31: 415–426.

Tarlatzis BC, Bontis J, Lagos S, et al. Pregnancies from in vitro fertilization and embryo transfer. *Hellenic Journal of Obstetrics and Gynecology* 1988; 1: 260–268.

Trotnow S, Kniewald T, Al-Hasani S, Becker H. Pregnancies obtained by oocyte aspiration, in vitro fertilization, and embryo transfer during clomid/HCG stimulated cycles (author's translation). *Geburtshilfe Frauenheilkd* 1981; 41:835-836.

van Os HC, Alberda AT, Janssen-Caspers HA, et al. The influence of the interval between IVF and embryo transfer and some other variables on treatment. *Fertility and Sterility* 1989; 51:360–362.

Yovich JL, Hamzah H, Massouras H. Transportability of in-vitro fertilization technology. *The Medical Journal of Australia* 1987; 146:657–658.

Zeilmaker GH, Alberda AT, van Gent I, et al. Two pregnancies following transfer of intact frozen-thawed embryos. *Fertility and Sterility* 1984; 42: 293–296.

Chapter 6

The Development of In-Vitro Fertilization in Israel

Zion Ben-Rafael

The past Shaping the Present Shaping the Future

In 1947, before I was born, and before the first issue of dedicated journals like *Fertility and Sterility* and *Human Reproduction* were published, Robert G. Edwards served as a young soldier in His Majesty the King of England's Army, as part of the British Mandate in Israel-Palestine. Little did anyone know then that, in that young soldier, was the seed of a great scientist – a Nobel Prize Laureate – who would affect the lives of an entire generation, as well as of those to come. He was not the first to write about IVF in animals, and he was not the first to try IVF in humans; however, Edwards and his colleague Steptoe were the first to achieve a successful birth – a birth that would change everything. Millions of infertile couples worldwide would be assisted, and the careers of tens of thousands of yet-unborn physicians – me included – scientists, embryologists, and an all-new dedicated industry, would be affected and shaped. A new inter-disciplinary field in medicine was born. Robert G. Edwards would receive the Nobel Prize, and the Controversies in Obstetrics Gynaecology and Infertility (COGI) Congress has humbly dedicated its opening lecture to this pioneer ever since. What seemed in the beginning to be a modest humanitarian medical solution for a few unfortunate infertile couples, grew in dimensions, and has the current disturbing potential, with the use of gene editing, to be the first step towards changing the essence of human beings.

Life of the Fertility Specialist Before the IVF Era – the Introduction of Gonadotropins in 1962

Before IVF was developed and matured, gynecologists were judged by their manual competences to perform a hysterectomy and, in perinatology, to perform rotational forceps deliveries. Infertility treatments were not considered anywhere to be the spear-head of the discipline. This was about to change.

The situation in Israel then was a bit different. Since the country's inception in 1948, infertility treatments were considered as almost a basic right, and were part of the health basket for every couple; and they were the focus of research and development in leading hospitals, institutes, and medical schools. Active infertility treatments were offered free-of-charge, though limited due to the poor means. Research on hormonal or mechanical infertility, pelvic tuberculosis, and ovulation induction were performed by many of the accomplished physicians who immigrated to (pre-State) Israel in the 1930s, sensing the risks in the pre-war Germany and Austria and leaving high-ranking positions at top universities to start new services in a new country. Among them, to mention just a few, were: Bernard Zondek, who first suggested that the pituitary gland secretes two gonadotropins, and later described both the existence of human chorionic gonadotropins (hCG), and also the "Zondek–Ascheim" pregnancy test. He chaired the Hadassah Medical Center in Jerusalem. Joseph Asherman characterized the intrauterine adhesions also known as "Asherman Syndrome", and he chaired the Tel Aviv Medical Center. Ervin Rabau was smart to call the head nurse in the Charité Hospital in Berlin to ask what SS cars were doing in front of his department. When she warned him that they were after him, he escaped from Germany and would soon chair Beilinson and then Sheba Medical Centers, and lead the Sheba group when the first world pregnancy with urinary gonadotropins and OHSS was described.

The next generation included Lunenfeld who set, with his colleagues, the cornerstone in ovulation induction by achieving the first human menopausal gonadotropins (hMG) pregnancy. Insler and Lunenfeld from Sheba Medical Center described the cervical mucous scoring system to monitor ovulation induction and timing of insemination. These and other early pioneers have carried on their shoulders generations of dedicated physicians: the IVF generation.

The many incoming immigrants and Holocaust survivors who lost their entire families received free access to treatments in Israel to try to rebuild their lives. Success was inadequate. Treatments were carried out with limited tools by a few dedicated physicians. Corrective operations of uterine anomalies and intra-uterine adhesions or tubal disease were far from perfect. Sperm donation was the main solution for bad quality sperm, since no other treatment worked for male factor infertility. Induction of ovulation started in the late 1950s.

In 1962, the world's first pregnancy with hMG was reported by Bruno Lunenefeld (Lunenfeld et al., 1962) in collaboration with Italian scientist P. Donini (Donini et al., 1964) from the pharmaceutical company Serono. Later it was also marketed by local pharma (TEVA) and became available free of charge for all infertile women in the country. The same Sheba group went further to describe what was known later as the threshold theory (Lunenfeld et al., 1961). The availability of this new tool brought a vivid scenario of ovulation induction (OI) treatments in referral hospitals for a plethora of indications, throughout the 1960s and 1970s. The Sheba Medical Center group participated with a number of other groups around the world in "writing the book" on OI and ovarian monitoring, with a full report of the Sheba experience much before it was a mainstay in infertility treatment (Rabau et al., 1967), and it also included a description of the perils, namely ovarian hyperstimulation syndrome (OHSS), including the first serious complication of OHSS (Mozes et al., 1965) and first classification (Melmed et al., 1969) that was adopted by the WHO, and successive classifications (Schenker and Weinstein, 1978; Golan et al., 1989) and torsion of ovaries. We, the first IVF generation in the country, inherited the two-decade acquaintance with intricate methods of controlled ovarian stimulation (COS). My MD thesis, at Sheba Medical Center, just before the first successful IVF, included the first follow-up of adolescent girls and boys born to amenorrhoeic women who conceived with hMG, indicating for the first time in a series that "amenorrhea was not hereditary" (Ben-Rafael et al., 1983) and retrospective analysis of the hMG clinic results, the treatment, independent pregnancies, and abortion rates.

Before 1978, the decade-long British, Australian, and American experiments with IVF ending in miscarriage (De Kretzer et al., 1973) or extrauterine pregnancy (Steptoe and Edwards, 1976) were barely known and had little impact on the learning or teaching of young residents in obstetrics and gynecology in Isreal. When the first IVF birth was announced using no ovarian stimulation, we still did not understand that the vast experience that we had accumulated in ovarian stimulation would be a cornerstone in the future IVF clinic. It took a few more years to witness the Australian success, and with clomiphene citrate (Trounson et al., 1981) induced ovarian stimulation to increase recruitment and the number of embryos, to realize that we were already well equipped with a crucial first step of IVF, i.e. COS.

Upon the announcement of the IVF birth of Louise Brown in July 1978 (Steptoe and Edwards, 1978), I was a second-year resident and served in the out-patient referral clinic of "hMG" at the Sheba Hospital. We treated tens of patients daily including those with classical PCOS, oligo-amenorrhea, mechanical factor infertility, and even mild male factor with hMG stimulation, tubal washing, or insufflations. Concomitant male factor infertility was rarely treated by varicocelectomy and, if insemination failed, donor sperm was offered, even for mild sperm problems. The so-called "Pergonal clinic" took place after working hours, during our free time, demonstrating our dedication but also the low priority in comparison to other perinatal, gynecological, and surgical activities. Nevertheless, we became very proficient in ovulation induction using longstanding means of monitoring of the time, like cervical mucus score, post-coital tests, 24-h urinary estrogen estimations, and digital pelvic palpation. Real-time ultrasound (US) was not introduced yet, and it took almost another decade to have the first vaginal US probe. We had to use imagination and often extrapolation of the results, if the assay, or urine collection, was incomplete or missed. We needed to exercise extreme caution not to fall into OHSS using digital palpation as a mean of estimating ovarian size, even in obese women. With a large population of amenorrhoeic patients, we knew that using the lowest possible effective dose would result in success with low complication rates. We knew that it was futile to increase the hMG dose before 5–6 days of treatment and before reaching a steady state and full response to the dose. We also knew that ovarian expansion in the late luteal phase (secondary OHSS) heralded the pregnancy a week before we could detect it with crude urinary pregnancy tests. Unfortunately, we also learned a great deal about the complications, like the higher likelihood of

133

ovarian torsion when OHSS and pregnancy occurred, and we described de-torsion as the surgical solution (Ben-Rafael et al., 1990), and we encountered a rare incredible case of triplet pregnancy in a didelphys uterus with a delivery interval of 72 days between two fetuses in the right uterus and the one in the left uterus (Mashiach, 1981).

First IVF Clinic in Israel is Launched

In 1979, shortly after the announcement of the birth of Louise Brown, the heads of the ObGyn Department at Sheba Medical Center, Professors David Serr, Bruno Lunenefeld, and Shlomo Mashiach sent Dr. Jehoshua Dor for training in Professor Roger Short's laboratory in Scotland. He returned after a few months recruiting from that laboratory an accomplished biologist Dr. Edwina Rudak, who was the cornerstone of the newly established laboratory and an important reason for the early go-ahead to start treatments in 1981, when no more than five or six groups around the world had programs. The first team of clinicians at Sheba included Shlomo Mashiach as Head of the Department, Jeoshua Dor who would be the first head of the unit, myself as the first resident in the program, and David Levran who joined after a short training in Australia. The Hadassah Hospital program, headed by Joseph Schenker, with head of the unit Neri Laufer, and Ehud Margaliot and Daniel Navot as residents, was simultaneously granted official governmental permission to begin treatments. The credit for the first delivery in Israel was achieved by the Sheba Medical Center on September 22, 1982. This was shortly after the UK and Australia, the Joneses in the USA in 1981, and in the same year as some other centers like those of René Frydman (and, later, Jean Cohen) in France, Lars Hamburger in Sweden, Wilfried Feichtinger in Austria, and later Victor Gomel in Canada in 1983, among others.

From 1984, more IVF centers were approved for treatments in almost all the major hospitals in the country, and then this was extended to all hospitals. The first private IVF clinic gained approval in 1987 and today nearly half of all IVF cycles are done in a few private IVF settings with governmental funding. I was proud, back at the start, to have achieved the first twin pregnancy, but it made me also realize that the technical part of laparoscopic ovum pick-up can be grasped quite easily, and that what was needed was to keep researching into the basic science behind the laboratory work and clinical practice. I achieved this in Philadelphia, upon

completion of my residency when I spent three years of research at the Hospital of University of Pennsylvania (HUP), a well-known institute of reproductive biology headed by Gerome F. Strauss in Luigi Mastroianni's department. The time spent in the laboratory with George Flickinger culminated in tens of clinical and basic publications back in the mid-1980s, when every study related to IVF was of interest. The University of Pennsylvania was a gold mine for research. Daily blood tests from IVF patients were saved, and every oocyte was photographed from every possible angle, and the department was very supportive of our research. We soon published a series of studies casting doubt on the use of high doses of FSH, indicating that lower doses of hMG (150 IU) were preferable over higher doses of 225 IU in terms of clinical parameters and pregnancy potential (Ben-Rafael et al., 1986, 1987; Benadiva et al., 1988a, b). We summarized our finding as follows: "all the above data suggest that the preferred initial dose in IVF stimulations protocols, should be 2 amps (150 IU) of hMG and that this dose should not be raised during stimulation. This low-dose regimen results in a better hormonal milieu, which positively influences the oocyte quality and the endometrial receptivity" (Levy and Ben-Rafael, 1995). However, the practice of using a higher dose of FSH in IVF continued to be the rule in most IVF programs for another decade before more doubt was raised.

Unfortunately, the most important practical message that could have been carried already from our vast "pre-IVF" experience in the late 1970s, i.e. to keep using the lowest effective dose of FSH for stimulation, was "lost in translation" in the IVF era. The first two decades of IVF stimulation seem, today, more like the "maximal dose finding mission" than the search for real sound medical and clinical conclusions. The initial annoyingly low success rates in IVF caused physicians to use high doses of FSH to achieve high numbers of eggs and multiple embryo transfers, resulting in high-order multiple pregnancies, which in turn resulted in late OHSS. The introduction of GnRH-a (gonadotropin-releasing hormone agonists) further allowed the use of even higher FSH doses for extended periods of time, with less monitoring and without premature ovulation or need for cancelation; and claiming better success rate (Fleming et al., 1988), which was probably due to the higher number of eggs. Application of aggressive protocols with a mega dose of 300–600 IU became the holy grail – a trend that was carried into the late 1990s with an alarming incidence of severe OHSS to epidemic levels, until improved laboratory methods and conditions, and better success rates encouraged the current trend of mild stimulation as published by Fauser's group (Heijnen et al., 2007), to which the single ET was added to prevent multiple pregnancies and late OHSS.

Technical Development

In the early 1980s, publications and conferences dealt with endless small technical issues that today would seem amusing: COS protocols, the size of the aspiration needle, aspiration pressure, type of ET catheter, gas mixture, and medium ingredients and preparation. Industry seized the commercial opportunities, industrialized every advance, and made it available to all.

Resistance to IVF among doctors and the public did not disappear quickly. The fear of deep changes in society were expressed, not only by ethicists, philosophers, and religious groups, who did not trust the new technique, but also by doctors who condemned the low success rate in comparison to other treatments, or even to no treatment at all.

In Israel, we were lucky to receive support from mainstream religious groups, who accepted IVF as another way of fulfilling the famous biblical command "procreate and multiply." With their consent, politicians had no problem giving the go-ahead, not only for IVF, but also for egg donation and embryo freezing soon after their introduction (Navot et al., 1986) (Levran et al., 1990). However, a couple in need of surrogacy were only served in the United States until an appeal to the supreme court brought about approval in the late 1990s. Nevertheless, the high cost of the procedure pushed many infertile couples to look "across the border" for less expensive surrogate solutions in Asia and Eastern European.

In the mid-1980s, after a short experience with trans-abdominal and trans-vesical US guided follicular aspiration, the first publication on transvaginal ovum pick-up was described by Feichtinger (Feichtinger et al., 1986), and simultaneously we received the first Israeli-produced vaginal ultrasound probe by Elscint, a local high-tech US producer that was later sold to GE. Transvaginal ultrasound-guided ovum pick-ups replaced laparoscopy, increased the yield of ovum pick-up and, with simplified ET without bed rest and better luteal support, made IVF simpler to master, patient-friendly and a more successful procedure, needing only a local, regional, or even no anesthesia.

Intracytoplasmic sperm injection (ICSI) was the next big development in ART/IVF (Palermo et al., 1992) that resulted in the expansion of IVF services for male factor infertility. Suddenly patients with severe oligo-terato-astenospermia (OTA), or patients with only a few testicular-extracted sperm, had a chance for success. ICSI laid to rest all other previous techniques like PZD (partial zona dissection) or SUZI (sub-zonal insertion) or medical treatments like "male Metrodin" (purified FSH), which were used with some success before. This, and the development of preimplantation genetic diagnosis (PGD) services, which gained popularity in the late 1990s, and screening (PGS), which remained controversial even after many years of use, have further increased IVF services.

OHSS in Israel

OHSS is a disturbing complication of COS that developed at alarming levels through the 1990s, but fortunately has markedly reduced in the new millennium. Abramov et al. (1998) documented an increase in the annual three-to-four fold incidence of severe OHSS in Israel. Over the ten-year period from 1987 to 1997, which exceeded the increase in total IVF activity (20-fold versus six-fold respectively) during the same period. This increase reflects very well the worldwide epidemic of OHSS, which required action. Fortunately, there was not a single fatality due to OHSS in the 73,492 cycles studied by these authors; however, there were some fatalities internationally. To justify the high doses of gonadotrophins during those years, doctors and authors in Israel and abroad relied on unproven methods of OHSS prevention such as albumin infusion, early ascites aspiration, follicular reduction, and re-aspiration of the corpora lutea, etc. Most of these, without any real proof of efficacy, have disappeared from the medical arsenal. We condemned albumin as inefficient in 1995 (Ben-Rafael et al., 1995; Orvieto and Ben-Rafael, 1998), but it continued to be used due to the lack of better methods. The main obstacle to developing preventive methods lies in the fact that severe OHSS cannot be predicted with high accuracy, even in high-risk cases, and the methods offered were all secondary preventive methods, i.e. only when the problem has already started. Of note is that neither high estradiol levels nor the number of large follicles or eggs bore a good relationship with OHSS. We published a case of OHSS with a block to estradiol production and levels <500 pg/ml (Levy et al., 1996). Others established that

135

OHSS was related to the mid-size and small and not to the large follicles (Blankstein et al., 1987). Clearly the number of small and midsize follicles, as the number of eggs, is related to the meticulousness of the ultrasound and thoroughness of oocyte aspiration.

It took almost 20 years from the beginning of IVF to reach widespread acceptance of mild stimulation, which made ESHRE claim that the trend of OHSS was reversed. The current idea of an "OHSS-free clinic" (Devroey et al., 2011) that uses COS with GnRH antagonist and GnRH-a as surrogate to hCG (which started in Israel and was reviewed by Kol et al., 2004) and "freeze-only" embryos arrived shortly after OHSS almost disappeared, mainly due to milder stimulation, single-embryo transfer, and better freezing options. Nevertheless, the element of "freeze only" for later transfer, when the endometrium is supposedly more natural, may have a potential *per se*, but awaits scientific proof from several ongoing studies before it can be applied on a larger scale.

Legislation and Regulation: The Sixth World IVF Congress

Israel was one of the first countries to regulate IVF by law in 1987; and the law went through several cycles of amendments as the field grew and matured. There were also set criteria and permission procedures for opening new units, along with regular periodic peer review audits to assure compliance and quality. Nevertheless, as with all scientific progress, the legislation was, as a rule, lagging behind the rapid development. In the late 1990s, when I was Chairman of the Obstetrics & Gynecology Department at the Rabin Medical Center (at both Hasharon and Beilinson Hospitals), the family of a young man who died in a road accident was willing to donate all his organs, with only one request: to collect and freeze his sperm to be used later by his spouse. Although never done before, it was obvious that there was no technical barrier. Posthumous collection was not yet regulated at the time and we needed urgent direction. We informed the Ministry of Health of the situation and the difficulties in denying their only personal wish. In the absence of regulations and this being the first case of this nature, we received the Ministry's consent, which limited the release of the sperm for later use by court order only. Posthumous sperm collection remains an issue to be regulated in many countries, indicating the many social, ethical, and legal issues it presents as, well as the question of whose right

is superior - the wife, the family, or the dead who left no will.

In 1989, Jerusalem hosted the Sixth World IVF Congress. As secretary, I was in charge of the organization and the program. The congress was the largest and most successful so far. Over 1800 participants from all over the world enjoyed four days of Jerusalem spring with a unique scientific program, including an opening session on the "Controversies on Ovulation Induction," which was the seed for a future congress on controversies and debates, namely the COGI Congress. A year before the congress, Jacques Cohen suggested giving a talk on assisted hatching, based on his observations on partial zona dissection (PZD). For more than a decade IVF units all over the world offered the technique as a service without any real proof to its efficacy. Chemical methods and expensive laser tools were developed to dissect the zona and the decades after saw the "rise and fall" of all these laser procedures. We critically debated and discussed PZD at each COGI congress for several years, since I never trusted the method as proven beyond doubt, until the method faded away. For about a decade our group had been using "fibrin sealant glue" (described by Feichtinger) for embryo transfer in cases of implantation failure. Since two of our prospective studies resulted in significantly better implantation rates in women older than 38 years, we suggested that the better results were due to "a PZD effect" of proteolytic activity of the protease that are active in dissolving the glue – an explanation that probably lost ground with the fading out of PZD. With the better success rates biological glue also disappeared from our practice.

The book of proceedings of the Sixth IVF World Congress, which I edited alone for about a year, contained over 100 chapters and 1000 pages by world leading authorities of the time. I invited three famous authors under the names of "J Cohen, J Cohen, and J Cohen" to contribute a special chapter to the book. Jacques Cohen from the USA, the late Jean Cohen from France, and Jack Cohen from the UK. The content of the chapter, which was about the plethora of acronyms that washed the shores of our discipline along with IVF, was less important.

Other Israeli Contributions

Israel is leading the world with the number of IVF treatments per capita, which will be discussed later. Accordingly, Israeli physicians have contributed to the literature in many ways, far beyond its population size.

Studies on the use of GnRH-a as surrogate to hCG, on oocyte donation, on the use of Metrodin for male infertility (before the ICSI era), on the use of fibrin sealant glue for ET, on the protocols for ovarian stimulation for PCOS and poor responders, as well as on the new classifications of OHSS, were published by Israelis and were among the first in the field. Obviously, the above is only a partial list. Hadassah & Haifa Medical Schools were among the first to embark on embryonic stem cell research in the late 1990s.

Several procedures, some of which are still in use and some still controversial, were published and gave ground to vivid discussions. Benjamin Bartoov, a basic scientist from Bar Ilan University, and his colleagues, introduced the motile sperm organelle morphology examination (MSOME) and intracytoplasmic morphologically selected sperm injection (IMSI) using high-magnification ($\times$ 6000) instead of the usual $\times$ 400 digital imaging microscope for microinjection into the egg (Bartoov et al., 2001). Despite being a logical development in the ICSI procedure, and being used by many clinics worldwide, the value of this adjunct treatment is still debated.

The method of endometrial scratching was introduced in Israel (Barash et al., 2003) more than 15 years ago, which seems to mimic the old-time D&C practice for infertile women before treatment that was also performed without any real proof. The use or abuse of the procedure is characteristic of many other clinical procedures and methods that are introduced without rigorous research; they remain in use in many clinics, and even when declared inefficient doctors continue to use them despite facing repeated failures.

One of the first handful of groups around the world that embarked on the preservation of fertility with ovarian tissue transplantation was the group from Sheba. Following the first success (Donnez et al., 2004), Meirow (Meirow et al., 2005) started his career at Hadassah and later was welcomed to my department at Rabin/Beilinson Medical Center, where he planned to do the first case. Finally, he joined the staff at Sheba Medical Center, where he had the first pregnancy after transplantation of cryopreserved ovarian tissue.

We were the first to alert against smoking (Elenbogen et al., 1991); today there are indications that the effects may be carried over to the next generation. Our group launched a never-ending intense discussion on the ill-effects of fibroids on implantation rates (Farhi et al., 1995).

Israel is also a country with very vivid high-tech and pharmacology research and development (R&D) industries. For many years Teva was a supplier of Pergonal. In recent years BTG (Biotechnology General Ltd, Rehovot, Israel), a company owned by Ferring, has produced the new Human Recombionant FSH, which Ferring launched recently under the name Rekovelle. Not as sophisticated, the vaginal suppository Endometrin was developed and marketed locally by a private pharmacist, Azaria Yosiffov, who later sold it to Ferring, and it is used worldwide. The medical laser industry started in Israel and the many local companies have contributed to the trials and errors in performing assisted zona hatching, which did not last long.

Social Freezing

The "new kid on the block" is social freezing. Late childbearing and the financial crisis of the Y-generation contribute in many European countries to a dramatic decline in birth rate and population. As physicians, we cannot solve the financial problem of this generation. We also cannot influence much, beyond providing education, the change in societal behavior, which is also due to longer life expectancy.

Nonetheless, reproductive specialists feel now that they have a partial solution to help ease the population shrinkage and delayed childbearing – i.e. social freezing. Over the past decade, the extension of "oncology related fertility preservation" and the increasing efficacy of oocyte vitrification have fueled the imagination of patients and doctors to think that freezing can be a solution for all young women who delay family planning to the fourth or fifth decades of life. It is a medical procedure that was born without any specific indication, hence it is not surprising to find that global corporates are offering it as a "work benefit" to make essential workers feel comfortable with delaying childbearing. Women who are trapped between the hammer of social changes and the anvil of aging ovaries are the target of aggressive marketing of the procedure, especially by private IVF units. Obviously, the fact that the patients pay the full price for an insurance-type procedure that the patient may never use creates a dilemma.

In Israel, as in other countries, there is mounting pressure for unmarried women to freeze their eggs, and others are calling on governments to support large scale "fertility preservation" for young women, at no charge. Theoretically poor responders could have been a perfect fit for the procedure, but we can't identify them at an early age before they started (Broekmans et al., 2009) and when it started it might be too late (Farhi et al., 1997). Moreover, the need for 20–30 eggs to secure success calls for freezing at an early age, while the request today is mainly by women older than 37 years, at which time they need ten metaphase II oocytes to reach 30% success, while below 35 years they can reach 60% with that number (Cobo et al., 2016). On the other hand, the younger the patient the lower the future usage will be, which lowers the cost effectiveness and, in private hands only, the cost effectiveness considerations will be secondary.

Why Does Israel Have a Record High Number of IVF Cycles *per Capita* and What Can Be Learned?

The number of IVF units *per capita* in Israel (population 1,350,000) always exceeded the mean in other parts of the world by a factor of three. Today it does not seem surprising anymore, as IVF has become so standard that you expect it to be done in your local neighborhood clinics. The birth rate in Israel is higher than in Europe, and yet still the number of children born after IVF in Israel is above 4% of all the children born. The number of annual cycles is astonishing and is probably double of the next country in line, Denmark. For example, while in fairly served countries the number of cycles is about 500–1000 per one million population (Collines, 2002) and in only a few is it over 2000 per million, in Israel the number is over 4000, and with frozen cycles is over 5000 per one million population. The reasons are multiple:

1. All citizens (and most non-citizens) have medical national insurance.
2. IVF is free of charge to all citizens.
3. Every patient, including single parents, can run unlimited attempts until achieving two healthy babies.
4. Some 80% of patients have a second private insurance coverage that offers treatments for a third healthy child.
5. Patients keep trying until the age of 44–45. After the age of 45, or if FSH is high, women are entitled to try oocyte donation.
6. Most families still want three children, despite delaying child bearing.
7. The number of single-parent families is high and they opt for only slightly smaller families.
8. The number of voluntarily childless women/families in Israel is low in comparison with Europe, which explains the high usage of IVF.
9. Same-sex couples have similar rights to benefit from IVF.

Israel already led the number of cycles, with about 1000–2000 per million population, in the 1980s, and this number was incomprehensible then. The number of cycles rose worldwide, and in some countries even into the 1000–2000 per million range, but it has not reached its balance yet. Although 4000–5000 cycle per one million population is extremely high, it indicates that if there is free access to IVF programs and, under the above assumptions, the number IVF cycles will keep growing substantially globally. So, if you are an IVF expert, you will not be out of business any time soon, especially in low usage countries.

References

Abramov Y, Elchalal U, Schenker J. Febrile morbidity in severe and critical ovarian hyperstimulation syndrome: a multicenter study. *Hum Reprod* 1998; 13: 3128–3131.

Barash A, Dekel N, Fieldust S, et al. Local injury to the endometrium doubles the incidence of successful pregnancies in patients undergoing in vitro fertilization. *Fertil Steril* 2003; 79:1317–1322.

Bartoov B, Berkovitz A, Eltes F. Selection of spermatozoa with normal nuclei to improve the pregnancy rate with intracytoplasmic sperm injection. *N Engl J Med* 2001; 345:1067–1068.

Benadiva CA, Ben-Rafael Z, Blasco L, et al. An increased initial follicle-stimulating hormone/luteinizing hormone ratio does not affect ovarian responses and the outcomes of in vitro fertilization. *Fertil Steril* 1988a; 50:777–781.

Benadiva CA, Ben-Rafael Z, Strauss JF III, Mastroianni L Jr., Flickinger GL. Ovarian response of individuals to different doses of human menopausal gonadotropin. *Fertil Steril* 1988b; 49:997–1001.

Ben-Rafael Z, Blankstein J, Sack J, et al. Menarche and puberty in daughters of amenorrheic women. *JAMA* 1983; 250:3202–3204.

Ben-Rafael Z, Strauss JF III, Mastroianni L Jr., Flickinger GL. Differences in ovarian stimulation in human menopausal gonadotropin treated woman may be related to follicle-stimulating hormone accumulation. *Fertil Steril* 1986; 46:586–592.

Ben-Rafael Z, Benadiva CA, Ausmanas M, et al. Dose of human menopausal gonadotropin influences the outcomes of an in vitro fertilization program. *Fertil Steril* 1987; 48:964–968.

Ben-Rafael Z, Bider D, Mashiach S. Laparoscopic unwinding of twisted ischemic hemorrhagic adnexa after in vitro fertilization. *Fertil Steril* 1990; 53: 569–571.

Ben-Rafael Z, Orvieto R, Dekel A, Peleg D, Gruzman C. Intravenous albumin and the prevention of severe ovarian hyperstimulation syndrome. *Hum Reprod* 1995; 10:2750–2752.

Blankstein J, Shalev J, Saadon T, et al. Ovarian hyperstimulation syndrome: prediction by number and size of preovulatory ovarian follicles. *Fertil Steril* 1987; 47:597–602.

Broekmans FJ, Soules MR, Fauser BC. Ovarian aging: mechanisms and clinical consequences. *Endocr Rev* 2009; 30:465–493.

Cobo A, García-Velasco JA, Coello A, et al. Oocyte vitrification as an efficient option for elective fertility preservation. *Fertil Steril* 2016; 105:755–764.

Collines J. An international survey of health economics of IVF and ICSI. *HR Update* 2002; 8:277–365.

De Kretzer D, Dennis P, Hudson B, et al. Transfer of a human zygote. *Lancet* 1973; 29(2):728–729.

Devroey P, Polyzos NP, Blockeel C. An OHSS-Free Clinic by segmentation of IVF treatment. *Hum Reprod* 2011; 26:2593–2597.

Donini P, Puzzuoli D, Montezemolo R. Purification of gonadotropin from human menopausal urine. *Acta Endocrin* 1964; 45:329.

Donnez J, Dolmans MM, Demylle D, et al. Birth after orthotopic transplantation of cryopreserved ovarian tissue. *Lancet* 2004; 364(9443): 1405–1410.

Edwards RG, Steptoe PC, Purdy JM. Establishing full term human pregnancies using cleaving embryos grown in vitro. *Br J Obstet Gynaecol* 1980; 87:737–756.

Elenbogen A, Lipitz S, Levran D, et al. The effect of smoking on E2 levels and aromatase activity in women undergoing IVF. *Hum Reprod* 1991; 6:242.

Farhi J, Ashkenazi J, Feldberg D, et al. Effect of uterine leiomyomata on the results of in vitro fertilization treatment. *Hum Reprod* 1995; 10:2576–2578.

Farhi J, Homburg R, Ferber A, Orvieto R, Ben Rafael Z. Non-response to ovarian stimulation in normogonadotrophic, normogonadal women: A clinical sign of impending onset of ovarian failure pre-empting the rise in basal follicle stimulating. *Hum Reprod* 1997; 12:241–243.

Feichtinger W, Kemeter P. Transvaginal sector scan sonography for needle guided transvaginal follicle aspiration and other applications in gynecologic routine and research. *Fertil Steril* 1986; 45: 722–725.

Fleming R, Haxton MJ, Hamilton MPR et al. Combined gonadotropin-releasing hormone analog and exogenous gonadotropins for ovulation induction in infertile women: Efficacy related to ovarian function assessment. *Am J Obstet Gynecol* 1988; 159:376–381.

Golan A, Ron-el R, Herman A, et al. Ovarian hyperstimulation syndrome: An update review. *Obstet Gynecol Surv* 1989; 44:430–440.

Heijnen EM, Eijkemans MJ, De Klerk C, et al. A mild treatment strategy for in-vitro fertilisation: a randomised non-inferiority trial. *Lancet* 2007; 369(9563):743–749.

Kol S. Luteolysis induced by a gonadotropin-releasing hormone agonist is the key to prevention of ovarian hyperstimulation syndrome. *Fertil Steril* 2004; 81:1–5.

Levran D, Dor J, Rudak E, et al. Pregnancy potential of human oocytes – The effect of cryopreservation. *N Engl J Med* 1990; 323:1153–1156.

Levy T, Ben Rafael Z. Low versus high dose human menopausal gonadotropin in an in vitro fertilization embryo transfer program. *J IVF Genetics* 1995;12:4.

Levy T, Orvieto R, Homburg R, et al. Severe ovarian hyperstimulation syndrome despite low plasma oestrogen concentrations in a hypogonadotrophic, hypogonadal patient. *Hum Reprod* 1996; 11: 1177–1179.

Lunenfeld B, Rabau E, Rumney G, Winkelsberg G. The responsiveness of the human ovary to gonadotrophin. *(Hypophsis III)*. Proceedings of Third World Congress Gynecology and Obstetrics, Vienna 1961; 1:220.

Lunenfeld B, Sulimovici S, Rabau E, Eshkol A. L'induction de l'ovulation dans les amenorrheas hypophysaires par un traitement combine de gonadotrophins urinaires menopausiques et de gonadotrophins chorioniques. *C R Société Française de Gynecologie* 1962; 32;346.

Mashiach S, Ben-Rafael Z, Dor J, Serr DM. Triplet pregnancy in uterus didelphys with delivery interval of 72 days. *Obstet Gynecol* 1981; 58:519–521.

Meirow D, Levron J, Eldar-Geva T, et al. Pregnancy after transplantation of cryopreserved ovarian tissue in a patient with ovarian failure after chemotherapy. *N Engl J Med* 2005; 353:318–321.

Melmed H, Mashiach S, Insler V, et al. The response of the hyposensitive ovary to massive stimulation with human gonadotrophins. *J Obstet Gynaecol Brit Commonwealth* 1969;76: 437–443.

Mozes M, Bogokowsky H, Antebi E, et al. Thromboembolic phenomena after ovarian stimulation with human gonadotrophins. *Lancet* 1965; 2:1213–1215.

Navot D, Laufer N, Kopolovic J, et al. Artificially induced endometrial cycles and establishment of pregnancies in the absence of ovaries. *N Engl J Med* 1986; 314: 806–811.

Orvieto R., Ben-Rafael Z. Role of intravenous albumin in the prevention of severe ovarian hyperstimulation syndrome. *Hum Reprod* 1998; 13:3306–3309.

Palermo G, Joris H, Devroey P, Van Steirteghem AC. Pregnancies after intracytoplasmic injection of single spermatozoon into an oocyte. *Lancet* 1992; 340: 17–18.

Rabau E, David A, Serr DM, Mashiach S, Lunenfeld B. Human menopausal gonadotropins for anovulation and sterility. Results of 7 years of treatment. *Am J Obstet Gynecol* 1967; 98:92–98.

Schenker JG, Weinstein D. Ovarian hyperstimulation syndrome: A current survey. *Fertil Steril* 1978; 30: 255–268.

Steptoe PC, Edwards RG. Reimplantation of a human embryo with subsequent tubal pregnancy. *Lancet* 1976; 24(1):880–882.

Birth after the reimplantation of a human embryo. *Lancet* 1978; 12(2):366.

Trounson A, et al. Pregnancies in humans by fertilization *in vitro* and embryo transfer in the controlled ovulatory cycle. *Science* 1981; 212:681–682.

Chapter 17

The Development of In-Vitro Fertilization in Latin America

Fernando Zegers-Hochschild

After Robert Edwards and Patrick Steptoe announced the birth of Louise Brown, back in 1978, many young and senior gynecologists all over the world, were fascinated by the possibility of implementing such a challenging technology to help infertile couples build their families with this revolutionary treatment. In those years, we saw this technology restricted to cases with severe and irreparable damage of the Fallopian tubes, severe male factors or endometriosis, where surgery could not reach the ovaries or restore a functional relationship between the ovaries and Fallopian tubes. Today, in-vitro fertilization (IVF) and the many technologies that followed, have much wider and diverse indications than in the early days.

In 1979, I was a WHO fellow at the University of Sheffield with Professor Ian Cooke and although no facilities were then available for gamete or embryo research, together with other young gynecologists, we dedicated an important part of our time to studying how Professor Edwards had managed to generate life in vitro, the difficulties in generating good culture conditions, especially the generation of pure water free from contamination and ions, was then a major task. We also learned the importance of timing laparoscopy in order to collect mature oocytes. In fact, an English colleague was performing diagnostic laparoscopies in a nearby hospital and although it was not possible for us to program patients according to their cycle, we managed to collect oocytes, but never mature oocytes. In those years, a consent form to allow for follicular aspiration at the time of a diagnostic laparoscopy was not something we had in mind. This would be unacceptable today; however, the concepts of bioethics were just starting and, looking back, we had no conscience of wrongdoing.

After finishing my fellowship in the UK and later in Ghent, Belgium, I returned to Chile in 1980, determined to start IVF locally; but it was not until 1982 that real attempts were made by two groups in Santiago, Chile, and simultaneously by one other group in Bogotá, Colombia. Most Latin American gynecologists and biologists were receiving training in Norfolk, Virginia, under the direction of Professor Howard Jones.

Perhaps it is worth sharing an anecdote, which marked my views on how to look at this new and ever changing technology. In early 1983, Bob Edwards invited me to spend five days at Bourn Hall; in fact the right way to say it would be that I got myself invited by Bob Edwards whom I had never met before. The first night, he invited me to dinner with him at Churchill College, where he was a senior fellow. The formalities before and during dinner were impressive, but what impressed me most was when we started drinking after dinner and finished a long conversation in his car, it must have been around 1 am and the car windows were fogged after hours of intense conversation. Bob Edwards then told me that we should be able to remove the inner cells from an embryo and redirect totipotential cells into forming a new pancreas in order to treat diabetes. This was in 1983 and I immediately reacted by saying that he had no right to change the fate of an embryo and re-direct its existence into forming spare parts. That first deep conversation marked the start of a long-lasting and rich relationship, and we met almost every year at the ESHRE meetings and always found a place to drink and keep reflecting on how science permeates society. I now realize that he was several decades in advance of everybody else.

Doing IVF in a university setting in Chile was, in those years, unthinkable. It was the time of our military dictatorship and the University of Chile was controlled by the army and had no resources; and the Catholic University had already reacted with outrage when Louis Brown's birth was first communicated. Although I was part of the University of Chile, in those years I collaborated with a research group at the Catholic University in order to describe ovum transport in the Fallopian tube. We used to program laparoscopic tubal ligations, and collect eggs from different segments of the oviduct at specific times after the LH surge. The biologists working on these projects would handle the oocytes and describe the time course of ovum transport and maturation. Their experience with human oocytes was very limited and no attempts were ever made to fertilize these nice looking oocytes recovered from the oviduct.

When in 1983 we started a systematic training in oocyte pick-up, we invited the two main biologists working in ovum transport at the Catholic University to work with us and establish an IVF team. They had to use fake names otherwise they would have been expelled from the university. For almost six months we were collecting eggs in different hospitals and they would stand in the operating theater with a dissecting microscope and practice identifying and handling oocytes as fast as possible. The first real attempts of IVF were made between 1983 and 1984; but it wasn't until 1985 that the two first IVF babies were born almost simultaneously: from a group by the name of Colombian Center of Fertility and Sterility (CECOLFES), which today remains as one of the largest IVF groups in Colombia; and a group associated with the Army Hospital in Chile

that disappeared with the return of democracy in 1989. By the end of 1985, my team at Clínica las Condes, a private hospital in Santiago, had the first birth of a baby generated after gamete intra-Fallopian transfer (GIFT) and remained as the only ART program in Chile for many years. A few years later, Peru and Argentina contributed with their first IVF babies.

The magnitude of this revolutionary and unexpected discovery of IVF is revealed by the length of time it took to achieve success in other parts of the world. It took a couple of years after the birth of Louise Brown in the United Kingdom for the first birth in Australia, four years for the USA, and six years to succeed in Latin America. The magnitude of this revolution is also reflected by its rapid spread around the globe. In less than 40 years, almost every country in the world has established IVF programs and approximately eight million babies have been born so far.

The contribution of Latin America to these eight million is unfortunately very small. In the last report by ICMART, Latin America represents only 4–5% of the approximately 400,000 babies born each year (Figure 17.1). Although the main barrier to access

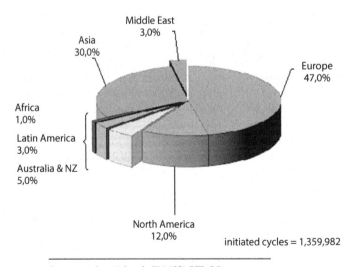

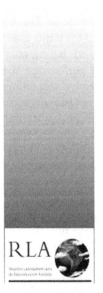

Regional distribution of ART cycles reported to the world registry (2012)

Middle East 3,0%
Asia 30,0%
Europe 47,0%
Africa 1,0%
Latin America 3,0%
Australia & NZ 5,0%
North America 12,0%

initiated cycles = 1,359,982

• Corresponde a ciclos de FIV, ICSI, FET, OD y otros

Figure 17.1 ART cycles reported to the World Registry 2012.

results from the fact that the vast majority of ART cycles performed in the region are out-of-pocket funded, the strong and permanent opposition of the Catholic Church has also been a difficult barrier to overcome, both for persons requiring treatment and also a barrier for the establishment of public policies in favor of the right of persons to found a family free of undue interference in their private lives.

The opposition of the Catholic Church to advances in sexual and reproductive health and rights started in 1968 with publication of the *Encyclical Humane Vitae*, in which Pope Paul VI established that the conjugal act (coitus) has both a unifying and a procreative meaning, and that mankind is not allowed to voluntarily dissociate these two meanings. This, of course, came as a result of the development of safe and efficient methods to regulate fertility, allowing sexuality to be devoid of its procreative consequence. On the other hand, IVF also falls into the same prohibition, since it dissociates these two meanings, thus allowing procreation not mediated by sexual intercourse.

We were in our third year of IVF, with abundant media exposure and criticism from the Catholic Church and from the most conservative political parties, which at least in Latin America are very much bound to the magisterium of the Catholic Church. Such was the situation when in 1987 Cardinal Joseph Ratzinger, later Pope Benedict XVI, released the document on Instruction on Respect for Human life "*Donum Vitae*" which condemned in the most severe way every form of assisted reproduction and reproductive donation. This was even before the existence of embryo freezing and pre-implantation genetic testing. Furthermore, irrespective of whether embryos would or would not die as a consequence of IVF, in this document the Vatican explicitly stated that those born of IVF were deprived of perfection: "In homologous IVF and ET, therefore, even if it is considered in the context of 'de facto' existing sexual relations, the generation of the human person is objectively deprived of its proper perfection: namely, that of being the result and fruit of a conjugal act."

In those years I was in permanent discussion with ecclesiastic authorities concerning the right of women and men to use science and technology to build their families. I remember, as if it was today, a debate I had on a television program with the Cardinal Archbishop of Santiago. During our debate he referred repeatedly to those born of IVF as "entities." I was so annoyed that abruptly interrupted his intervention with a strong knock in the table that separated the two of us and told him…

Tell me Cardinal, do you really think that if I sit two babies on this table in front of you, one born after sex mediated procreation and the other after IVF, you will be able to tell me which is perfect and which is not? Would you dare say that one resulted from God's will while the other does not? Your intervention Cardinal is atrocious.

Fortunately the program went rapidly to commercials and we never met again, but that was only the start of an exhausting and arduous sequence of confrontations, especially when embryo freezing was implemented. In 1995 our program was closed because of embryo freezing and in the city of Buenos Aires, Argentina, a "guardian" was appointed as protector of the cryopreserved embryos, so they would not be eliminated. This strong and many times undercover influence by the Catholic Church is seen in a variety of aspects relevant to sexual and reproductive rights. Chile is still one of the five countries in the world where all forms of abortion are penalized by law. Apart from Malta, the other three countries are El Salvador, Nicaragua, and Dominican Republic. Today a law project is being discussed in Chile to de-penalize abortion in cases where women's lives are at risk, in cases of rape, and where the foetus has lethal malformations. The arguments used by the conservative legislators against this law are almost the same as those expressed in the past against IVF, embryo freezing, etc. They are based on the right to life of embryos and fetuses as if they were persons.

Perhaps the most significant and evident interference of the Catholic Church in the development of public policies and laws on IVF is exemplified by Costa Rica. As in most countries in Latin America, Costa Rica started IVF in the late 1980s and early 1990s. After ten years of a successful program, the Constitutional Court, dominated by the extreme conservative wing and the Catholic Church, banned every form of IVF, under the argument that IVF destroyed embryos or generated embryos, which were meant to die as a result of treatment. It took two years to take this decision, which discriminated against women suffering from infertility, to the Inter American Court of Human Rights; and in 2012, the Court ruled against Costa Rica (Inter American Court of Human Rights, 2012) obliging the country, not only to compensate infertile couples who became childless due to this prohibition,

143

but it also obliged Costa Rica to restore IVF in the Social Security System in order to provide equitable access to treatment to those in need. Today, Costa Rica has restored IVF and is the third country in Latin America to have a law regulating universal access to ART.

It is reasonable to say that although IVF is now available in almost every country in the region, access to treatment is difficult, mainly because of the costs involved, which in a majority of countries is out-of-pocket funding. It is also important to recognize that, in many countries, the lack of appropriate and inclusive public policies favoring equalitarian rights to use science and technology for fertility care is the result of the strong barrier of the Catholic religion, which, as mentioned before, opposes all expressions of what are internationally recognized as sexual and reproductive rights.

In a different dimension, Latin America has also been an example of regional collaboration among countries and institutions. We initiated the first regional IVF registry in 1990 as a voluntary registry, which included 19 institutions from 12 countries, and reporting 2415 initiated ART cycles (Zegers-Hochschild et al., 2011). For the past 27 years, we have reported global results for Latin America every year and the latest report records 65,534 initiated cycles performed in 158 institutions in 2014 (Zegers-Hochschild et al., 2017).

In 1995, after five years of the Latin American Registry (RLA), the clinical directors and one biologist from each of the participating institutions met for the first time near Valparaiso on the coast of Chile. We had very little idea of what we wanted to achieve, but we knew that we needed to meet, to share each others' perspective and to decide how to make our region better, and how we might increase the participation of new centers in our voluntary registry. After all, being part of a regional registry can make your identity more visible, but at the end of the day we felt that building a strong network could achieve many more objectives apart from registering regional outcomes. We agreed that there were many institutions that needed technical support, but several senior centers complained that their data were combined with data of other institutions from their same country, giving them worse results and a less prestigious reputation. We then decided that the "open arm" policy followed until then should evolve into a more selective process, whereby only accredited centers would be entitled to belong to the registry. We all agreed to have an accreditation program whereby a biologist and a clinician from a different country would

visit each center and evaluate the veracity of the data reported, as well as the facilities, protocols for maintenance of incubators, water purification for the generation of culture media, and a variety of quality control programs. At the same time, we decided that it would be unfair for many new institutions to be forced to receive an accreditation team without due preparation; so it was decided to start regional workshops, meant primarily to establish quality control protocols for IVF laboratories and have hands-on workshops for biologists. In order to implement this regional education and certification program, Latin America was divided in five subregions and a regional director was elected for each of these regions. Regional directors were elected with the vote of one clinician and one biologist from each participating center. Their responsibility was to stimulate the reporting of all centers belonging to their region. It was also their responsibility to coordinate the education program, organize regional workshops, and prepare centers for the accreditation program. It is worth recognizing the invaluable collaboration of Dr. Richard Rawlings from Chicago, a member of the American College of Pathologists, who for many years devoted his time, knowledge, and care in organizing numerous workshops that ultimately contributed to enhancing the quality of services provided by centers all over Latin America. He also contributed with local biologists in the development of the first accreditation program.

For the certification program, every center voluntarily agreed to open their facilities and records to an external accreditation team, formed by a clinician and a biologist from a different country. Centers were either certified and could therefore report to the registry, or certified with conditions, which needed to be met within a fixed period of time; others were rejected, sometimes because their files did not reflect what they were reporting or because the personnel involved or the facilities were less than acceptable. We believe this accreditation program has generated enormous benefit to women seeking treatment. Centers reporting to the RLA appear in the list of certified institutions in the webpage (www.redlara.com) and consumers can at least identify those who are internationally certified. We believe that both the education and accreditation programs have helped Latin America to grow in terms of efficacy and safety; and much collaboration has been observed, especially among biologists, who are part of this network.

Twenty-two years have passed since we started the education and accreditation program and both activities have grown and diversified. Today, regional and sub-regional workshops continue to take place on a regular basis, and it is more than just QC of laboratories. Today, hands-on workshops are carried out for embryo biopsy, time-lapse imaging, and gamete and tissue freezing; but the original model remains, whereby sub-regions organize workshops and convey representatives of all centers from that region. These are unique opportunities to learn and to make friends among scientists and clinicians from neighboring countries. Many biologists travel between countries helping new centers when they have poor results.

Today, apart from the workshops, the education program includes an e-learning module, with complementary hands-on activities provided at certified centers in the region. More than 200 biologists, laboratory technicians, and clinicians have been certified by REDLARA after completing their online and hands on educational course.

The Latin American registry of ART has also evolved over time. When we started in 1990, we reported the data of 19 centers from 12 countries. In those years, data were collected manually, but since the late 1990s, each center has an individual code, which is used to report online to a central office located in Santiago, Chile. In 2010 we made a huge move forward from software collecting quite sophisticated summary data to a completely new cycle-based registry, thus becoming the only multinational registry collecting individualized data from ovarian stimulation until birth or abortion. Figures 17.2 and 17.3 show the database we have up until now, first as summary data and now in a cycle-by-cycle modality, with the number of babies born by country.

The Latin American registry is a voluntary reporting program whereby centers willing to participate need to open their facilities to an accreditation team. I would say it is quite remarkable that today, 175 centers from 15 countries in the region voluntarily report on a regular basis. Regional reports are published yearly in the journal *RBM Online* and the latest correspond to procedures initiated in 2014 and babies born up to September 2015 (Zegers-Hochschild et al., 2017).

Until today, every two years, the Latin American Network of Assisted Reproduction organizes workshops, which include clinicians and biologists from all centers in the region. Many prominent scientists have participated in our workshops and generously shared their knowledge with their peers in Latin America, but I would like to recall one special occasion. We

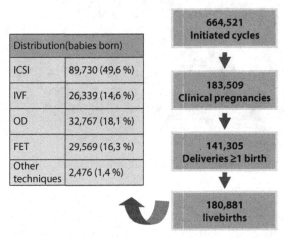

**Number of initiated cycles, pregnancies, deliveries, and livebirths by procedure.
RLA 1990–2015**

Distribution(babies born)	
ICSI	89,730 (49,6 %)
IVF	26,339 (14,6 %)
OD	32,767 (18,1 %)
FET	29,569 (16,3 %)
Other techniques	2,476 (1,4 %)

664,521 Initiated cycles

183,509 Clinical pregnancies

141,305 Deliveries ≥1 birth

180,881 livebirths

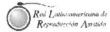

Figure 17.2 Number of initiated cycles, pregnancies, deliveries, and live births reported to the Latin American Register of Assisted Reproduction 1990–2015.

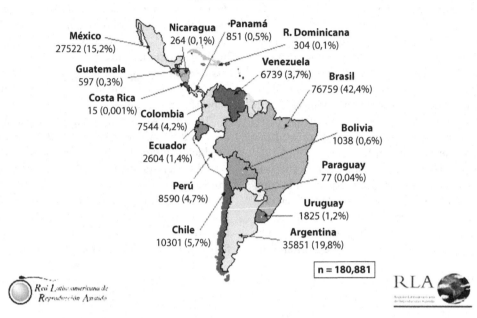

Figure 17.3 Showing the number of babies born during the 25 year period 1990–2005.

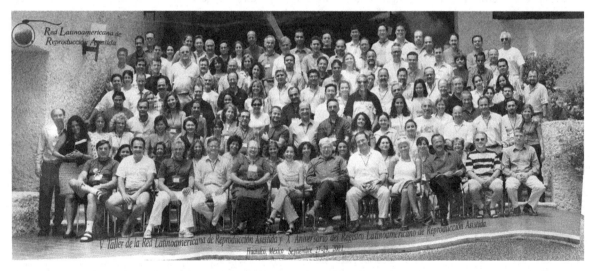

Figure 17.4 Attendees at the meeting of the Latin American Registry of Assisted Reproduction, in Huatulco, Mexico, September 27–29, 2001, with Bob Edwards center front.

had organized a workshop in Huatulco, a beautiful beach side in Mexico, for September 27–29, 2001. Bob Edwards was our guest speaker and many other invitees failed to assist because of the September 11 terrorist attack in New York, but Bob arrived on time and he was as simple and friendly as always. What we did not know until the very last moment was that September 27 was his 76th birthday, which we celebrated the next day. We were astonished that he would spend this special day teaching and sharing his life experience with professionals and friends in Latin America (Figure 17.4).

Latin America is moving in the same direction as the rest of the world, trying to balance efficacy and safety by reducing the number of embryos transferred. The mean number of embryos transferred in 2015 was 2.0, with 23% of women being 40 years of age or more; and more than 80% of treatments covered by out-of-pocket funding. These two conditions, age and source of funding, determine to a great extent the way ART is practised in Latin America. It is very unlikely that we will follow the same direction as the Nordic countries or Australia, with a majority of single embryo transfers; but there is no doubt that, at its own pace, Latin America is moving in the right direction, keeping efficacy in spite of drastic reductions in the number multiple births.

On behalf of our region, I surely represent the thoughts of the majority of professionals and consumers in expressing our deep appreciation to all those who have shared their wisdom with no other intention than the dissemination of knowledge for the good of humanity.

I personally believe that Bob Edwards' willingness to share his knowledge and adventurous thoughts without restriction, was unlimited and a characteristic we all cherish, and made him a unique and great man. Many people in Latin America argue that IVF has taken procreation out of the hands of God. It is my belief that this revolution is not an attempt against those who believe that children result from God's will; on the contrary, in the same way that an abundant harvest can only happen after thorough preparation of the soil, also, having children, for many women results only if thorough and technologically sound work is undertaken with the help of science, and hopefully peace and the wisdom to understand its limitations.

References

Inter-American Court of Human Rights case of Artavia Murillo et al. ('in vitro fertilization') v. Costa Rica judgment of November 28, 2012 (http://www.corteidh.or.cr/docs/casos/articulos/seriec_257_esp.pdf)

Zegers-Hochschild, F, Schwarze, J-E, Crosby, JA, Borges de Souza, M. Twenty years of Assisted Reproductive Technology (ART) in Latin America. *JBRA Assist. Reprod.* 2011;15:19–30.

Zegers-Hochschild, F, Juan Enrique Schwarze, JE, Javier A Crosby, JA, Carolina Musri, C, Urbina, MT, on behalf of the Latin American Network of Assisted Reproduction (REDLARA). Assisted reproductive techniques in Latin America: the Latin American Registry, 2014. *Reproductive BioMedicine Online* 2017; 35(3):287–295 http://dx.doi.org/10.1016/j.rbmo.2017.05.021

The Development of In-Vitro Fertilization in India

Rina Agrawal and Elizabeth Burt

Introduction

Subfertility is not a condition unique to the developed world, and difficulties in conceiving affect couples worldwide. Treatment options for subfertility tend to lend themselves to controversy and ethical debate; however, this is with good reason, given the sensitive nature of the work and responsibilities that clinicians hold. This is true even in highly regulated countries where public consultation, government legalisation, and regular audit of clinical work occur. The licensing and legislation infrastructure is only beginning to catch up with the advance of fertility treatment in several countries.

India is a prime example where a developing country has a rapid pace of expansion, globalization, and opportunity. It has achieved one of the fastest market growths within this sector. If regulations significantly lag behind clinical practice, then we can expect some degree of professional misconduct and commercial exploitation. This is having a significant impact on the framework of fertility practice in India.

In this chapter, we examine the incidence of subfertility in India, the origins of fertility treatment, and the legalization and current regulatory landscape in this rapidly developing and populous country, which is tipped to complete 260,000 ART cycles per year by 2020.

Subfertility in India

It is estimated that subfertility of various etiologies affects 27.5 million couples in India. The nation faces comparable environmental and lifestyle challenges to other countries and an increasing prevalence of both female and male subfertility across a diverse population (Kumar et al., 2014). This includes factors such as delayed marriages, delayed childbearing, an increasing female work force, a higher prevalence of the use of contraception, and lifestyle factors such as obesity, smoking, and alcohol use. Furthermore, there is now an increased incidence of sexually transmitted infections (Bhilwar et al., 2015) and Polycystic Ovarian Syndrome (Balaji et al., 2015) affecting female fecundity. Many couples therefore require fertility treatment (15%), although only approximately 1% of them currently seek help. The barriers to treatment are multifactorial, including the balance between social tradition driving the wish for treatment and parenthood and the stigma of infertility exposed by those seeking treatment. This is compounded further by the prohibitive costs for treatment and the disruption to daily living the treatment necessitates. Gender inequality is more pronounced in India and subfertility increases the social pressures on women, especially in the most rural areas. Not being able to conceive generates relationship and extended family tensions, and subfertility increases the incidence of violence against women and divorce rates.

Reproductive Medicine in India

India quickly followed the United Kingdom with the second baby born via IVF in 1978, but the news was shrouded in contention and debate. After the birth of Louise Brown in the UK on July 25, 1978, baby Durga was born a few months later in India on October 3 of the same year. The parents of the Indian baby forbade publication of their clinical care and the birth of their daughter, which led to the integrity of the work being challenged. This had substantial repercussions for Dr. Subhas Mukerji who led the pioneering work and established a scientific landmark in Indian reproductive medicine. The news of the baby was told in the media, but not documented in medical journals or shared with the scientific community in the conventional manner, which denied Dr. Subhas Mukerji the credit for his successful endeavor. Following news of the baby and the claims that she was born via IVF technology, the Indian government set up an enquiry to investigate, but concluded that the claims were fabricated and false. The Indian government then prevented Dr. Mukerji from further publication or attending scientific conferences to present and defend his work. He was barred from reproductive medicine and transferred to an insignificant role in ophthalmology in a smaller sub- district of India. Surrounded by dishonor, disbelief and humiliation, sadly, Dr. Subhas Mukerji committed suicide on June 19, 1981.

Dr. Anand Kumar played two pivotal roles in the history of IVF in India. Firstly, his scientific team in Mumbai, along with the clinical lead, Dr. Indira Hinduja, took the credit for the first Indian baby born with IVF on August 6, 1986. Secondly, and somewhat ironically, years later, Dr. Kumar also led a noble campaign supporting Dr. Mukerji's claim for precedence. Dr. Kumar reviewed the steps and process of Dr. Mukerji's work through detailed analysis and revision of his presentations and publications, and published a paper documenting Dr. Mukerji's work chronologically. His aim was to provide the evidence for restoring Dr. Mukerji's professional reputation and substantiating his rightful place as the creator of the second baby born through IVF technology in the world. The Indian Council of Medical Research (ICMR) added its poignant acknowledgement in 2002, 21 years after Dr. Mukerji's death.

Current Scenario

India is a heterogeneous country with old traditions and social constructs nestling alongside "new" western ideology and technology. This has inevitably led to conflict in acceptability and apparent contradictions in moral conduct. On the one hand, there is a conservative and private approach to reproductive medicine and, on the other, there is the overt fertility "tourism" trade that is occurring in India. Owing to the concentration of fertility clinics in major Indian cities (55%), coupled with the high price of treatment, many Indian couples are unable to access services; this exemplifies the inequalities in awareness and provision of treatment. However, the comparatively lower price of treatment than in many other parts of the world makes India a very attractive destination for many foreign patients. Thus, finding the balance between medicine and commercialism is a challenge for the Indian government and the regulatory bodies of the fertility practices in India.

India has hit the headlines over several issues related to IVF treatment, some welcome and some less so. Compared with other countries, India has a greater degree of moral autonomy, which has led to some practices and outcomes drawing criticism from around the world. There have been cases which have emphasized the distinction between what is "possible" and what is "right." With new regulations being put in place, standardized procedures will start to harmonize concepts for professional practice, but currently there is no official code of practice.

In some clinics, the opportunity to be a mother is offered to older post-menopausal women, and in other clinics multiple embryos are placed in the uterus. This raises serious ethical dilemmas. India was the focus of attention in May 2016 with news of the birth of a baby to a 72-year-old woman. This may be a record, but it was not an isolated event, as pregnancies in women long past menopausal age are reported to be relatively common in some clinics. This case, however, provoked worldwide attention, and caused questions about the appropriate use of reproductive technology and potentially exposed Indian clinics to public criticism. The motives of such parents varied, but the stigma of being "barren" was often cited as a justification for treatment, thus completely overruling responsible medical care and the interests of any children. A new Bill (see below) intends to ban the use of treatment for females over the age of 50, in line with policy in many other countries.

India is keeping pace with other countries in all aspects of reproductive medicine. In 2002, it was the second country to perform a complete orthotopic ovarian transplant for a female with Turner Syndrome (Mhatre et al., 2005). On May 18, 2017, it completed its first uterine transplant at the Pune Galaxy Care Laparoscopy Institute. India has also been at the forefront of surrogacy practice, which is discussed further below.

National Registry

IVF and reproductive treatment is commercially very appealing. This has led to a massive expansion within the women's health care sector, but the organization of clinics and their regulation is on an *ad hoc* basis. By 2020 it is predicted that India's clinics will be performing 260,000 cycles per year. Worryingly, clinics can be opened with minimal scrutiny of the treatments on offer or the qualifications and skill of those providing care. The ICMR and Indian Society of Assisted Reproduction (ISAR) have appreciated that this may compromise patient safety; success rates and procedures are therefore being put in place to rectify this

149

weakness. They have advocated the adoption of an accreditation and licensing system similar to that of the UK.

Previously there has been no official central data collection for assisted reproductive treatments and, as a consequence, keeping track of the number of cycles, success rates, and treatments offered by the clinics in India is suboptimal. This lack of surveillance motivated the implementation of a national registry to aid data sharing and clinical transparency, not only nationally but also internationally (e.g. International Federation of Fertility Societies – IFFS). Recognition of variations in practice globally, appreciating the diversity in pathologies affecting effectiveness, analysing the incidence of complications, and gaining exact figures on pregnancy outcomes will benefit both the reproductive medicine community and especially the patients. There have been concerns regarding issues such as the number of embryos transferred, inappropriate handling of gametes and misuse of technology for sex selection. With registration, practices can be held accountable, treatment can be monitored to ensure that only ethically sound treatment is carried out and that there is adequate safety with treatment carried out to the highest quality.

With the aim of formal information sharing, the National ART Registry of India (NARI) was founded in 2001 by the ISAR. This in turn supplies information to the global registries such as International Committee for Monitoring Assisted Reproductive Technologies (ICMART) (Malhotra et al., 2013). Engagement with the registry is advantageous for both the clinic and the patients. There is an ongoing concern though that not all fertility centers are registered, with only about 30% in compliance, as there is no enforcement, and participation is voluntary. The awaited Assisted Reproductive Technology (Regulation) Bill will, however, make it compulsory for ART clinics to register.

Following the creation of the registry, there has also been the publication of several important documents, including the *National Guidelines for Accreditation, Supervision and Regulation of ART Clinics in India* and *Ethical Guidelines for Biomedical Research on Human Subjects* published in 2005 and 2006 respectively by ICMR.

Current Legalisation

In-vitro fertilization and fertility treatment present many ethical and legal challenges. Respect for the law is paramount, but also to the sensitivities of native culture and society in reproductive medicine. Although the fundamentals are universal, the permutations and interpretations vary in different countries. Understanding how fertility treatment may affect issues such as legitimacy, parentage, and inheritance is of great cultural significance.

When donor eggs or sperm are used as part of treatment it is vital that the prospective parents and the donor understand the legal situation in order to give informed consent. Donors have no parental rights over the child and their information is kept confidential. Under Indian law, insemination using donor sperm does not constitute adultery because sexual intercourse does not occur, and if an Indian married couple have artificial insemination and conceive a child she or he is considered legitimate. The act of insemination itself though, is not considered sufficient to consummate the marriage and therefore there is still the possibility of the marriage being subject to annulment. If this were to occur after successful treatment resulting in pregnancy, the child would be considered illegitimate with the associated adverse societal consequences.

Reproductive Medicine Bills

There are two parliamentary Bills within India concerning reproductive medicine. The Assisted Reproductive Technology (Regulation) Bill has had various editions from 2009 until 2015 and the current draft is awaiting government approval, as in 2017. The vision of the Bill is to transform the current fragmented provision into cohesive care, with sustainable practice and standardized organization, protocols, and pricing. Care should be provided by competent practitioners, following evidence-based medicine. There is a clear exclusion of preimplantation genetic diagnosis for non-medical sex selection, which is currently reported to be carried out, and provides clear guidance for the use of embryos for research purposes. Ultimately, the aims of the Bill are to provide comprehensive monitoring and supervision for all aspects of reproductive medicine.

Initially incorporated into the Assisted Reproductive Technology (Regulation) Bill, but subsequently separated, was the Surrogacy Bill, which was expedited and released in November 2016. Since surrogacy was first legalized in India in 2002, there was increasing awareness and anxiety over the development of the surrogacy "industry." This has accelerated the need for strict rules and expectations for this niche of reproductive medicine. Amid significant international press coverage, non-altruistic surrogacy has been banned, and now only family members can act as surrogates for relatives. Surrogacy will be available only for Indian couples who are childless, have proven subfertility, and have been married for more than five years. They must have certificates both of essentiality and eligibility issued to prove this. There is no provision for couples in same-sex relationships or for single individuals. Surrogates must be married, already have their own children and can be reimbursed only for medical costs and insurance. They can act as a surrogate only once and they must have a medical certificate ensuring physical and psychological wellbeing. The clinics need to be fully registered and clinical details must be archived for at least 25 years. Failure to comply with this jurisdiction will incur a custodial sentence and a significant fine.

This is welcome news for many, and sets to eliminate the corporate edge from this very beneficial medical intervention. The objectives of the Bill are to remove the financial incentive and replace it with responsible medical care. Not all, however, view the policy favorably.

The original surrogacy arrangement had benefits for both the surrogate and the intended parents, and although not perhaps viewed as an ideal situation, it provided advantages for many families. This is a situation where it should be questioned if it is appropriate to impose Western idealistic ideas in a heterogeneous culture and on potentially vulnerable patients. It has been voiced that the intention of doing good and preventing perceived harm may, in fact, cause harm. For many Indian women, paid surrogacy has provided an avenue and opportunity to provide a better life for their own family. Equally, for many visiting couples the option of surrogacy in India has given them hope of having a child, which is denied in their own country. Any practice of surrogacy that may adversely affect the health of women or the welfare of children should not, of course, be condoned, but it has been suggested that banning "commercial" surrogacy may, in fact, open up more illicit activity and its well-known risks.

Conclusion

India has maintained a fast tempo of growth and technological advancement in IVF and other fertility treatments, comparable to its peers in other countries. It is apparent that the current state of practice has not been achieved without significant dedication, turmoil, and collaboration. The moral compass of IVF can, at times, be hard to navigate but India has strived to provide reputable, world-class fertility treatment.

Acknowledgments

I am grateful to Professor Roger Gosden (Virginia, USA) and Professor Duru Shah (President of Indian Society of Assisted Reproduction) for their valuable help during the preparation of this manuscript.

I would also like to thank my colleagues in India, Professor C. N. Purandhare, Dr. Hrishikesh Pai, Dr. Nandita Palshetkar, Dr. Narendra, Dr. Jaideep Malhotra, Dr. Rishma Pai, and Dr. Shanta Kumari for their helpful advice.

References

Balaji S, Amadi C, Prasad S, et al. Urban rural comparisons of polycystic ovary syndrome burden among adolescent girls in a hospital setting in India. *Biomed Res Int* 2015;2015:158951.

Bhilwar M, Lal P, Sharma N, Bhalla P, Kumar A. Prevalence of reproductive tract infections and their determinants in married women residing in an urban slum of North-East Delhi, India. *J Nat Sci Biol Med* 2015;6(Suppl. 1):S29–34.

Kumar S, Murarka S, Mishra VV, Gautam AK. Environmental & lifestyle factors in deterioration of male reproductive health. *Indian J Med Res* 2014;140 Suppl:S29–35.

Malhotra N, Shah D, Pai R, Pai HD, Bankar M. Assisted reproductive technology in India: A 3 year retrospective data analysis. *J Hum Reprod Sci* 2013;6:235–240.

Mhatre P, Mhatre J, Magotra R. Ovarian transplant: a new frontier. *Transplant Proc* 2005;37:1396–1398.

Chapter 19

The Development of In-Vitro Fertilization in China

Daimin Wei, Jianfeng Wang, Yingying Qin, and Zi-Jiang Chen

Abstract

China has the largest population in the world. Having children is viewed as a matter of cardinal significance in traditional culture. Nonetheless, a large number of couples are suffering from infertility. The advent of IVF has fundamentally changed the infertility treatment as well as the fate of these couples. As an estimate, more than 700,000 cycles of IVF are completed in more than 500 IVF centers in China each year. Techniques such as intracytoplasmic sperm injection (ICSI), in-vitro maturation (IVM), and preimplantation genetic diagnosis (PGD) or screening (PGS) have been widely used in clinics. New techniques, such as single-cell DNA amplification, mitochondrial replacement, and gene editing, are continually being developed. High-quality randomized controlled trials are being conducted to generate evidence for practice. Meanwhile, under the regulations set by government, the IVF techniques in China have more and more Chinese characteristics.

Background

In Chinese traditional culture, having children is one of the most important tasks for young couples. There is an old saying concerning behaviors that are regarded as not being filial, i.e. not supporting parents when they are old, not giving them a decent burial and not producing offspring, and the last one is the worst. Now China feeds the largest population in the world. The prevalence of infertility is estimated at about 12% in couples of reproductive age. Possible explanations for this increasing prevalence may lie in pollution, mental stress, delay of childbearing age, and some other factors. Therefore, the population suffering from infertility is very large. Infertility brings about much pressure to young couple, even their whole family. They are hungering for children to avoid a family breakdown. They may seek any possible treatment, like herbs, acupuncture, and wizards, before turning to modern assisted reproductive technology (ART); this is especially true of rural patients.

The application and popularization of ART has fundamentally changed the treatment of infertility in China and all over the world. The research on in-vitro fertilization (IVF) in China began about ten years later than that in the UK. However, its development has become very rapid since the 1980s. Up to 2016, 541 reproductive medicine centers offer clinical services to those in need, with a 40–50% pregnancy rate per transfer cycle. The cycles of oocyte retrieval exceeded 700,000 annually. The number of babies born from ART has accounted for 1% of all newborns. With the two-child policy implementation since 2015, a second boom in IVF cycles has occurred. By rough estimate, the number of oocyte-retrieval cycles may be over 900,000 per year. Meanwhile, numerous Chinese scientists and physicians have been working on revealing the mysteries of reproduction and developing new techniques that have contributed greatly to the development of IVF in the world.

The Development of IVF in China

IVF was initially performed in the 1980s in China. The year of 1978 saw the world's first IVF baby Louise Brown born. In the same year, China's government adopted the policies of "reform and opening-up." Since then, academic communication between China and the world has been increasing. The news of the birth of Louise Brown greatly encouraged Chinese doctors. They were determined to produce Chinese IVF babies. The research environment at that time was very tough: lack of funds, poor equipment, and no easy access to academic references. Counterviews went against developing IVF because they felt it unnecessary with such a big population in China, and it was against the policy of family planning. Professor Lizhu Zhang and her team succeeded in oocyte retrieval during laparotomy for treating pelvic diseases in 1984 and succeeded in in-vitro fertilization and embryo culture in 1985. After twelve failures to achieve a pregnancy after embryo transfer, they succeeded on the thirteenth try in a 38-year-old woman with bilateral tubal occlusion. The first IVF baby in mainland of China was reported in 1988 by Professor Lizhu Zhang from Peking University Third Hospital, Taiwan China in 1985, and Hongkong China in 1986. Subsequently, IVF was performed and succeeded in Changsha, Guangzhou, and Jinan. Since 1995, IVF centers have been established all over the country. The number of IVF centers has doubled every year. With the further development in the economy, the demand for high-quality life and reproductive health is increasing. The attitude towards IVF has changed from denial and doubt to acceptance, and more and more infertile couples are willing to receive IVF to achieve pregnancy. Nowadays, the number of IVF centers in China is approximately 540. Every center is crowded with patients every day. IVF has enabled millions of couples to become parents.

The Techniques of IVF

Ovarian Stimulation

Ovarian stimulation has typically been used to multiply the number of oocytes maturated in vivo since the 1980s. Ovarian stimulation has greatly improved the success of IVF. Many protocols have been developed to optimize ovarian response, such as GnRH agonist long and short protocol, GnRH antagonist protocol, and mild stimulation protocol. Nonetheless, poor ovarian response (POR) is still a challenge in a certain number of patients. In China, Professor Yanping Kuang tried a double stimulation protocol during the follicular and luteal phases, called the "Shanghai protocol," in patients with poor ovarian response and obtained good-quality blastocysts and live births (Kuang et al., 2014). The Shanghai protocol provided an alternative option for POR patients and challenged the concept that ovarian stimulation typically started from the early follicular phase.

However, ovarian stimulation is not always safe. Ovarian hyperstimulation syndrome is a severe iatrogenic complication and potentially lethal. Some patients, such as women with polycystic ovary syndrome, are at high risk of OHSS during ovarian stimulation. In-vitro maturation as an infertility treatment involves a process of retrieval of immature oocytes, maturation in vitro, in-vitro fertilization, and then embryo transfer. In China, the first live birth through the IVM technique was born in 2001 from Zi-Jiang Chen's team from Shandong Provincial Hospital of Shandong University (Li et al., 2002). With the refinement of culture media, the success rate of IVM has been increasing. Meanwhile, the safety of IVF, especially the long-term safety of offspring, is still of concern, and further studies are needed (Li et al., 2006).

Intracytoplasmic Sperm Injection (ICSI)

Severe male infertility was virtually untreatable until the application of ICSI. The first baby through ICSI in mainland of China was born in 1996 in the First Affiliated Hospital, Sun Yat-sen University by Professor Guanglun Zhuang's team. At the beginning, ICSI was preferentially used instead of IVF in order to get high rate of fertilization and the percentage of ICSI even reached 50%. However, concerns on the safety of ICSI were raised gradually later (Hansen et al., 2002; Kurinczuk and Bower, 1997). In 2003, the Chinese government issued regulations on assisted reproductive technology, in which the indications for ICSI were clearly stated: severe oligo- or/and asthenospermia, obstructive azoospermia, spermatogenesis dysfunction, immune infertility, failure of fertilization in IVF, abnormal sperm acrosome, and the need for preimplantation genetic diagnosis or screening. At present, the percentage of ICSI has been reduced to 20–25%. While current evidence on the safety of ICSI is reassuring (Han et al., 2010, Yan et al., 2011), its long-term safety on offspring should be followed up.

Cryopreservation Technique

By the introduction of ovarian stimulation, multiple oocytes and embryos were obtained. Embryo cryopreservation enables physicians to preserve the surplus embryos for later transfer and thus to avoid the risk of multiple pregnancies. With the refinement of the technique, cryopreservation has become an integral part of ART. Cryopreservation of embryo and gametes are already routine clinical procedures.

Sperm cryopreservation started much earlier than embryo or oocyte cryopreservation because the sample is convenient to get and easier to freeze. In China, the first human sperm bank was established in the 1980s. Up to 2016, there are 23 sperm banks all over the country. The government in China has implemented regulations on the use of donor sperm, which should be used only for couples with non-obstructive azoospermia, severe oligo- and/or astheno- and/or terato-spermia but declining ICSI, paternal severe inheritable disease, or couples who failed to get a live baby due to maternal–fetal blood group incompatibility. Sperm frozen for fertility preservation has also been increasingly carried out in people who are undertaking chemotherapy or radiotherapy, or who are engaging in special careers.

Initially, the freezing of embryos was used to preserve surplus embryos after fresh embryo transfer or for medical indications such as a high risk of OHSS. The first baby from frozen embryo transfer in mainland of China was born in 1995 in Peking University Third Hospital by Professor Lizhu Zhang's team. In early years, embryos were frozen at the zygote or cleavage-stage by the slow cooling method. Nowadays more and more centers perform blastocyst freezing with the improvement of technique and optimization of culture. Zi-Jiang Chen and her colleagues reported the first live birth from blastocyst transfer in China in 2002 in Shandong Provincial Hospital of Shandong University. Blastocyst cryopreservation allows selection of embryos before freezing and increases the rates of survival and pregnancy after thawing. Since the 2000s, the application of vitrification has been widely used and has replaced the slow cooling method in most IVF centers. Vitrification contributes to the increased pregnancy rate in frozen embryo cycles. Coinciding with the requirement for reducing the number of embryos transferred, more surplus embryos need to be cryopreserved. Frozen embryo transfer has recently been suggested to be associated with better pregnancy outcomes compared with fresh embryo transfer (Maheshwari et al., 2012; Weinerman and Mainigi, 2014). Elective freeze-only and frozen embryo transfer is attracting increasing attention. Zi-Jiang Chen's team conducted a multicenter randomized controlled trial in 1508 women with polycystic ovary syndrome and observed that frozen embryo transfer resulted in a higher live birth rate, lower risks of OHSS and pregnancy loss, but an increased risk of pre-eclampsia, compared with fresh embryo transfer (Chen et al., 2016). Whether frozen embryo transfer is superior to fresh embryo transfer in other IVF populations is still under investigation. There is a series of ongoing randomized controlled trials (NCT02712840, NCT02746562, NCT02471573, NCT02570386, ChiCTR-IOR-14005406, ChiCTR-IOR-14005405) to compare frozen versus fresh embryo transfer. ChiCTR-IOR-14005406 and ChiCTR-IOR-14005405 are being conducted by Zi-Jiang Chen's team; the former to compare fresh versus frozen cleavage-stage embryo transfer in ovulatory women, and the latter to compare single fresh versus frozen blastocyst transfer in women with good prognosis (ChiCTR-IOR-14005405). Hopefully, sufficient evidence will be obtained to prove whether elective frozen embryo transfer in lieu of fresh embryo transfer should be performed in the future.

Oocyte cryopreservation provides the opportunity of fertility preservation for women who are going to undergo radio- or chemotherapy, and those who want to postpone childbearing. The slow freezing method was initially used and the success rate was quite low. Vitrification has also greatly improved the survival rate of oocytes after thawing (Kuleshova et al., 1999). The first live birth from vitrified oocytes in China was born in 2005 by Zi-Jiang Chen's team (Chen et al., 2006). Nowadays, the application of oocyte cryopreservation has been more and more popular for both medical and social indications.

Gamete Intrauterine Transfer (GIUT)

Gamete transfer is an infertility treatment involving the process of retrieval of oocytes and sperms, in-vitro mixture, and then transferring into the female peritoneal cavity, Fallopian, or uterine cavity. Tubal ampulla is the place of fertilization in spontaneous conception; therefore, scientists invented the gamete intra-Fallopian transfer (GIFT) technique. The first live birth from GIFT in China was born in 1988 in Peking University Third Hospital by Professor Lizhu Zhang's team. The first live birth from *transvaginal* GIFT in China was reported by Professor Zi-Jiang Chen in 1997. However, GIFT requires patients have at least one patent tube and involves the surgical procedure or complex transvaginal procedure for intra-Fallopian gamete transfer. Estes had reported live births from implantation of an ovary onto the cornua uteri (Estes, 1925). The results suggested that the uterine cavity can also serve as a place for fertilization. Professor Zi-Jiang Chen and her colleagues investigated gamete intrauterine transfer (GIUT) in 1989 and succeeded the first live birth in the world (Su, 1992). With the higher success rate of IVF, the application of GIUT is not very common. At present, GIUT is utilized in some special patients with repeated failure with in-vitro fertilization or patients with repeated poor-quality embryos. Some live births have been achieved.

Preimplantation Genetic Diagnosis or Screening (PGD/PGS) and Gene Editing

The first live birth from PGD in China was in 1998. PGD mainly helps those couples with a chromosomal abnormality or monogenic disorders. In China, deafness is one of the major congenital defects, with 30,000 deaf newborns annually. Approximately 60% of neonatal deafness is due to a genetic defect. In 2015, the first healthy baby in China using PGD from parent carriers with GJB2 mutations was born by Zi-Jiang Chen's team in Shandong University, which was honored as one of the top ten breakthroughs in medicine in China in 2015. Up to 2016, a total of 13 PGD centers have been certificated by the government. With the popularization and maturity of comprehensive chromosome screening such as whole exome sequencing (WES), array-comparative genome hybridization (aCGH), and quantitative polymerase chain reaction (qPCR), the accuracy and coverage of PGS has also been improved significantly. In 2017, the committee of The Chinese Society of Reproductive Medicine published an expert consensus regarding the indications for PGS, which includes: recurrent spontaneous miscarriage for three or more times, two or more spontaneous miscarriages with at least one abortus having confirmed abnormality in karyotype or genes, repeated implantation failure, and advanced maternal age (>38 years). PGD/PGS for sex selection is strictly prohibited in China.

Recently, Professor Qiao and her collaborators of Peking University Third Hospital have developed a new amplification method, i.e. multiple annealing and looping-based amplification cycles (MALBAC), which enables DNA amplification from a single cell (Hou et al., 2013). With MALBAC, they have performed genome analysis of blastomeres from cleavage-stage embryos (Huang et al., 2014). PGD using MALBAC based sequencing technique can simultaneously detect single-gene mutations, aneuploidy, and perform linkage analysis in a cost-effective way (Yan et al., 2015).

The application of PGD provides a more accurate method for embryo selection. Nonetheless, not all patients will benefit from PGD. Some patients may experience the disappointing fact that none of their embryos is normal after suffering the enormous psychological and economical pressure of an IVF/PGD cycle. With the rapid development of gene-editing technology, especially the wide use of clustered regularly interspaced short palindromic repeat (CRISPR)/CRISPR associated 9 (Cas9) system, scientists have already successfully used CRISPR/Cas9 for gene editing in animal zygotes. In 2014, Professor Huang and his colleagues were the first to use CRISPR/Cas9 for correcting β-thalassemia disease mutation in early human embryos derived from 3PN fertilization (Liang et al., 2015). Still, more and further studies are needed before it can be used clinically. This work attracted broad attention from all over the world and provoked a heated debate on whether gene editing should be used on human embryos. Later in 2015, an international summit on Human Gene-Editing was held in Washington. A consensus was reached that human embryo gene editing should not be used for pregnancy at present.

Mitochondrial Replacement and Gamete Donation

Mitochondria are membrane-bound organelles contain a small amount of DNA that is maternally inherited. Mutations in the mitochondrial DNA (mtDNA) cause disorders with severe clinical symptoms, such as Leber hereditary optic neuropathy and mitochondrial encephalomyopathy. Replacement of defective mitochondria with non-pathogenic mtDNA from normal donor oocytes is considered as an effective approach for mitochondrial diseases. Mitochondrial replacement can be accomplished by maternal spindle transfer (MST), pre-pronuclear transfer (PPNT), pronuclear transfer (PNT), and polar body transfer (PBT). PPNT was firstly used in a human embryo successfully in 2017 by Zi-Jiang Chen's team from Shandong University (Wu et al., 2017). On the basis of PPNT, the same group from Shandong University further improved the method of second polar body transfer (PB2T) (Wu et al., 2017). According to the policy issued by the government of China in 2003, cytoplasm or nuclear transplantation is still prohibited for human infertility treatment. Therefore, those derived embryos were not transferred into the uterus.

Sperm donation has been widely used in China with the maturity of sperm cryopreservation. As mentioned above there are now more than 20 human sperm banks in China. The Chinese government rules that donated sperm from one donor can be used to fertilize no more than five women.

In contrast to sperm donation, oocyte donation is much tougher in the clinic. The first live birth from donated oocytes in mainland of China was in 1992 in Peking University Third Hospital by Professor Lizhu Zhang's team. The "Regulation of Human Assisted Reproductive Technology" issued in 2003 ruled that oocyte donation from relatives or volunteer women who don't undergo the in-vitro fertilization procedure is forbidden. Oocyte donation is permitted only in women who are undergoing IVF or ICSI because of infertility and are willing to donate their surplus oocytes. Similarly, the donated oocytes from one donor could be used in no more than five women to conceive. The number of oocyte donors is many fewer than sperm donors because of the invasiveness of the oocyte retrieval procedure and also because women seem to cherish their limited number of oocytes. There is a huge demand for donated oocytes for patients with premature ovarian failure, genetic diseases or oocyte maturation disorders, and for a "one-child died family" with advanced maternal age. It often will take over five years, even ten years, to wait for donor eggs.

The first live birth from donated embryos was in 1988 in Xiangya Medical College of South Central University. Interestingly, this baby later joined the team that created him when he grew up and became a physician in the same Reproductive Medicine Center. In 2003, the regulation on assisted reproductive technology of China prohibited embryo donation in China.

Surrogacy

Surrogacy is a solution for patients with congenital uterine anomalies, or severe intrauterine adhesions. The first live birth from surrogacy in mainland of China was born in 1996 in Peking University Third Hospital by Professor Lizhu Zhang's team. The Reproductive Medicine Center of Shandong University performed 16 cases of surrogacy and delivered healthy babies during 1996–2000 (Cui et al., 2016). In 2001, the Chinese government issued regulations on ART and prohibited surrogacy. However, there is great demand for surrogacy in China. Prohibition of surrogacy leads to the development of "underground grey markets." By searching a public internet database, more than 120 surrogacy agents can be found in China (Cui et al., 2016). More reasonable rules allowing surrogacy under fine surveillance are anticipated in China.

In summary, IVF and derived technologies have helped millions of couples to become parents in China. On the whole, with the special characteristics of Chinese culture and ART regulation by government, the development of IVF has been rapid and healthy. Chinese scientists and physicians have contributed to promote the development of reproductive medicine, both in the fields of basic research and in clinical practice, both domestically and internationally. The prospects for IVF in China are promising.

References

Chen ZJ, Li Y, Hu J, Li M. Successful clinical pregnancy of cryopreserved human oocyte after vitrification. *Nat Med J China* 2006;29: 2037–2040.

Chen Z-J, Shi Y, Sun Y, et al. Fresh versus frozen embryos for infertility in the polycystic ovary syndrome. *N Engl J Med* 2016;375: 523–533.

Cui L, Li L, Adashi EY, Chen ZJ. Surrogacy: a family-building option in search of legitimacy. *Bjog* 2016;123 Suppl 3: 65–68.

Estes WL. Implantation of ovary. *Ann Surg* 1925;82: 475–482.

Han JL, Chen H, Niu ZH, et al. [A 10-year survey on birth defects after in vitro fertilization-embryo transfer in Shanghai]. *Zhonghua Fu Chan Ke Za Zhi* 2010;45: 124–127.

Hansen M, Kurinczuk JJ, Bower C, Webb S. The risk of major birth defects after intracytoplasmic sperm injection and in vitro fertilization. *N Engl J Med* 2002;346: 725–730.

Hou Y, Fan W, Yan L, et al. Genome analyses of single human oocytes. *Cell* 2013;155: 1492–1506.

Huang J, Yan L, Fan W, et al. Validation of multiple annealing and looping-based amplification cycle sequencing for 24-chromosome aneuploidy screening of cleavage-stage embryos. *Fertil Steril* 2014;102: 1685–1691.

Kuang Y, Chen Q, Hong Q, et al. Double stimulations during the follicular and luteal phases of poor responders in IVF/ICSI programmes (Shanghai protocol). *Reprod Biomed Online* 2014;29: 684–691.

Kuleshova L, Gianaroli L, Magli C, Ferraretti A, Trounson A. Birth following vitrification of a small number of human oocytes: case report. *Hum Reprod* 1999;14: 3077–3079.

Kurinczuk JJ, Bower C. Birth defects in infants conceived by intracytoplasmic sperm injection: an alternative interpretation. *BMJ* 1997;315: 1260–1265; discussion 1265–1266.

Li Y, Chen Z-J, Zhao L, et al. A live birth from oocyte in vitro maturation. *National Journal of Andrology* 2002;1: 70–71.

Li Y, Feng HL, Cao YJ, et al. Confocal microscopic analysis of the spindle and chromosome configurations of human oocytes matured in vitro. *Fertil Steril* 2006;85: 827–832.

Liang P, Xu Y, Zhang X, et al. CRISPR/Cas9-mediated gene editing in human tripronuclear zygotes. *Protein Cell* 2015;6: 363–372.

Maheshwari A, Pandey S, Shetty A, Hamilton M, Bhattacharya S. Obstetric and perinatal outcomes in singleton pregnancies resulting from the transfer of frozen thawed versus fresh embryos generated through in vitro fertilization treatment: a systematic review and meta-analysis. *Fertil Steril* 2012;98: 368–377, e361–369.

Su Y CZ. The success of gametes intrauterine transfer. *Chinese Journal of Obstetrics and Gynecology* 1992;27: 1995–1996.

Weinerman R, Mainigi M. Why we should transfer frozen instead of fresh embryos: the translational rationale. *Fertil Steril* 2014;102: 10–18.

Wu K, Chen T, Huang S, et al. Mitochondrial replacement by pre-pronuclear transfer in human embryos. *Cell Res* 2017;27: 834–837.

Wu K, Zhong C, Chen T, et al. Polar bodies are efficient donors for reconstruction of human embryos for

potential mitochondrial replacement therapy. *Cell Res* 2017(Aug);27(8): 1069–1072.

Yan J, Huang G, Sun Y, et al. Birth defects after assisted reproductive technologies in China: analysis of 15,405 offspring in seven centers (2004 to 2008). *Fertil Steril* 2011;95: 458–460.

Yan L, Huang L, Xu L, et al. Live births after simultaneous avoidance of monogenic diseases and chromosome abnormality by next-generation sequencing with linkage analyses. *Proc Natl Acad Sci U S A* 2015;112: 15964–15969.

The Development of In-Vitro Fertilization in Africa

Willem Ombelet

Introduction

Infertility is a universal health issue and it has been estimated that 8–12% of couples worldwide are infertile, with 9% currently cited as the probable global average and remarkably similar between more and less developed countries (Boivin et al., 2007; Ombelet et al., 2008). On the other hand, in some areas of Sub-Saharan Africa it seems that up to 30% of couples are infertile (Nachtigall, 2006).

In Africa the consequenses of involuntary childlessness are usually much more dramatic and can create broader problems compared to Western societies, particularly for women. Negative psychosocial consequences are often severe and childless women are frequently stigmatized, isolated, ostracized, disinherited, and neglected by the entire family and even the local community (Daar and Merali, 2002; Dyer et al., 2005; Van Balen and Bos, 2009) (Figure 20.1). This may result in physical and psychological violence, polygamy, even suicide. Because many families in developing countries completely depend on children for economic survival, childlessness has to be regarded as a social and public health issue, and not only as an individual medical problem. According to the results of a systematic analysis by Dyer and Patel (2012), infertility may impose impoverishing health costs as well as economic deprivation secondary to social consequences.

Substantial geographical differences are noted and these differences can be explained by different environmental, cultural, and socioeconomic influences (Boivin et al., 2007). In Sub-Saharan Africa, infection is the cause of infertility in over 85% of cases among women, compared to 33% worldwide (Cates et al., 1985; Nachtigall, 2006). Approximately 70% of pelvic infections are caused by sexually transmitted diseases (STDs) while the other 30% are attributable to pregnancy-related sepsis (Ericksen and Brunette, 1996). Similarly, many cases of male-factor infertility are caused by previous infections of the male genitourinary tract.

The most important reason for childlessness in Africa is the high incidence of STDs – which affects both men and women – and pregnancy-related infections due to unsafe abortions and home deliveries in unhygienic circumstances, mainly in rural areas. The high prevalence of genital infections in developing countries is commonly compounded by a complete lack of diagnosis, together with incomplete, inappropriate, or no intervention at all (Ombelet et al., 2008).

Severe male infertility due to STDs and female infertility due to tubal block can only be treated by "expensive" assisted reproductive technologies (ART), which are either not available or only within reach of those (the happy few) who can afford it, mostly in private settings. According to the results of a cross-sectional online survey in Kenya (Murage et al., 2011) almost 90% of patients have to self-fund their IVF treatment, with costs amounting to approximately 4000 USD per cycle.

The African continent has seen less development in IVF technology in recent decades than has been seen in other parts of the world (Inhorn and Patrizio, 2015). The high cost associated with IVF/ICSI is the main barrier preventing many from benefiting from this technology in so far that in Sub-Saharan Africa it is calculated that less than 2% of the population have access to IVF. There is hardly any funding from public institutions or insurance companies.

Despite the high infertility prevalence and the severe economical consequences of childlessness in developing countries, infertility care remains a low priority area for local health care providers and community leaders. It has been marginalized and neglected by health care authorities despite its high prevalence and unmet need (Fathalla et al., 2006; Ombelet, 2011).

Table 20.1 summarizes the factors associated with the problem of accessibility to infertility care in Africa.

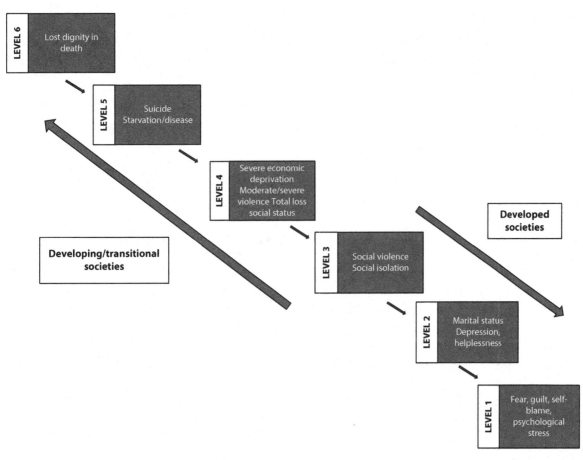

Figure 20.1 Continuum of the consequences of infertility and childlessness: In developed countries, the consequences of infertility rarely extend beyond level two; in developing countries, at least in Asia and Africa, the consequences of infertility are infrequently as mild as level three (Daar and Merali, 2002).

The History of IVF in Africa

Up to 2001 there was little or no interest at all in subfertility prevention and treatment in Africa, with the exception of Egypt and South Africa. Almost all scientific papers on the issue of childlessness and the need for infertility care in Africa were published by anthropologists, sociologists, and epidemiologists describing the huge sociocultural, psychological, and economical consequences of being childless, especially for women (Dyer et al., 2004, 2005; Van Balen and Bos, 2009).

As a result of a meeting entitled "Medical, Ethical and Social Aspects of Assisted Reproduction," organized by the World Health Organization in 2001, the following recommendations were made: (1) infertility should be recognized as a public health issue worldwide, including developing countries; (2) policy makers should give attention to the needs of infertile patients; (3) infertility management should be integrated into national reproductive health care programs; and (4) ART has to be complementary to other ethically acceptable sociocultural solutions to infertility.

In 2006, ESHRE founded a "Special Task Force" dedicated to infertility in developing countries. The organization of the expert meeting on the topic of "Developing Countries and Infertility" in Arusha, Tanzania, December 2007, was the first project of this Task Force and was organized in cooperation with the "Genk Institute of Fertility Technology." As a result of this expert meeting it was concluded that the major

Table 20.1 An overview of the number of IVF units in the different continents

	2017 Population	%	Number of IVF units	%	Number of IVF units/ million population
World	7,515,284,153	100%	3321	100%	0.44
Asia	4,478,315,164	59.60%	689	20.70%	0.15
Africa	1,246,504,865	16.70%	131	3.90%	0.10
Europe	739,207,742	9.90%	1638	49.30%	2.21
South America	426,548,298	5.80%	303	9.10%	0.71
North & Central America	540,473,499	7.30%	447	13.50%	0.82
Oceania	40,467,040	0.50%	113	3.40%	2.82

Box 20.1 Twenty-two out of the 54 African countries have at least one IVF unit

Algeria	1	Benin	1
Burkina Faso	1	Burundi	1
Cameroon	1	Egypt	52
Ethiopia	1	Gabon	1
Ghana	9	Kenya	3
Libyan Arab Jamahiriya	2	Mauritius	1
Morocco	2	Niger	2
Nigeria	12	South Africa	38
Sudan	2	Tanzania	1
Togo	2	Tunisia	7
Uganda	4	Zimbabwe	1

African countries with an IVF unit: 22.

Total of IVF units in Africa 2017: 145.

(source: IVF Worldwide: http://www.ivf-worldwide.com).

Box 20.2 Thirty-two out of the 54 African countries (59.2%) have no IVF unit

Angola	Botswana	Cape Verde
Central African Republic	Chad	Comoros
Congo	Djibouti	Equatorial Guinea
Eritrea	Gambia	Guinea
Guinea-Bissau	Kiribati	Lesotho
Liberia	Madagascar	Malawi
Mali	Mauritania	Mayotte
Mozambique	Namibia	Nauru
Rwanda	Sao Tome and Principe Senegal	Seychelles
Sierra Leone	Somalia	Swaziland
Western Sahara	Zambia	

African countries without an IVF unit: 32.

(source: IVF Worldwide: http://www.ivf-worldwide.com)

challenge would be **to reduce costs of laboratory procedures,** namely fertilization and culture of eggs and embryos, and to decrease the costs associated with ovarian stimulation for IVF. It was also mentioned that more research on **social, cultural, ethical, religious, and judicial aspects of infertility** in poor-resource countries is needed.

The Unmet Need for Accessible and Affordable IVF

Table 20.1 gives an overview of the number of IVF units in the different continents. Boxes 20.1 and 20.2 describe the availability of IVF centers in the different African countries. It was calculated before that there should be 1500 IVF cycles per million people to meet the population demand (Fauser et al., 2002; Figure 20.2). To compare, in Belgium we have a reimbursement policy for six IVF cycles per patient in a lifetime, the financial burden for the patients is minimal. According to the most recent 2014 data, 16,500 IVF/ICSI cycles were performed for a population of 11 million, exactly what we predicted many years ago. The African population is actually estimated to be 1.2 billion; therefore 1.8 million IVF cycles should be done to meet its current population demand. According to the published data less than 1.5% of the African population has access to assisted reproduction (Figure 20.2).

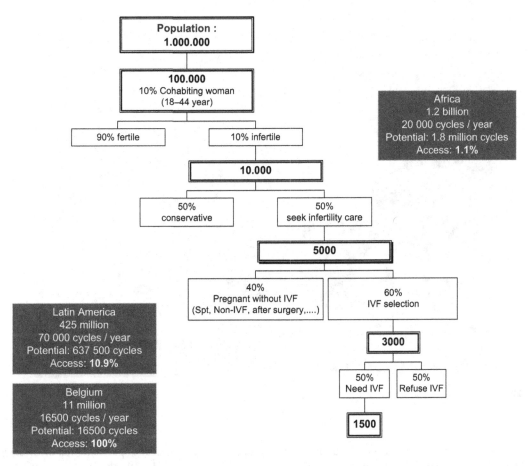

Figure 20.2 Access to IVF procedures: estimated need of IVF cycles per million (population) (Fauser et al., 2002). Calculation for Belgium (reimbursement of six IVF cycles per woman), Latin America and Africa.

(If 10% of the population consist of cohabiting women aged 18–44 years, taking into account that 10% of these have a fertility problem, among them 50% will seek infertility care. Of the remaining 5000 infertile couples 2500 would qualify for IVF due to persistent infertility and 500 because of tubal factor or severe male infertility. Assuming that only half of them will accept proceeding with IVF, the assumed need for IVF would at least be 1500 procedures per annum per million population.)

African ART Registration

In the latest World Report on Assisted Reproductive Technology (Adamson et al., 2017), data from Africa represented only 1% of global ART activity although the African population actually contributes 16.7% of the world population.

It is difficult to find out how many centers are nowadays performing IVF in Africa, but the number is growing day by day. The African countries with the highest number of IVF centers are Egypt, Ghana, Kenya, Nigeria, and South Africa. According to the latest SARA (South African Registry for Assisted Reproductive Techniques) report 4995 ART cycles were performed in 2014 in 15 IVF centers; this means

that even in South Africa only 6.4% of the need for ART was met.

ANARA (African Network and Registry for Assisted Reproductive Technology) was established in 2015 as a research network and platform for communication and information, sharing the practice and outcomes of ART in sub-Saharan Africa. ANARA is modelled on the successful Latin American Network and Registry for Assisted Reproductive Technology (RLA). ANARA has its own data collection software and the software is free for participating ART centers. The software collects case-by-case data, which is the superior method of ART data collection when compared to retrospective summary data. ANARA collects data from two settings: (1) directly from participating

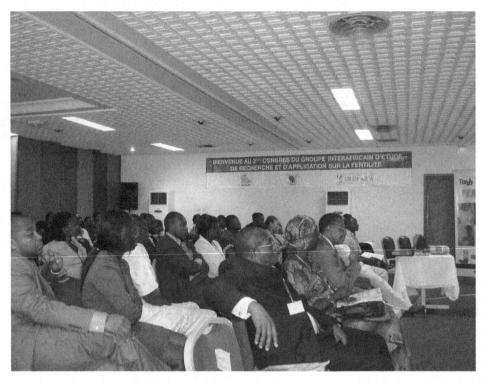

Figure 20.3 February 2010: second meeting of GIERAF in Douala (Cameroon).

ART centers in countries that have adopted the ANARA software for national data collection or where no national registry exists; and (2) from national ART registries in countries that collect their own national data through a different software program. The registry arm of ANARA collects and disseminates data on the availability, effectiveness, and safety of assisted reproductive technology in Africa. On the occasion of the RCOG World Congress in March 2017 in Cape Town, the ANARA Director Silke Dyer presented the 2012 ART data, which were collected from 30 African IVF centers (South Africa 13, Nigeria 7, Tunisia 3, and one center each from Morocco, Ghana, Togo, Benin, Cameroon, Mali, and Ivory Coast). A total of 9471 aspirations were noted with a very acceptable pregnancy rate of 30.7% per aspiration.

Regional and national fertility organizations have expressed their support for ANARA very recently. This includes GIERAF (Groupe Inter Africain d'Etude, de Recherche et d'Application sur la Fertilité), which was founded in 2009. GIERAF aims to promote: (1) prevention of the avoidable causes of infertility; (2) the training of practitioners in the field of reproduction;

and (3) exchanges and partnerships with scientific societies concerned with the problems of medicine and the biology of human reproduction. Eleven countries are involved: Bénin, Burkina Faso, Cameroon, Congo, Ivory Coast, Gabon, Mali, Niger, Democratic Republic of Congo, Senegal, and Togo (Figure 20.3). They recently presented the 2013 data on 523 oocyte aspirations with a live birth rate per transfer of 26.9% for IVF and 29.0% for ICSI (Moîse Fiadjoe, personal communication, 2017).

Although the future for ART registration in Africa looks bright, one should be aware of the fact that a substantial number of African IVF clinics still don't share their data.

Accessible and Affordable IVF: Attempts at Lowering the Costs of IVF

According to a calculation made by C. Huyser (Pretoria, South Africa) the average percentage of the major cost-drivers of an IVF cycle at an active private practice in South Africa in 2012 were the following: 8% of costs are allocated for clinic fees, 28% to medication, 29%

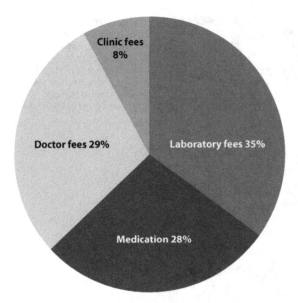

Figure 20.4 Cost analysis per IVF procedure in private centers in South Africa (Huyser and Boyd, 2013).

FACTS
- Prevalence of infertility: similar to Western countries
- Negative consequences of childlessness are much stronger
- Prevention and alternative methods are not always successful
- ↑ Secondary infertility due to STDs and unsafe abortions/deliveries
- HIV and infertility: ↑ prevalence of HIV in infertile couples
- HIV and infertility: very different in how the issue has been treated by the international community
- Access to IVF in Africa: less than 1.5%
- **Arguments contra** global access to infertility care
  Overpopulation
  Limited resources
  Problem of funding: "the battle for money" between initiatives on reproductive health care
- **Arguments pro** global access to infertility care
  ↑ Demand from developing countries
  ART techniques can be simplified
  Social justice and equity

VIEWS
- A need for ↑ reproductive health care education
- A need for ↑ prevention programmes
- Raising awareness: support of media and patients networks needed
- Implementation of more and accessible infertility centers
  → Urgent need for simplified, safe and effective methods (diagnostic procedures and ART)
- Prevention of complications is crucial: OHSS, multiple pregnancies
- Facilities to handle complications have to be available, including facilities for surgery

VISION
- Simplified methods of infertility care will be available in the near future
- The demand from Africa to introduce ART will increase
- The implementation of accessible infertility centers should be part of an integrated reproductive care program including family planning and contraception, maternal care, and reproductive health
- Foundations, NGOs, and international societies have to be convinced about the value of this project

(ART = Assisted Reproductive Technologies, STDs = Sexually Transmitted Diseases, OHSS = Ovarian Hyperstimulation Syndrome, NGOs = Non-Governmental Organizations)

to clinicians' fees and consultations, and 35% for laboratory fees (for use of equipment and the laboratory, disposables, culture media, and staff expenditures) (Huyser and Boyd, 2013)(Figure 20.4).

Box 20.3 gives an overview of the actual situation regarding access to infertility care in Africa.

Suggested strategies to reduce the cost of infertility care and infertility treatment are as follows.

Simplifying the Diagnostic Methods: a Simplified "One-Stop Clinic for the Diagnosis of Infertility"

Standardized investigation of the couple at minimal costs is possible and undoubtedly will enhance the likelihood that infertile couples, both men and women, will come to the infertility centers. How to organize a one-stop diagnostic clinic has been described before (Ombelet et al., 2011). A questionnaire will be provided to both partners and can be adapted to the local situation in the specific locations and countries. Screening for infections and STDs can be done by using low-cost affordable screening tests. Since tubal obstruction associated with previous pelvic infections is the most important cause of infertility in many African countries, hysterosalpingography and/or hystero-salpingo-contrast-sonography are affordable techniques to detect this problem, easy to perform and

without major costs. A standard gynecological and fertility ultrasound scanning of the uterus and the ovaries can easily be done. Combining these techniques with an accurate medical history will identify the majority of women's infertility causes, such as ovulatory disorders, uterine malformations, and tubal infertility.

Male factor infertility can be evaluated by a simple semen analysis. Semen analyses can also be performed by well-trained paramedics, another important advantage for developing countries.

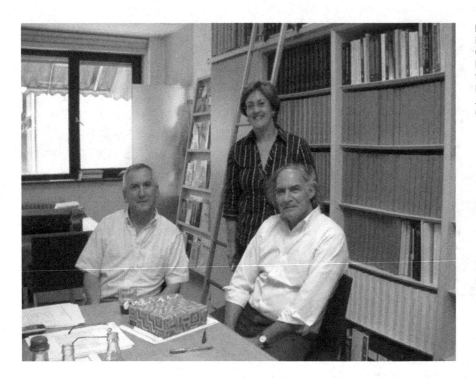

Figure 20.5 Meeting in 2009 in Genk with Willem Ombelet, Carin Huyser (University of Pretoria, South Africa), and the inventor of The Walking Egg simplified culture system, Jonathan Van Blerkom (University of Colorado, USA).

Owing to the high prevalence of uterine factors (Ashermann disease, intrauterine polyps, myomas, etc.), investigating the cavity is very crucial. Office mini-hysteroscopy to investigate intrauterine abnormalities has been simplified in its instrumentation and technique, so that it can become a non-expensive diagnostic technique accessible for every gynecologist, provided there has been appropriate training (Ombelet and Campo, 2007). All the procedures of the one-day diagnostic clinic can be performed by a small team of health care providers within a short period of time in an inexpensive setting (Ombelet and Campo, 2007). The consequences of the results for the management of the couple have to be discussed with them on that same day. More studies are needed to assess the reproducibility of "one-stop infertility clinics" in African countries.

Low-Cost Mild Ovarian Stimulation Protocols for IVF

In order to make infertility care more affordable in developing countries, **effective, cheap, and safe stimulation schemes** for in-vitro fertilization (IVF) need to be established. A review of the literature clearly shows the value and effectiveness of mild ovarian stimulation protocols in ART settings (Verberg et al., 2009). The use of clomiphene citrate (CC) or tamoxiphene, very cheap oral drugs, in combination with low-dose recombinant FSH or hMG (gonadotrophins), has been proven to be an optimal alternative with acceptable results, minimal side effects, and a very low complication rate (Verberg et al., 2009; Ferraretti et al., 2015). Monitoring of follicular development in an IVF cycle, as well as the timing of the hCG administration can be done solely on sonographic criteria with basic inexpensive ultrasound equipment thereby avoiding the need of expensive endocrine investigations.

Simplified IVF Laboratory Procedures

Another major challenge is **to reduce costs of laboratory procedures**, namely fertilization and culture of eggs and embryos for IVF. Different options and approaches have been developed or are presently being field-tested with promising results.

As part of The Walking Egg Project (Figure 20.5) we developed a new simplified method of IVF culturing, called the TWE lab method (Van Blerkom et al., 2014). With this new system, specifically designed for low resource settings, we can avoid the high costs of medical gases, complex incubation equipment, and infrastructure typical of IVF laboratories in high resource settings. For insemination of the eggs, we use only 1000–10,000 motile washed spermatozoa per oocyte, with very promising results, which makes this technique usable for more than 70% of the actual IVF/ICSI population (Genk data, not published).

Since development from insemination to transfer is undisturbed and in the same tube until embryo transfer, we can avoid many problems frequently occurring in regular IVF laboratories, such as unwanted temperature changes, air quality problems, etc.

Up to October 2017 a total number of 105 healthy babies have been born after using this technique with a low prevalence of low-birth weight and prematurity. According to our preliminary results, the perinatal outcome of babies born after using the simplified Walking Egg IVF culture system is reassuring.

Intravaginal fertilization and culture is another simplified method that has been used for many years (Mitri et al., 2015). A tube filled with culture medium containing the oocytes and washed spermatozoa is hermetically closed and placed in the vagina. It is held intravaginally by a diaphragm for incubation for 44–50 h, with very promising results.

Hurdles and Misunderstandings Surrounding the Implementation of Assisted Reproduction in Africa

The biggest obstacle in implementing health policies that consider infertility as a problem in Africa is the widespread belief that infertility is not a pressing problem in poor developing countries where fatal and contagious diseases remain uncontrolled. Because infertility as such is not directly life-threatening, it remains an entirely neglected problem in most African countries, despite the devastating social, psychological, economic, and personal consequences of being childless. Above this, inadequate or complete lack of rules and regulations concerning treatment conditions and commercial interests may lead to unethical practices in some African centers. Two arguments are always cited when talking about the issue of "infertility care" in resource-poor countries.

The "Limited Resources" Argument

Can expensive techniques be justified in countries where poverty is still an important issue and where health care systems still struggle with the immense problem of infectious diseases such as malaria,

tuberculosis, gonorrhoea, and HIV? The strong competition for funding is a reality in most African countries, leaving little space for expensive infertility treatment. Most health care providers argue that the limited resources should only be given to programs focussing on reducing STDs, postpartum and postabortion complications, rather than offering high-technology treatments to infertile couples: Prevention and education rather than cure. Nevertheless, it has been proven that HIV is three times more prevalent in infertile couples when compared to fertile controls in the same population (Dhont et al., 2011). HIV and infertility share the same determinant of high-risk sexual behavior. Public solutions are being applied for HIV; for infertility the solution is mainly found in the private sector. It is striking that budgets for HIV research are huge and the information on HIV is easily available while the contrary is true for infertility.

The "Overpopulation" Argument

The argument of **overpopulation** suggests that, in countries where overpopulation poses a demographic problem, infertility management should not be supported by the government.

It is well known that the world population is expected to increase to more than 9 billion by 2050. This increase will be most prominent in the poorest areas, such as Sub-Saharan Africa and South East Asia. Therefore, the idea of infertility treatment in Africa often evokes a feeling of discomfort and disbelief. A large part of the world population claims that helping infertile couples in these areas contradicts the interests of the countries and the world at large. However, this narrow approach contradicts human rights in general and reproductive rights in particular.

On the other hand, many developing countries have already succeeded in dropping their global fertility rate (number of children per woman) and United Nations data clearly show that in the majority of developing countries the mean fertility rate has already dropped from more than 5 to 2.6 and is expected to decline to 1.92 by mid-century, i.e. below the replacement level of 2.1. This doesn't mean that family-planning programs are not important anymore. Infertility care should be part of the concept of family planning, emphasizing that family planning is not only the prevention of unwanted pregnancies, but also includes promoting the chance of pregnancy in cases of involuntary childlessness. The expected population growth

165

in developing countries cannot be attributed to high fertility rates in the first instance anymore. As in most developed countries, an improved life expectancy will be the most important factor considering world population growth. Even in the least developed countries life expectancy is going to rise from an average of 51 years currently to 67 years in 2045–2050, which highlights the important issue of population aging.

Even if infertility treatment could be made more accessible in African countries it would probably account for less than 1% of all deliveries. Increasing efforts on family planning and health education should readily overcome this small contribution to the fertility rate.

Major Challenges and Hurdles in African Settings

Although more than 98% of the population in Africa cannot afford IVF because it is too expensive or because of a lack of IVF centers, establishing local low cost IVF programs seems to be a low priority, even from local health care providers, despite claims to the contrary. Our first experience with The Walking Egg project in Sub-Saharan Africa showed that considerable opposition from established and expensive IVF centers can be expected against low resource settings, but above this it has become apparent that, despite claims for a huge unmet need for IVF services made by well-intentioned individuals, medical institutions and government officials, they are not really ready or waiting for a viable option to be provided at the moment. Beside this, many hurdles can be expected when implementing low resource settings in Africa.

In almost all African countries there is a lack of well trained fertility specialists, embryologists, and IVF nurses. They are mostly trained for a short time in India and elsewhere, but in many cases the expertise is not good enough to ensure adequate experience in the field of assisted reproduction (Adageba et al., 2015). African training programs for the various key personnel in ART centers are lacking and are available only in Egypt and South Africa.

The lack of a reliable supply of good quality drugs, culture media, and other important consumables is another serious constraint when running or setting up an IVF center. In Ghana, drug supplies are sometimes erratic and most relevant consumables such as egg-retrieval needles, transfer catheters, Petri dishes, and culture media have to be imported from different countries. Subsequently, delays in delivery are frequently seen and high import duties contribute significantly to the cost of treatment (Adageba et al., 2015). Prices for drugs related to assisted reproduction vary a lot between different African countries; they are often even more expensive compared with Western countries.

Because the companies involved in the setting-up of new IVF centers are often based in foreign countries, many centers regularly face problems with maintenance of the equipment because it is expensive to bring in experienced service technicians/engineers from abroad.

In many African countries a stable power supply is not available, leading to frequent, even daily, power outages and fluctuations, although a stable power supply is a necessary requirement in the IVF laboratory. To run a successful IVF program requires standby generators, batteries, and powerful Uninterruptable Power System (UPS) systems to guarantee optimal laboratory conditions (Adageba et al., 2015). This surely also contributes to the costs.

The Walking Egg Project

The Walking Egg non-profit organization (npo) was founded in 2010 by scientists and an artist. Right from the start The Walking Egg has opted for a multidisciplinary and global approach to the problem of infertility and in cooperation with the Special Task Force (STF) on "Developing Countries and Infertility" of the European Society of Human reproduction and Embryology (ESHRE) and the WHO. The project aims to raise awareness surrounding childlessness in resource-poor countries and to make infertility care in all its aspects, including assisted reproductive technologies, available and accessible for a much larger part of the population. By simplifying the diagnostic and IVF laboratory procedures and by modifying the ovarian stimulation protocols for IVF, assisted reproductive techniques can be offered at affordable prices in the near future.

The Walking Egg also aims to integrate infertility care within the concept of family planning, emphasizing that family planning is not only the prevention of unwanted pregnancies, but also includes promoting the chance of pregnancy in case of involuntary childlessness. The ultimate goal of The Walking Egg is to work towards a world with less suffering caused by infertility. Figure 20.6 describes the setting-up of a

(a)

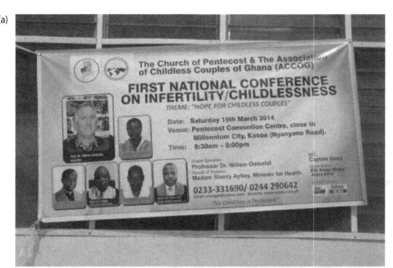

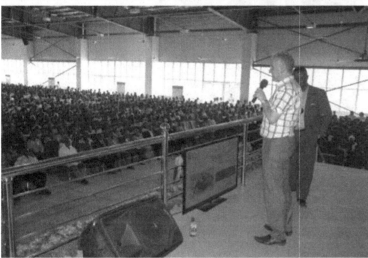

(b)

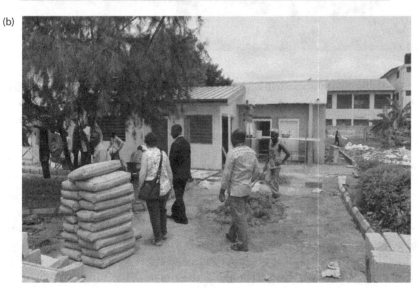

Figure 20.6 History of the implementation of the first Walking Egg center in Africa in Accra, Ghana. (a) Lecture about The Walking Egg project on the occasion of a meeting in Accra, Ghana, organized by the Church of Pentecost and ACCOG (Childless Couples of Ghana). The Pentecost Church decided to fund the implementation of a Walking Egg center in Accra. (b) Building up a Walking Egg center. (c) The final result. (d) Training in hysteroscopy of the Accra team in Genk (Belgium). (e) Starting up the first IVF trials with a batch of selected couples: Oocyte retrieval and laboratory performance. (f) On August 7, 2017, the first TWE baby was born in Accra.

(c)

Figure 20.6 (*cont.*)

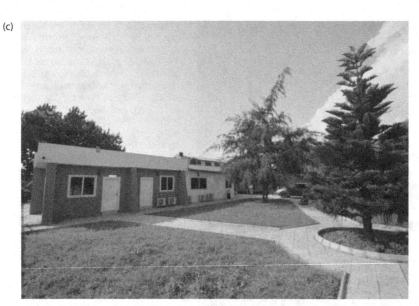

(d)

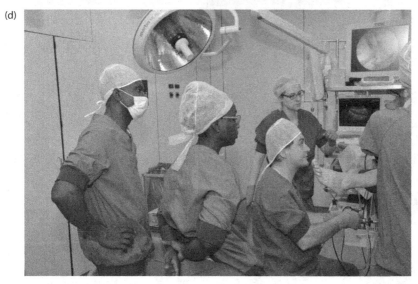

Walking Egg center in Accra, Ghana, including fund-raising, building the center, training by the team in Genk, batching of treatment cycles, and the birth of the first baby on August 7, 2017. The Walking Egg npo emphasizes the importance of preventing infertility as part of integrated reproductive health programs and the need to improve the quality of (low tech) infertility care in the public health sector by means of standard-ized guidelines, training of health staff and improved counselling (Gerrits and Shaw, 2010).

As evidence-based, affordable solutions begin to drive global guidance within both public and private health care systems, access to care for infertile couples will become one of the largest emerging fields in global medicine. We hope and believe that infertility care will be one of the more predominant components of future reproductive health care practice in Africa.

Conclusion

The magnitude of childlessness in African countries has dimensions beyond its prevalence. Although repro-ductive health education and prevention of infertility are number one priorities, the need for accessible diag-nostic procedures and new reproductive technologies is very high. Utilization of IVF is still very influenced

(e)

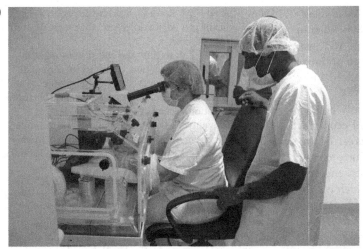

Figure 20.6 (cont.)

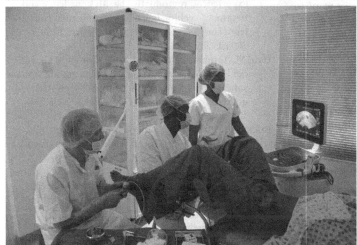

(f)

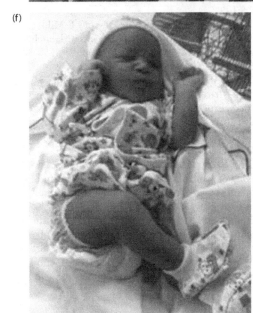

by affordable access to ART, which is related to insurance or public funding. Especially in Sub-Saharan Africa, the success and sustainability of ART will depend to a large extend on our ability to optimize these techniques in terms of availability, affordability and effectiveness.

Accessible infertility treatment can only be successfully introduced if socio-cultural and economic prerequisites are fulfilled and governments can be persuaded to support their introduction. We have to liaise with the relevant authorities to discuss the strengthening of infertility services, at the core of which lies the integration of infertility, contraceptive, and maternal health services within public health care structures.

Registration of data and quality control programs are extremely important if African countries want to become valuable players in the world of assisted reproduction. After a fascinating period of 40 years of IVF, only a small part of the African population benefits from these new technologies. The time has come to give equitable access to effective and safe infertility care in resource-poor countries as well.

In a world that needs vigorous control of population growth, concerns about infertility may seem odd, but the adoption of a small family norm makes the issue of involuntary infertility more pressing. If couples are urged to postpone or widely space pregnancies, it is imperative that they should be helped to achieve pregnancy when they so decide, in the more limited time they will have available.

Mahmoud Fathalla, *Former Director UNDP/ UNFPA/UNICEF/WHO/World Bank Special Programme of Research, Development and Research Training in Human Reproduction*

References

Adageba RK, Maya ET, Annan JJ, Damalie FJ. Setting up and running a successful IVF program in Africa: Prospects and challenges. *J Obstet Gynaecol India* 2015;65:155–157.

Adamson GD, DeMouzon J, Dyer S, et al. ICMART world report 2013. *Hum Reprod* 2017;32 Supplement 1 (i64–i65).

Boivin J, Bunting L, Collins JA, Nygren KG. International estimates of infertility prevalence and treatment-seeking: potential need and demand for infertility medical care. *Hum Reprod* 2007; 22:1506–1512.

Cates W, Farley TM, Rowe PJ. Worldwide patterns of infertility: is Africa different?' *Lancet* 1985; 2(8455):596–598.

Daar AS, Merali Z. Infertility and social suffering: the case of ART in developing countries. In Vayena E, Rowe PJ and Griffin PD (Eds.) *Current Practices and Controversies in Assisted Reproduction*. World Health Organization, Geneva, Switzerland, 2002.

Dhont N, Muvunyi C, Luchters S, et al. HIV infection and sexual behaviour in primary and secondary infertile relationships: a case-control study in Kigali, Rwanda. *Sex Transm Infect* 2011;87:28–34.

Dyer SJ, Patel M. The economic impact of infertility on women in developing countries – a systematic review. *Facts Views Vis ObGyn* 2012;4:102–109.

Dyer SJ, Abrahams N, Mokoena NE, van der Spuy ZM. "You are a man because you have children": experiences, reproductive health knowledge and treatment-seeking behaviour among men suffering from couple infertility in South Africa. *Hum Reprod* 2004;19:960–967.

Dyer SJ, Abrahams N, Mokoena NE, Lombard CJ, van der Spuy ZM. Psychological distress among women suffering from couple infertility in South Africa: a quantitative assessment. *Hum Reprod* 2005;20: 1938–1943.

Ericksen K, Brunette T. Patterns and predictors of infertility among African women: a cross-national survey of twenty-seven nations. *Soc Sci Med* 1996;42:209–220.

Fathalla MF, Sinding SW, Rosenfield A, Fathalla MM. Sexual and reproductive health for all: a call for action. *Lancet* 2006;368:2095–2100.

Fauser BC, Bouchard P, Coelingh Bennink HJ, et al. Alternative approaches in IVF. *Hum Reprod Update* 2002;8:1–9.

Ferraretti AP, Gianaroli L, Magli MC, Devroey P. Mild ovarian stimulation with clomiphene citrate launch is a realistic option for in vitro fertilization. *Fertil Steril* 2015;104:333–338.

Gerrits T, Shaw M. Biomedical infertility care in sub-Saharan Africa: A social science review of current practices, experiences and viewpoints. *Facts Views Vis ObGyn* 2010;2:194–207.

Huyser C, Boyd L. ART in South Africa: The price to pay. *Facts Views Vis Obgyn* 2013;5:91–99.

Inhorn MC, Patrizio P. Infertility around the globe: new thinking of gender, reproductive technologies and global movements in the 21st century. *Hum Reprod Update* 2015;21:411–426.

Mitri F, Esfandiari N, Coogan-Prewer J, et al. A pilot study to evaluate a device for the intravaginal culture of embryos. *Reprod Biomed Online* 2015;31:732–738.

Murage A, Muteshi MC, Githae F. Assisted reproduction services provision in a developing country: time to act? *Fertil Steril* 2011;96:966–968.

Nachtigall RD. International disparities in access to infertility services. *Fertil Steril* 2006;85:871–885.

Ombelet W. Global access to infertility care in developing countries: a case of human rights, equity and social justice. *Facts Views Vis Obgyn* 2011;3:257–266.

The Walking Egg Project: Universal access to infertility care – from dream to reality. *Facts Views Vis Obgyn* 2013;5:161–175.

Ombelet W, Campo R. Affordable IVF for developing countries. *Reprod Biomed Online* 2007;15:257–265.

Ombelet W, Cooke I, Dyer S, Serour G, Devroey P. Infertility and the provision of infertility medical services in developing countries. *Hum Reprod Update* 2008;14:605–621.

Van Balen F, Bos HMW. The social and cultural consequences of being childless in poor-resource areas. *Facts Views Vis Obgyn* 2009;1:106–121.

Van Blerkom J, Ombelet W, Klerkx E, et al. First births with a simplified culture system for clinical IVF and ET. *Reprod Biomed Online* 2014;28:310–320.

Verberg MF, Macklon NS, Nargund G, et al. Mild ovarian stimulation for IVF. *Hum Reprod Update* 2009;15:13–29.

The Development of In-Vitro Fertilization in Russia

Vladislav Korsak and Anatoly Nikitin

Some of the early discoveries in reproductive biology were made in Russia. It started with Karl Ernst von Baer (1792–1876), a Prussian–Estonian embryologist who discovered the mammalian ovum and the notochord, and established the new science of comparative embryology alongside comparative anatomy. In 1827 he described his discovery of the mammalian ovum (egg) in his *De Ovi Mammalium et Hominis Genesi* (*On the Mammalian Egg and the Origin of Man*), thereby establishing that mammals, including human beings, develop from eggs.

In 1897, V. S. Gruzdev, a Russian obstetrician and gynecologist, who worked in St. Petersburg, published an article about studies on fertilization of eggs obtained from a female rabbit's follicles that he transferred to the animal's egg tube in sperm suspension (Gruzdev, 1897). Based on his experience, he concluded that fertilization adequacy is connected with the degree of the egg maturity. In the article he mentioned that D. O. Ott had been the first in Russia to conduct experiments on artificial insemination of rabbits.

In 1934, the Russian researcher O. V. Krasovskaya reported on in-vitro fertilization of rabbit eggs. In 1936, she published three articles about a successful transfer of rabbit embryos after IVF (Krazovskaya, 1936).

From 1955 to 1959, G. N. Petrov, a postgraduate student under the supervision of Professor B. P. Khvatov, in Crimean State Medical Institute, Simferopol, studied fertilization of human eggs obtained from ovaries that had been removed due to gynecological diseases. The first publication was in the *Book of Abstracts of the Institute Symposium* of June, 1955, pp. 14–15: "On fertilization and embryonic fission of a human ovicell." It is known that G. N. Petrov transferred some embryos that he had obtained to women. A newspaper of the time published an article about a pregnancy that had terminated in the early stage. However, there are neither case reports nor documents about it. Petrov himself never spoke about it.

The first report in the world about in-vitro cultivation of a fertilized and splitting human egg was the above-mentioned "On fertilization and embryonic fission of a human ovicell" (Crimea, Simferopol, 1955); see Figure 21.1. A comprehensive article about the results of the study was published in 1958 (Petrov, 1958).

In 1959, G. N. Petrov defended a thesis "The Process of *In Vitro* Fertilization of Some Mammalian and Human Eggs."

Professor P. G. Svetlov (of the D. O. Ott Institute, St. Petersburg) disputed Petrov's results, pointing out that Petrov's "fission of fertilized eggs" looked more like degenerative oocyte fragmentation (Svetlov and On, 1959).

From a present-day perspective it is clear that Professor Svetlov is right. Petrov did not have culture media, he did not know about sperm capacitation, nor about the importance of carbon dioxide. He did not have access to foreign scientific publications. We value the work of Professor B. P. Khvatov and G. N. Petrov's team for their research ideas and their commitment to obtaining a result in the circumstances prevailing behind the Iron Curtain at the time – a complete absence of information about similar work abroad.

Laboratory scientists at the Laboratory of Clinical Embryology at the All-Union Maternal Health Centre in Moscow, headed by Professor B. V. Leonov, and at the Laboratory of Human Early Embryogenesis at the D. O. Ott Research Institute of Obstetrics and Gynecology in St. Peterburg (then Leningrad), headed by Professor A. I. Nikitin, who started working at the end of the 1960s, were pioneers of IVF in Russia. The first child born after IVF in Russia, a girl, was born in Moscow in March 1986; the second child, a boy, was born in St. Petersburg in November 1986 (Lukin et al., 1988; Nikitin, 1989).

Commercialization of IVF in Russia

Commercialization of IVF in Russia was a direct consequence of the "perestroika" reforms initiated by

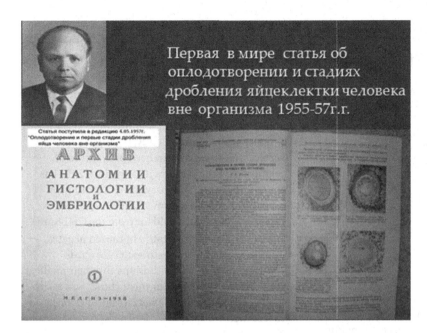

Figure 21.1 The first report on in-vitro cultivation of a fertilized and splitting human egg (Crimea, Simferopol, 1955).

M. Gorbachev in 1985. The centrally planned economy disappeared together with the USSR. An economic collapse, hyperinflation, and total deficit – that's what a new Russia had inherited from the communist regime. In medicine, there were just enough funds for emergency care; financing of research decreased radically and almost stopped in many areas. Qualified doctors and researchers were leaving the country ("brain drain"); those who stayed here and got scanty salaries started looking for sideline jobs. Part-timers from among university professors and researchers with academic degrees joined the ranks of night watchmen, yard keepers, kitchen workers, and outdoor salespeople. Yet at the time of the economy crash the new Russian Constitution formalized equal rights of government and private property. Commercial activity was allowed and commercialization started in all spheres of economy.

Private medical clinics appeared in Russia at the very beginning of the 1990s. IVF clinics were among the first, founded by professionals who had formerly worked in state institutions. In the USSR, only four state institutions had IVF departments: two in Moscow (with B. V. Leonov and V. M. Zdanovsky as Heads of Departments), one in Leningrad (later St. Petersburg; A. I. Nikitin) and one in Kharkiv (F.V. Dakhno).

IVF specialists from Moscow (V. M. Zdanovsky, E. A. Kalinina, A. P. Lazorev, and K. N. Kechiyan) and from Leningrad (A. Nikitin) created the first five private ART centers in Russia. All but one are still functioning today.

In December 1992, Yury Verlinsky received authorization to open an affiliate of Chicago Reproductive Genetics Institute in St. Petersburg. Thus the sixth private commercial institution, named the International Centre of Reproductive Medicine (ICRM), appeared. At the same time, a private clinic was opened in Samara (V. I. Karnaukh).

According to the first RAHR ART Register report, in 1995 there were already 12 clinics in Russia, eight of them private clinics (67%) that performed 80% of ART cycles. The share of government centers started growing with an improvement of the economic situation during the past 10 years. However, commercial centers still lead both in number and in volume of rendered ART services. In 2015 (the latest report of the RAHR ART Register), the share of commercial centers was 65.3%, and they performed 66.3% of all ART cycles.

With the end of state distribution of goods and services, the market was opened, and almost all internationally known companies working in ART came to Russia and are still supplying their products here. Russian ART centers are equipped as well as Western clinics, they use the same medications and consumables, and perform absolutely all ART programs. According to EIM ESHRE, in 2014 Russia accounted

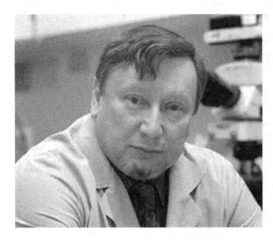

Figure 21.2 Yury Verlinsky (1943–2009).

for the second highest number of ART cycles (94,985) in Europe. In 2015, the RAHR ART Register was informed of 111,972 cycles. Russia is approaching the **millionth** ART cycle. Treatment efficacy in Russian ART programs is comparable with average European results and even slightly higher.

Yury Verlinsky's commercial programs notably contributed to the development of IVF in Russia and in the former USSR Republics (Figure 21.2). Under his supervision, the Director of RGI programs in Russia, M. Anshina, and ICRM staff participated in the establishment of commercial centers/clinics in Sochi, Krasnoyarsk, Tyumen, Minsk (Belarus), and Kiev (Ukraine). ICRM in St. Petersburg was the first center in Russia to achieve cycles of preimplantation diagnosis for cystic fibrosis in 1994; the first pregnancy after ICSI in 1995; the first pregnancy under the surrogacy program; and the establishment of the first Donor Egg Bank.

In 1991, IVF specialists initiated the establishment of the Russian Association of Human Reproduction (RAHR). RAHR is a non-governmental association of professionals working in different areas of reproductive medicine. The RAHR budget is formed with annual membership fees, charitable contributions of RAHR members, ART centers and clinics, and income from holding conferences. Yuri Verlinsky was involved in the RAHR activities from 1992 until his death in 2009. While only 30–50 enthusiasts gathered together at the first conferences, more than 1300 professionals met at the XXVI Conference of RAHR in 2016 to celebrate the 30th anniversary of IVF in Russia (the birth of the first "in-vitro" child), the 25th anniversary of RAHR, and the 20th anniversary of the RAHR ART Register.

And yet, since "commercialization" means market and competition, together with advantages, there appeared disadvantages of the process.

- Expenditures of private centers associated with facilities, preparation and procurement of equipment, labor costs, high market price for consumables, drugs, etc., significantly raised the cost of and, consequently, the price for, ART services. Not everyone in need of this kind of medical care could afford it (only since 2013 has the Compulsory [Statutory] Health Insurance (CHI) covered the treatment; in 2017, 60,000 cycles will have been paid for from the CHI fund).

- Inaccessibility of the treatment caused negative attitudes of some people in society towards commercial medical institutions and their medical staff. "They cash in on our misfortune" was easily perceived by a former Soviet citizen who was used to free medical care.

- The necessity to survive in a competitive environment brought about many negative developments, like deceit, officials' protectionism, qualified labor pirating, bribes, and a protection racket in the 1990s, and many other things that the West had long left behind.

- Having no opportunity to finance medicine as required, the government first allowed the creation of cooperatives on the premises of state medical institutions with the participation of their staff, and then allowed these institutions to provide paid services. Naturally, it immediately turned out the following way: free services with two weeks' waiting tine, paid services available right now, without delay. Thus, at the expense of the population, the issue was decided with state institutions' maintenance and staff salaries. It caused unfair competition at the services market, but the quality of medical care became the crucial thing in the struggle for existence. Private medicine survived and is developing.

- The number of ART clinics that have been established in Russia during the past two decades, and the number of cycles performed, are shown in Figures 21.3 and 21.4.

Summarizing the above, it can be said that commercialization of IVF in Russia:

- not only saved IVF during the heaviest economic crisis of the 1990s, but boosted this area of medicine in Russia;

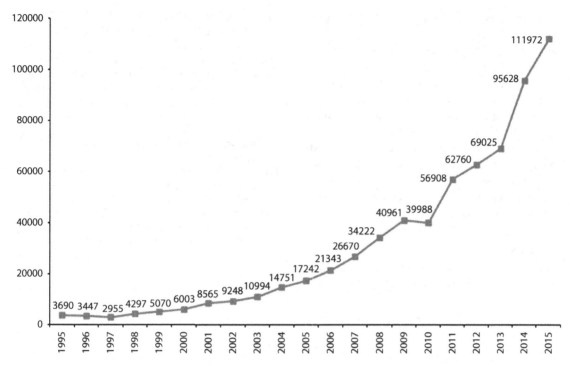

Figure 21.3 The number of cycles of IVF/ART in Russia, 1995–2015.

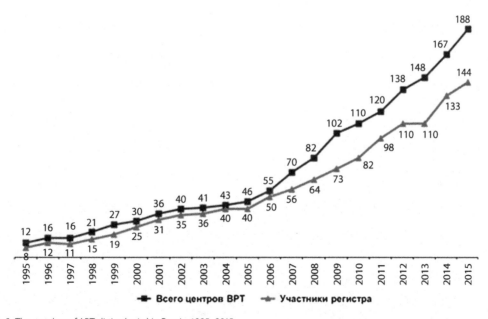

Figure 21.4 The number of ART clinics (units) in Russia, 1995–2015.

- made it possible to get high quality, effective ART services in Russia;
- owing to the high success rates achieved in commercial centers, in 2007 the Government came to a decision to pay for infertility treatment using ART, first through specific federal and regional programs and, starting in 2013, out of the funds of the Compulsory Health Insurance;
- encouraged existing highly skilled ART specialists to stay in Russia and new professionals to appear;
- made it possible to create RAHR – a community of real professionals in the sphere of medical assisted reproduction (MAR).

References

Gruzdev VS. An experiment with artificial fertilization of mammalian eggs. *Vrach* 1897;42:1199–1203.

Krasovskaya OV. A transfer of a rabbit egg in the other animal's uterus. *Arch Anat Hystol Embryol* 1936;15:135–145.

Lukin VA, Leonov BV, Kalinina EA, et al. A successful outcome of pregnancy resulting from in vitro egg fertilization and embryo transfer in woman's uterine cavity. *Obstetr and Gynek* 1988;4:38–41.

Nikitin AI, Kitaev EM, Savitsky GA, et al. IVF fertilization in humans with further successful embryo implantation and childbirth. *Arch Anat Hystol Embryol* 1989;2: 39–43.

Petrov GN. In vitro fertilization and first stages of embryonic fission of a human egg. *Arch Anat Hystol Embryol* 1958;35:88–93.

Svetlov PG. On G.N. Petrov's article "In vitro fertilization and first stages of embryonic fission of a human egg". *Arch Anat Hystol Embryol* 1959;36:79.

22

The Application of In-Vitro Fertilization in the Management of the Infertile Male

David M. de Kretser

It is always important to understand the statistics relating to couples who wish to have children. Eighty-five percent of normal couples usually achieve a pregnancy within one year of trying. If investigations indicate there is a fertility problem in the male or female, there is still a chance of a spontaneous pregnancy occurring, but, as the duration of infertility increases, the chances of a pregnancy occurring decrease (Bhasin et al., 1994).

In-vitro fertilization (IVF) was a major development in the technologies available to assist infertile couples to have their own children. Initially, the focus was on the female partner who had obstructed Fallopian tubes as the management of anovulatory infertility had been resolved by the availability of the human gonadotrophins, follicle stimulating hormone (FSH), and luteinizing hormone (LH), for the induction of ovulation. In fact, the experience in the use of gonadotrophins to stimulate ovulation was of great assistance in determining the best way of using FSH and LH in IVF to stimulate multiple ovarian follicular development in preparation for oocyte collection to enable in-vitro fertilization.

Clearly, the availability of several oocytes for IVF enhanced the possibility of having embryos available to be transferred to the uterus. It also raised the adverse possibility of high-order multiple pregnancies if the transfer of multiple embryo was successful, an outcome that increased as experience in IVF led to improvements.

The possibility of using IVF in the management of male infertility emerged as only small numbers of sperm were required to fertilize oocytes in vitro. It was during a casual conversation with Gab Kovacs over sandwiches in the Tuesday evening Reproductive Medicine Clinic at Prince Henry's Hospital, that I suggested that maybe males with subfertility and decreased numbers of motile sperm could achieve fertilization in vitro, since only small numbers of motile sperm were required. In fact, techniques to isolate the most active motile sperm were developed, which enhanced

outcomes. This led to Monash IVF establishing a "Male Factor Group," which I chaired, with Chris Yates (a PhD student and embryologist) becoming the male factor scientist, Jillian McDonald the nurse co-ordinator, and Gab Kovacs the IVF clinician. I took a sabbatical for two months and selected the couples that might benefit from amongst my large infertility practice.

Although IVF offers a potential way for infertile men to achieve a pregnancy with their partner, there should always be a full assessment of the male to ascertain the cause of his infertility. Some causes, such as decreased sperm counts due to decreased FSH and LH levels, were amenable to treatment with those hormones when they became available as injectable preparations. Treatment to restore sperm counts to normal in men with hypo-gonadotrophic hypogonadism can take several months, as the time taken to produce sperm from spermatogonia in humans is approximately 70 days, a time frame that cannot be speeded up (Clermont et al., 1961). The spermatogonia, primary and secondary spermatocytes, and spermatids cannot be induced to "speed up" their development. The spermatogonia, primary and secondary spermatocytes, and the final stage of the transformation of a round cell into a sperm with its condensed nucleus, progress at rates that are fixed for each germ cell type. The different germ cells progress at different rates that are fixed or degenerate and are phagocytosed by the Sertoli cells.

The potential of using sperm from men with low sperm counts, poor sperm motility, and those with an increased percentage of abnormally shaped sperm to achieve a pregnancy became a reality. It was possible to separate the highly motile sperm for incubation with the oocytes and some degree of selectivity could be obtained.

Initially, the "swim-up" technique was used, as described by Lopata in 1976, followed by a centrifugation–migration technique, with the sperm pellet being re-suspended and motile sperm isolated from the uppermost portion of the suspension. Later, by adding Ficoll (Pharmacia, Sweden), a density gradient interface was achieved, allowing only motile spermatozoa to pass across it. Albumin columns, glass wool columns, and Percoll gradients were all utilized as sperm selection techniques, the aim being to obtain the best sample to add to the oocyte(s) (Yates et al., 1989).

The use of microdrops for insemination was then adopted, using low volumes of semen with reasonable quality. This achieved good results in mild to moderate male factor subfertility (Ombelet, 2006).

The availability of this technical development led Graeme Southwick and Peter Temple-Smith in Australia to surgically aspirate seminiferous tubules with the largest diameter under an operating microscope and to isolate the small numbers of sperm obtained for IVF, thus achieving pregnancies. The first case of obstructive azoospermia successfully treated by surgical sperm retrieval and IVF was for a man who had a previous vasectomy. Graeme Southwick (plastic surgeon/microsurgeon) and Peter Temple-Smith (research scientist) were part of the surgical team that retrieved small numbers of sperm, which were then used in IVF. This resulted in the birth of "Baby Joseph" in 1985 (Figure 22.1).

The possibility of using sperm microinjection techniques was first suggested as early as 1984, when Alan Trounson wrote: "The possibility of microsurgical fertilization procedures are also being investigated in our laboratory" (Trounson, 1984). Trounson and colleagues reported success in mouse oocytes with subzonal sperm injection (SUZI) (Lacham et al., 1989) and the technique was replicated in humans, with the first human birth using SUZI being reported in Singapore in 1988 (Ng et al., 1988). This technique had a very low success rate.

A further major technical development, namely that of intra-cytoplasmic sperm injection (ICSI), became a reality when it became possible, with the use of fine injecting pipettes, to insert a single sperm into the cytoplasm of an oocyte. The development of ICSI and the first successful birth in Brussels, is described in detail in Chapter 9. The ICSI technique first came to the awareness of the Australian scientific community at a Serono Symposium held in Adelaide, in December 1992, when Professor Andre Van Steirteghem presented the Brussels experience and stated that the results were far superior then those achieved with SUZI (McLachlan, 1997).

Why was there a need to use these technologies to help men with poor fertility to successfully father children? The problem arose from the fact that in only

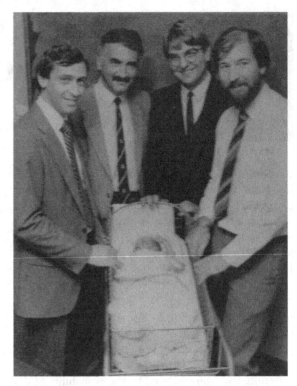

Figure 22.1 Baby Joseph. The first baby born after surgical removal of sperm from the epididymis using IVF. From left to right, Graeme Southwick (microsurgeon), Gab Kovacs (IVF clinician and obstetrician), Chris Yates (IVF scientist), and Peter Temple-Smith (research scientist).

10–20% of such men was it possible to diagnose the cause of their infertility, and in many instances there was no cure. It was certainly possible to indicate to a man that his sperm count was below normal levels, or that only a small percentage of his sperm were motile, or that many of his sperm were abnormally shaped. The latter usually indicated that the sperm were unlikely to be able to fertilize an egg.

Until IVF and then ICSI were utilized, there was no treatment for the majority of these men.

Nevertheless, there is now usually a full assessment of the male partner. Most doctors consulting subfertile men have a set of testicular sizes, known as an orchidometer, with which to compare the patient's testicular size. Normal testes range between 15–35 ml in size after puberty is complete.

Some men having such an assessment may have no sperm in their ejaculate. It would then be required by the doctor to determine if the testes were manufacturing sperm but since there was an obstruction in the epididymis or vas, the sperm were prevented from getting into the ejaculate. If the testes were of normal size then the likelihood of an obstruction is high whereas small testes would suggest abnormal development with very poor sperm production.

Should an obstruction be diagnosed, there a two possible approaches. The first would be to biopsy the testes to confirm spermatogenesis was normal. A surgical exploration for the epididymis would enable definition of the presence of an obstruction and the possibility of a microsurgical reconstruction. The second option is to obtain sperm from the testes by biopsy. This can be either by a needle biopsy under local anesthetic (pioneered by Gordon Baker and Ian Craft in London), or by open testicular biopsy. The latter has been further refined by using an operating microscope to identify distended tubules, which were the most likely regions of the tubules from which to harvest small numbers of sperm (Chapter 26). This is possible even if sperm counts in the ejaculate were severely depleted, e.g. less than 100,000 sperm.

However, if the biopsy shows germ cell arrest when spermatogenesis ceases at a particular point, e.g. the primary spermatocyte stage wherein meiosis has not been completed, the chances of finding small areas where sperm are still being produced is very small.

In the context of IVF, even very small number of sperm can be successfully used by ICSI and hence sperm samples can be stored until required for future IVF or ICSI.

The management of couples with infertility arising from a male cause frequently results in the use of IVF since treatment options to restore sperm counts are limited. Certainly, obstructions in the epididymis and vas deferens are capable of surgical management to bypass the obstruction using microsurgery. If unsuccessful, sperm taken from the testis itself can be used for ICSI.

References

Bhasin S, de Kretser DM, Baker HW. Pathophysiology and natural history of male infertility. *J Clin Endocrinol Metab*1994; 79: 1525–1529.

Clermont Y, Huckins C. Microscopic anatomy of the sex cords and seminiferous tubules in growing and adult male albino rats. *Am J Anat* 1961;108:79–97.

Lacham O, Trounson A, Holden C, Mann J, Sathananthan H. Fertilization and development of mouse eggs injected under the zona pellucida with single spermatozoa treated to induce the acrosome reaction. *Gamete Res* 1989;23:233–243.

McLachlan RI. The use of assisted reproductive technology for the treatment of male infertility. In: Kovacs GT (Ed.) *The Subfertility Handbook: A Clinician's Guide.* Cambridge University Press, 1997, pp.124–138.

Ng SC, Bongso A, Ratnam SS, et al. Pregnancy after transfer of sperm under the zona. *Lancet* 1988;2:790.

Ombelet W. Assisted reproductive technologies . In: Schill W, Comhaire F, Hargreave T (Eds.) *Andrology for the Clinician*. Springer, Berlin, 2006, pp. 578–584.

Trounson A. In vitro fertilization and embryo preservation ion. In: Trounson A, Wood C (Eds.) *In Vitro Fertilization And Embryo*. Churchill Livingstone, Edinburgh, 1984, pp.111–130.

Yates CA, Thomas C, Kovacs GT, de Kretser DM. Andrology, male factor and IVF. In: Wood C, Trounson A. (Eds.) *Clinical in Vitro Fertilization*, Second Edition. Springer-Verlag, 1989, pp. 95–112.

The Development of Preimplantation Genetic Diagnosis for Monogenic Disease and Chromosome Imbalance

Leeanda Wilton

The Beginning – Development of Embryo Biopsy

Some of the first reported attempts at sampling cells from embryos were in the 1950s by Andrzej Tarkowski, the eminent Polish scientist, who studied the development of single mouse blastomeres in vitro. When I was a young post-doc, Andrzej visited the lab where I was working and I was privileged to spend time with this quietly-spoken, respectful, brilliant man discussing the biology of embryonic cell allocation and commitment, an understanding of which was crucial to the development of embryo biopsy. He gave me a personally annotated copy of his PhD thesis, which remains one of my treasured possessions (Figure 23.1). In 1968, Gardner and Edwards biopsied trophectoderm cells from rabbit blastocysts and looked for the sex chromatin body, which is only found in cells from females, in the biopsied material. Transferred embryos were of the predicted gender, but unfortunately this biopsy approach was not successful in human embryos.

It took until the mid-1980s before scientists, notably Anne McLaren, began seriously considering that embryo biopsy and preimplantation genetic diagnosis (PGD) could be developed into a clinical technique. I started working in this field in 1985, and although successful embryo biopsy had been achieved in animal embryos many years earlier, there had been no studies demonstrating an effective biopsy technique where the embryo survival rate was high, which was an obvious prerequisite if clinical application were ever to be achieved. In fact, the possibility that one could remove a single cell from an embryo, whilst keeping the embryo alive, and then perform an accurate genetic diagnosis on that one cell was thought by many to be a fool's errand. We took the approach of removing a single cell from a four-cell embryo believing this would be a good compromise between having sufficient material and time to perform a diagnosis and minimizing

the cellular loss of the embryo (Wilton and Trounson, 1986, 1989). In the UK, Marilyn Monk, along with Alan Handyside, used a mouse strain that was a model for Lesch–Nyhan syndrome because of a deficiency in the hypoxanthine phosphoribosyl-transferase enzyme (HPRT). They were able to diagnose HPRT deficiency in embryos by biopsying one or two cells at the eight-cell stage (Monk et al., 1987). Audrey Muggleton-Harris had cleverly sampled trophectoderm cells that were just hatching from the zona pellucida and she, too, demonstrated the diagnosis of HPRT deficiency via blastocyst biopsy using Monk's assay. A useful review of some of this early work can be found in Harper (2009).

Such proof-of-principle studies were extremely valuable, but if clinical PGD was ever to be realized it was essential to demonstrate that embryo biopsy could be performed with a very high success rate, that is that almost no embryos were destroyed during the procedure and that embryo viability was maintained. Hence, from the mid 1980s much of the focus on the development of PGD technologies was on embryo biopsy, using animal embryos as a model for humans. My own work in this period was part of my post-doctoral position at the Centre for Early Human Development (CEHD), directed by Alan Trounson. We started using micromanipulation, which was very novel at the time (Figure 23.2). This was prior to the development of intra–cytoplasmic sperm injection (ICSI) and micromanipulation techniques were only just beginning to be applied to mammalian embryos. It seems so simple now, but back then embryo biopsy was very challenging. There were no instruction manuals or publications to follow and there were no commercial manufacturers of micropipettes so I made all the pipettes myself. This painstaking work involved pulling glass capillaries and then using a micro-beveller to grind the glass tip of the biopsy pipette to a point that would pierce the zona pellucida. A microforge was used to gently heat the tip

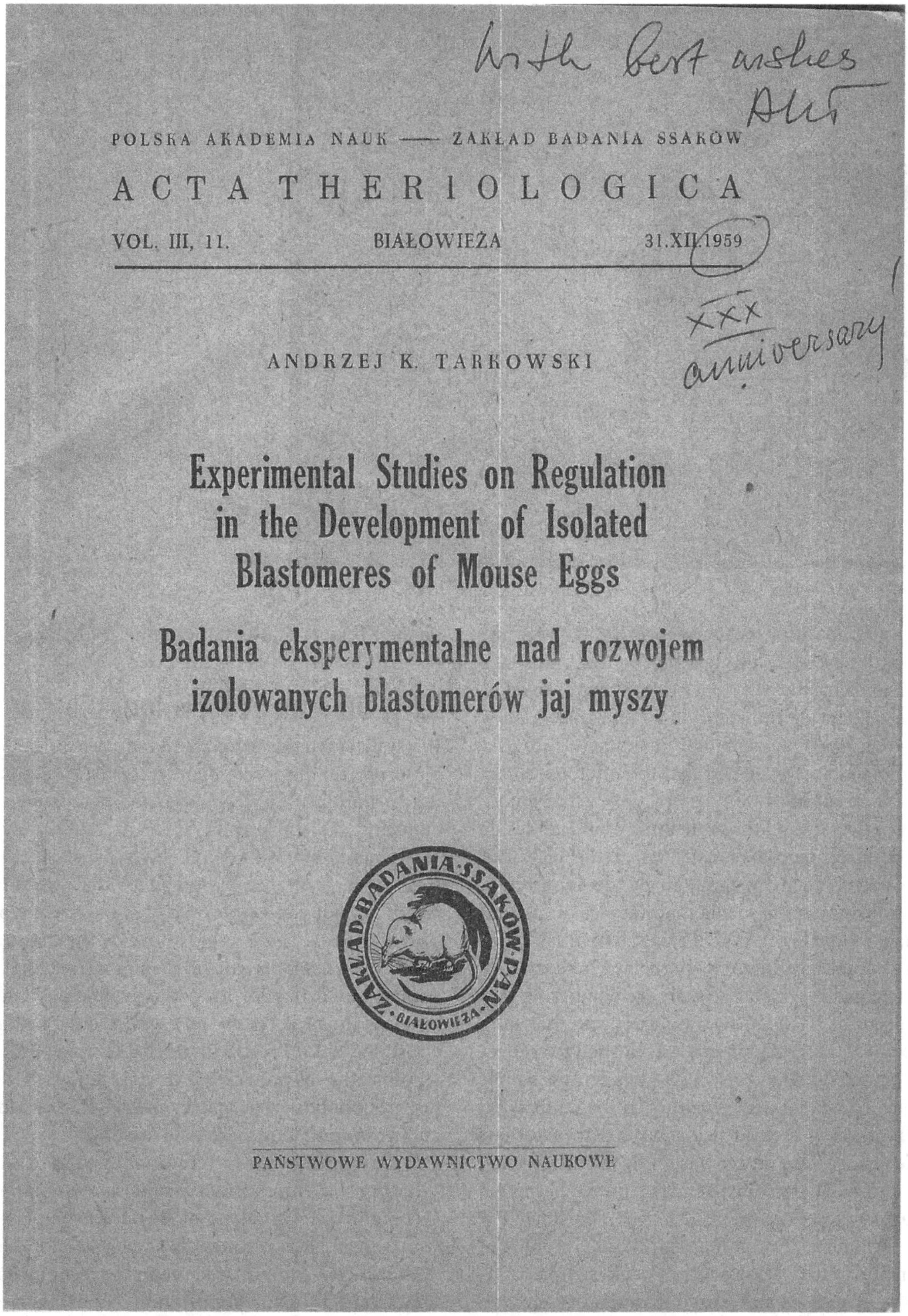
With best wishes

POLSKA AKADEMIA NAUK —— ZAKŁAD BADANIA SSAKÓW

ACTA THERIOLOGICA

VOL. III, 11. BIAŁOWIEŻA 31.XII.1959

XXX anniversary

ANDRZEJ K. TARKOWSKI

Experimental Studies on Regulation in the Development of Isolated Blastomeres of Mouse Eggs

Badania eksperymentalne nad rozwojem izolowanych blastomerów jaj myszy

ZAKŁAD·BADANIA·SSAKÓW·P.A.N. ·BIAŁOWIEŻA·

PAŃSTWOWE WYDAWNICTWO NAUKOWE

Figure 23.1 My treasured copy of the seminal thesis of the late Professor Andrzej Tarkowski, given to me on the 30th anniversary of its publication.

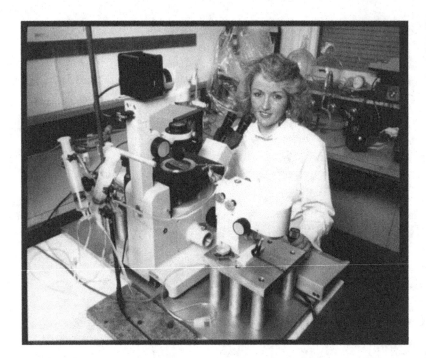

Figure 23.2 The author, sitting at the micromanipulation set-up, in about 1986 at the Centre for Early Human Development, Queen Victoria Medical Centre, Melbourne.

of the pipette to soften the sharp edge. It was a very fine compromise between having a pipette that was sharp enough to pierce the zona, but not so sharp as to damage the cells inside the embryo. I spent many, many hours each week painstakingly manufacturing glass micropipettes and it seemed that too often an unfortunate bump or knock would destroy all of that work.

In London around the same time, Alan Handyside was perfecting biopsy of embryos at the eight-cell stage, made easier by temporarily de-compacting embryos using culture media that was free of calcium and magnesium. In the United States, John Buster proposed a completely different approach where patients could become pregnant naturally (remembering that the majority of PGD patients would not have infertility problems) and then the uterus was flushed to recover a blastocyst. Although this was a tantalizingly simple approach compared with obtaining embryos through IVF, the risks of a child being born with a serious genetic disease if the lavage was unsuccessful were too great, and PGD after uterine lavage never became a clinical technique.

In Melbourne it took me many, many months of trial and error to develop a technique to sample a single blastomere from an embryo that retained embryo viability. Because we were using mouse embryos, I was able to thoroughly test viability right through to live

birth, a luxury that is not possible when developing novel technologies using human embryos.

Early Diagnostic Techniques

In parallel with this work, there were two other aspects of the project that were ongoing. Firstly, I was attempting to multiply the DNA available for diagnosis by culturing the single cells. This was moderately successful and I was able to reliably grow about 20 cells from a single mouse blastomere, which we thought might be enough to perform a PCR-based gene/mutation diagnosis. This was very novel at the time and in 1986 I presented this work at the annual meeting of the Australian Society for Reproductive Biology and was awarded the prize for the best work from a young scientist. Little did I realize that reliable single-cell DNA amplification by polymerase chain reaction (PCR) was just around the corner, which obviated the need for cell culture for mutation analysis at least.

Additionally, we were very interested in being able to perform a chromosome diagnosis on embryos by looking at the karyotype of single cells. I partnered with Ismail Kola who was also a post-doctoral fellow at the CEHD. Molecular karyotyping techniques, like fluorescent in-situ hybridization (FISH) and comparative genomic hybridization (CGH) were yet to be invented, so we had to rely on traditional karyotyping and metaphase preparation by mitotic arrest and cell spreading onto microscope slides. Ismail had developed a very clever method of applying this blood karyotyping system to just a single cell. We used embryos from a Robertsonian translocation model mouse strain, which had a fusion of two acrocentric chromosomes meaning the embryos were at high risk of being trisomic. Embryos were biopsied at the four-cell stage and the single blastomere karyotyped to predict the ploidy of the embryo, which we managed to do with 100% accuracy. This resulted in the first diagnosis of a chromosome abnormality in a preimplantation embryo (Kola and Wilton, 1991).

Public Controversy in Victoria

We always knew that the prospect of embryo biopsy and preimplantation genetic diagnosis was going to be ethically controversial. To his credit, Alan Trounson was insistent that we were open about the work in an effort to educate the general public. We held public meetings and invited the press to discuss what we were doing. We received vocal and strong opposition from many directions. We were not surprised that conservative religious groups and "Right to Life" organizations were opposed to our work, and we received some rather nasty, often anonymous, correspondence. I recall one occasion, in about 1986, where I was giving a talk about the possibilities of PGD at a public forum in Melbourne. Members of the Right to Life organization picketed the meeting and, throughout my entire presentation, paraded up and down at the back of the room waving placards objecting to what I was saying! This was very disconcerting for a young post-doc and I do recall wondering (just briefly) if I had made a mistake getting into this field. We also received disapproval from left-leaning feminist organizations in Australia who, in the 1980s, were opposed to IVF in general. What was unexpected was that we received significant criticism from some members of the scientific community, particularly those who worked in clinical genetics and prenatal diagnosis in Melbourne. In essence they believed it would never be possible to perform a genetic diagnosis on just one cell.

By about 1988, we had developed reliable and reproducible embryo biopsy and genetic diagnosis using mouse embryos and we were ready to begin testing the procedures using surplus human embryos. Human IVF and embryo research were controversial in many parts of the world, and our home state of Victoria had

been the first in the globe to enact legislation governing the practice of IVF that included the establishment of the Standing Review and Advisory Committee on Infertility (SRACI) in 1984, which was a statutory body made up of ethicists, theologians, lawyers, and others, who could make decisions independent of government (see Chapter 28). There had been much publicity about the prohibition of human embryo research in the legislation, but what was less well publicized was that this prohibition applied to embryos that were more than 14 days old and that embryo research prior to 14 days was permissible, with the approval of SRACI. We submitted a carefully crafted proposal to SRACI, requesting permission to use surplus two- or three-day-old human embryos to replicate our extensive mouse experiments. This approval was granted. Unfortunately for us, this came at a politically sensitive time when there was a forthcoming critical by-election. Opponents of embryo research were very active in lobbying government and they came out in force for this election campaign. Somehow news of our approval to perform human embryo research became public and the sitting member of the government announced that there would be no "brave new world" in the State of Victoria. So despite having fulfilled all stringent scientific and ethical requirements to get our research approved, we were advised by members of the government not to proceed with the work. This was extremely frustrating. We had believed PGD had the potential to make a huge difference to many people's lives and we were very invested in bringing it to fruition. However, it was difficult to see how this could ever happen in what had become a very restrictive research environment in the State of Victoria.

Development of Single Cell Fluorescent In-Situ Hybridization (FISH)

Right around this time I accepted an offer to take up a position as Research Fellow at the Institute of Zoology at Regent's Park in London, to work on the application of reproductive technologies, such as IVF and embryo cryopreservation, to the preservation of endangered species. I also saw it as an opportunity to continue the human PGD research that we had wanted to do in Victoria in the regulated, but less restrictive, human embryo research environment that existed in the United Kingdom at that time. I contacted Professor Robert Winston, head of the Hammersmith IVF unit, and suggested that, rather than work in opposition, with my impending arrival in London we could work together. I was very grateful for the enthusiastic response not only from Robert, but from Alan Handyside and the rest of the Hammersmith team. They were very keen for me apply our techniques of karyotyping single mouse blastomeres to human embryos. This proved to be much more difficult than anticipated as human embryos did not behave in the same way as the very well-studied, synchronous, and uniform mouse embryos. The cell cycle of mouse embryos was very regular and it was easy to anticipate when the next cell division would occur. We would add colchicine to the single cell, to induce metaphase arrest, at a very defined time before the next cell division was expected. This turned out to be very difficult to predict in human embryos as the cell cycle was often long and irregular, and the blastomeres within one embryo often had asynchronous cell division. This meant long exposure to colchicine, which we knew would produce very shortened chromosomes that would be difficult to karyotype. I spent many, many hours at the research labs of the Hammersmith IVF unit, gently teasing out cells from embryos and spreading single human blastomeres on microscope slides, trying to obtain interpretable metaphase chromosomes (Figure 23.3). It was not going well.

On one occasion, Alan Handyside happened to walk past as I tossed yet another slide of clumped, unreadable chromosomes into the bin. He suggested that, rather than discarding them, perhaps we could send them to a PhD student, Darren Griffin, who was at University College London under the supervision of Dr. Joy Delhanty. Darren's project was to implement

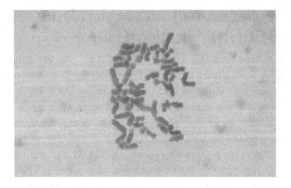

Figure 23.3 One of the very few (if not the only) set of readable metaphase chromosomes I was able to obtain from a single human blastomere whilst at the Hammersmith Hospital IVF unit in the late 1980s.

the (then) very novel technology of fluorescent in-situ hybridization (FISH), a method for enumerating one or two chromosomes in cells without the need for metaphase spreads. Darren had been working on this for some months without a great deal of success in getting FISH signals of sufficient quality to be interpretable. So I gave some of my failed slides to Darren and I recall that a couple of days later he called me, very excited, to say that the FISH had worked remarkably well. He had obtained very clear, bright signals – a huge leap forward from his previous results. We rushed to test more cells, hoping that it was not just luck and that we could repeat the results. We did – almost every time. It turned out that the method I had been using to karyotype single blastomeres produced very clean DNA spreads that were free of the cellular detritus that had been plaguing Darren's attempts at FISH. Very soon after we published our first results (Griffin et al., 1992) and the methodology was so successful that we very quickly moved to clinical PGD cases using FISH and were the first in the world to publish this (Griffin et al., 1993). Darren and I have often reflected since of the serendipitous nature of how this came about. We were both slogging away in different labs on different projects, neither having much success. But the joining of forces, because of a passing comment from Alan Handyside, unwittingly solved our problems.

The initial iterations of single blastomere FISH were technically challenging. The process was completely manual and quite laborious and hybridization times were long, at least overnight. For the early clinical cases I recall that Darren, in particular, had to work long into the night. We only had two fluorochromes, red and green, so could identify only two chromosomes simultaneously. Our first cases were sex selection using FISH for the X and Y chromosomes to identify female embryos from couples who carried serious X-linked diseases like muscular dystrophy and hemophilia. We knew this wasn't ideal because 50% of the female embryos selected for transfer would carry the condition and 50% of the embryos discarded because they were male would have been completely healthy. But this was the best that we could offer for PGD at the time.

Although we chose to analyze the X and Y chromosomes, FISH probes existed for many other human chromosomes. In the lab next door, Bridget Schrurs, a student of Alan Handyside, was using a FISH probe for chromosome 18 to analyze the complement of this chromosome in individual blastomeres from normally fertilized human embryos. This very interesting study, published in 1993, gave us the first signs that human embryos could be chromosomally mosaic, that is that cells within one embryo could have different numbers of a given chromosome. I returned to Melbourne in late 1992 as the Director of Embryology at Monash IVF and I immediately established a PGD laboratory and performed Australia's first clinical cases of PGD for medically indicated gender selection.

At the same time, Santiago Munné, working in Jacques Cohen's laboratory at the Cornell University Medical Center in New York, went a step further and developed a multiprobe FISH protocol that enabled simultaneous analysis of chromosomes X, Y, 18 and 13/21 on human embryos. Over the next few years, Santi and his group published many seminal studies describing chromosome complements in human embryos and provided the first extensive description of chromosomal mosaicism in early human embryos (Munné et al., 1994).

Around this time the late Yuri Verlinsky and colleagues in Chicago, USA, were also using multiprobe FISH to study early human development (Verlinsky et al., 1995). Yuri favored a different approach to obtaining diagnostic material for PGD and pioneered biopsy of the first polar body, the redundant extrusion from the oocyte that contains a haploid set of chromosomes. This was an indirect approach as it was presumed that, if the first polar body was missing a chromosome, then the oocyte had the extra copy. An obvious advantage of polar body biopsy is that no embryonic material is sampled. However, there are also significant disadvantages, particularly that only maternal abnormalities can be detected, although this was less of a problem for chromosomal analysis as most aneuploidies were thought to originate during meiosis I in the oocyte. It was not long before biopsy of the second polar body was added to this protocol to provide a more comprehensive diagnosis and to account for any errors that had occurred at the second meiotic division.

These early studies, particularly from the Chicago and New York groups, demonstrated a much higher than expected frequency of chromosomal aneuploidy in human oocytes and preimplantation embryos, even when just a few chromosomes were analyzed. It was well known that aneuploidy was the predominant cause of spontaneous miscarriage and that fetal aneuploidy was strongly linked to advanced maternal age. So it was a natural progression to suggest that aneuploidy could be a cause of implantation and pregnancy failure after IVF, especially for older women, and that PGD and

chromosome analysis might improve IVF pregnancy rates and outcomes. Philosophically, though, this was a big shift in thinking in PGD circles. For the first time it was being suggested that PGD could be used not just for couples whose families were affected by heritable genetic diseases, but by infertile couples to potentially improve their chances of a healthy live birth. The first report of the clinical use of aneuploidy testing in this way was by Verlinsky et al. (1995). They used FISH probes for chromosomes X, 18 and/or 13/21 to analyze the first and sometimes second polar bodies of oocytes from patients undergoing IVF treatment and reported successful pregnancies. The first report of pregnancies after PGD and aneuploidy testing on human embryos was from a collaboration between Luca Gianaroli and Christina Magli from Bologna, Italy, and Santi Munné (Gianaroli et al., 1997). They focussed on poor-prognosis couples, defined as those who had experienced multiple failed IVF cycles or where the woman was older and they performed cleavage stage embryo biopsy followed by FISH for chromosomes X, Y, 13, 18, and 21.

The early attempts at PGD for aneuploidy (PGD-A), often also called preimplantation genetic screening (PGS), investigated chromosomes that were known often to be abnormal in spontaneous abortions and miscarriage or to result in late term fetal mortality or disability at birth, that is chromosomes X, 13, 18, and 21. Early studies from Munne, Verlinsky, and Joyce Harper and Joy Delhanty in London, were demonstrating that early embryos also harbored higher than expected frequency of aneuploidy of many other chromosomes, but these were probably so lethal that affected embryos never resulted in clinically recognizable pregnancies and so had not been observed. At this time, FISH probes existed for almost every chromosome, but there were a limited number of fluorochromes so this restricted the number of probes that could be used simultaneously. New strategies were developed that involved stripping the FISH signals and then performing a second round of FISH using new probes for additional chromosomes (Munne et al., 1998). This allowed analysis of 8–10 chromosomes, usually including X, Y, 13, 16, 18, 21, and 22, on a single blastomere, and by the early 2000s most labs were offering PGD with aneuploidy testing for at least eight chromosomes. Cleavage stage biopsy of a single cell from a day-3 embryo was the most common approach and this continued to be the technique of choice for many years. The only real shift came with the more routine use of blastocyst biopsy from about 2010. Blastocyst biopsy had the advantage of providing more cellular material for analysis and many comforted themselves with the, in my view, spurious idea that blastocyst biopsy was safer because non-fetal cells were being sampled, as the trophectoderm was thought to contribute only to extra-embryonic membranes. Disadvantages of blastocyst biopsy include that diagnostic results are confounded by chromosomal mosaicism within the biopsy itself, and that some viable, euploid embryos develop more slowly to the blastocyst stage and so would not be included in the testing cohort. Nevertheless, blastocyst biopsy has been increasingly favored in recent years.

Towards Complete Karyotyping: Metaphase CGH

Ongoing research studies were demonstrating that aneuploidies that were rarely seen in spontaneous abortuses could be observed in early human embryos, and there was an incentive to analyze more chromosomes. Although FISH had been expanded it was always going to be limited by the few fluorochromes available. Increasingly scientists began to consider alternative technologies that might enable the analysis of all 24 chromosomes in a single cell.

In 1996, I was recruited to Melbourne IVF to establish a PGD program, but also to start a research program to achieve what I saw as the "holy grail," that is, complete single-cell karyotyping in PGD. We were fortunate to be very close to the Murdoch Childrens Research Institute, headed by Professor Bob Williamson whom I knew because of his interests in PGD for cystic fibrosis in London some years earlier. We were all familiar with the technique of comparative genomic hybridization (CGH), which had been developed to analyze chromosomes in solid tumors without the need for traditional karyotyping. Bob recruited one of his stellar molecular cytogeneticists, Lucille Voullaire, to the project, and together Lucille and I set forth on a quest to apply CGH to single cells to obtain a complete molecular karyotype. I knew that my good friend Dagan Wells was on a similar journey in London, and Dagan very generously let Lucille and me visit his lab to exchange ideas. Both groups took the approach of testing non-embryonic single cells known to have an aneuploidy. The whole genome was amplified and labeled with a green fluorochrome and then co-hybridized onto metaphase chromosomes on a microscope slide with known normal DNA labeled with a red fluorochrome. The red–green fluorescence

ratio of the metaphase chromosomes was indicative of the copy number of the particular chromosome in the original test cell. In 1999, Dagan was the first to publish successful single-cell CGH using cells with a known trisomy. Soon after, Lucille and I published successful CGH on single blastomeres from good quality normally fertilized embryos. We saw aneuploidies of every chromosome, even those that were never seen in spontaneous abortuses, confirming that PGD for aneuploidy really needed to cover all chromosomes and that complete molecular karyotyping was the way forward. We confirmed that chromosomal mosaicism was relatively common and that several embryos had multiple aneuploidies in every cell despite being scored as high quality, highlighting that embryo morphology was a poor predictor of chromosomal normality (Voullaire et al., 2000). Some months later, Dagan published a similar study with remarkably similar results. We were confident about the CGH and moved relatively quickly to clinical application. In 2001, we reported the birth of a healthy baby girl after PGD using CGH (Wilton et al., 2001). This was the first baby in the world born from an embryo that had been fully karyotyped prior to transfer (Figure 23.4).

I was delighted to be awarded the ESHRE Established Scientist award in 2001 for this work. We continued with clinical application and in 2003 published a report of PGD with CGH on 20 patients who had previously suffered implantation failure. Analysis of human embryos using CGH expanded earlier FISH studies and confirmed that human embryos, at least those from IVF patients, harbored many aneuploidies that were not covered by the cocktail of FISH probes

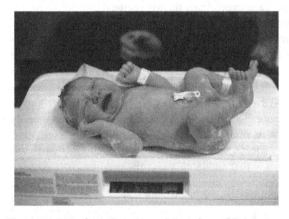

Figure 23.4 The first baby in the world born from a fully karyotyped embryo after Lucille Voullaire and I had applied CGH to a biopsied blastomere at the cleavage stage.

that most other centers were using. Additionally, unlike FISH, CGH provided information along the entire length of each chromosome so, as well as aneuploidies, large segmental errors could also be detected. We knew that complete karyotyping was the way forward, but CGH was a laborious and time-consuming technology that required significant expertise (for review see Wilton and Wells, 2014). Additionally, it took about five days to get results which was longer than the day-3 biopsied embryos could be retained in culture, so we had to freeze all embryos while the results were being analyzed. Dagan's group circumvented this problem by performing CGH on polar bodies, which allowed extra time for analysis. However, this too was problematic because paternal and post-zygotic aneuploidies were missed. Also, testing both first and second polar bodies doubled the already substantial workload required to get a result.

The technically difficult nature of CGH meant that it was not commonly used and most PGD labs, including my own at Melbourne IVF, continued to use FISH for 8–10 chromosomes throughout the first decade of the 2000s to perform aneuploidy testing on the embryos of IVF patients.

Array CGH

A significant improvement in CGH technology occurred in the late 1990s when the template metaphase chromosomes were replaced with an array of thousands of cloned DNA fragments of known genomic location, often derived from bacterial artificial chromosomes (BAC), many of which had become available as a result of the Human Genome Project. Like metaphase CGH, for arrayCGH fluorescently labeled amplified DNA was compared to known normal DNA. But the analysis was automated as the red–green fluorescence ratios of the BACs were analyzed in an array scanner and bioinformatics used to determine chromosome balance. As was so often the case, the challenge for those working in PGD was to modify techniques to meet the very specific requirements of working with single cells. One of the first reports of array-CGH on single cells and blastomeres came from a collaboration between the laboratories of Karen Sermon and Joris Vermeesch in Belgium (LeCaignec et al., 2006). Karen and I had been good friends for many years and we established a joint project for a much larger analysis of human blastomeres. Karen kindly allowed me to spend a couple of weeks with her team in Brussels learning

the microarray CGH methodology. Additionally, a number of commercial companies were developing kit-based methods of performing array-CGH. One of the most successful of these was BlueGnome, a small company in Cambridge, UK, set up by Nick Haan and Graham Snudden. I recall meeting Nick at an ESHRE meeting in 2010 and he invited me to their Cambridge labs to learn their single-cell array-CGH technology called 24sure, which utilized a microarray consisting of many thousands of BACs located approximately 1Mb apart across the genome. Two colleagues whose opinions I greatly respected, namely Carmen Rubio from IVI in Valencia, Spain, and Gary Harton from Fairfax, USA, had trialled the BlueGnome system and were impressed. I very quickly set the system up at Melbourne IVF and within a few months we had fully validated it and were performing our first clinical PGD cases using array-CGH. It was very successful and the automated nature meant that analysis took a few hours compared with days with metaphase CGH. The entire process from embryo biopsy to aneuploidy results could easily be completed overnight. Within a matter of a few months we went from performing about 100 cases per year of PGD-A to 700 per year.

Around this time, other methods of complete molecular karyotyping, notably single nucleotide polymorphism (SNP) arrays, were being honed for use in PGD-A, by Nathan Treff in New Jersey, USA, and Matthew Rabinowitz and his team at Natera Inc., in California, USA. SNPs are heritable variations in individual nucleotides that occur throughout the genome and can be mapped to a very specific location. A SNP array consists of short oligoprobes that target these polymorphisms and the pattern of SNPs can be used to determine copy number of individual chromosomes. SNP arrays are of much higher resolution than a CGH array used for aneuploidy detection and provide significantly more information, although this often confounded and confused analysis rather than adding value. It is fair to say that the BlueGnome 24sure system was the most widely used throughout the world primarily, in my opinion, because of its ease of use and because all components and consumables were available in kit form, making it easy to establish.

In addition to SNP arrays, Nathan Treff also pioneered the use of quantitative PCR for aneuploidy detection in embryos.

In the past few years, the use of array CGH for aneuploidy testing in PGD has been superseded by next generation sequencing (NGS). NGS is an advance on earlier sequencing methods because it enables thousands of short sequencing reactions to occur simultaneously. Bioinformatics is used to reassemble the genome sequence. In PGD the sequencing power is spread across a number of samples in parallel to provide sufficient information to provide whole chromosome copy number and imbalance of large segments of DNA. The process is fast and highly automated. Studies have shown that NGS results are highly concordant with array-CGH. NGS does not seem to be any more accurate than array-CGH and is not higher resolution, but its automated nature means that over time it is likely to be less expensive. One advantage, though, is it seems to be better able to predict chromosomal mosaicism in a sample than array-CGH. This is particularly relevant for those testing multiple cell samples like blastocyst biopsies.

Translocation Testing

Patients who carry a balanced chromosomal rearrangement, and so are at high risk of producing embryos with an unbalanced chromosomal complement, are also able to use PGD to avoid the risk of transmission of this abnormality. Diagnostic techniques for this type of PGD have largely followed developments for aneuploidy testing. Carriers of Robertsonian translocations are at risk of transmitting whole chromosome aneuploidies and these have been relatively straightforward to detect using the large centromeric FISH probes specific to the chromosomes involved in the translocation. Detection of imbalance caused by reciprocal translocations has been more difficult. In 1995, Clare Conn in Joy Delhanty's UCL lab used two locus-specific probes either side of one of the chromosome breakpoints and an additional probe located anywhere on the other chromosome involved in the translocation. This enabled all unbalanced forms of the translocation to be identified. Locus-specific probes are much smaller than the centromeric ones, making the single cell FISH more challenging. Signals were smaller and weaker and hybridization times had to be significantly longer, increasing the risk of non-specific background hybridization. Nevertheless, this was the method of choice for many subsequent years, until the introduction of array-CGH. The whole chromosome imbalance caused by Robertsonian translocations was easily detected by array-CGH. Additionally, because the BACs covered the genome and were about 1Mb apart, translocations involving large segments of chromosomes could

also be detected with exactly the same technology. For reciprocal translocations BlueGnome produced a specialized array, named 24sure+, which had almost twice the number of BACs with the additional ones being concentrated at the telomeres to improve the ability to detect imbalance of terminal segments. Of course, the enormous advantage of using a microarray for translocation PGD was that aneuploidies of every chromosome could be identified, not just those involved in the translocation as we had been restricted to through the FISH years. Additionally, array-CGH was much more robust and reliable. In my lab at Melbourne IVF, I noted that as soon as we switched to diagnosing translocations by array-CGH the number of embryos affected by the translocation apparently doubled. What this really showed was that we were erring on the side of caution and over-calling errors when using FISH, most often because of background noise signals. Like aneuploidy testing, testing for imbalance of large segments is now being done using NGS in many labs.

Single-Gene PGD

The whole concept of PGD was initially proposed to identify embryos affected with serious genetic diseases for couples who carried heritable mutations for monogenic disorders. This was first achieved by Alan Handyside in 1990 when he used PCR to amplify repeated sequences on the Y-chromosome of single cells biopsied from embryos from couples who carried X-linked diseases (Handyside et al., 1990). This was sex-selection, not specific mutation detection, and embryos predicted to be female were selected for transfer based on the absence of Y-chromosome material. It was soon realized that there were other explanations for the absence of Y-material including amplification failure, loss of the cell or absence of a nucleus in the biopsied cell. After a misdiagnosis in one of the early cases, Handyside switched to using FISH, which, as described earlier, Darren Griffin and I were working on almost in the lab next door. FISH not only identified the presence of both the X and Y chromosomes but enumerated them, meaning sex chromosome aneuploidies such as Turner syndrome (XO) could be diagnosed. The first report of successful PGD for an autosomal monogenic disease was in 1992 by Alan Handyside collaborating with Mark Hughes, who was based in Texas, USA, and they used a nested PCR technique to detect the deltaF508 cystic fibrosis mutation in single biopsied blastomeres from couples who were carriers of the mutation (Handyside et al., 1992). Soon after, Yuri Verlinsky's group also reported PGD for cystic fibrosis by analyzing polar bodies and blastomeres. There is no doubt that single cell PCR was particularly challenging and subject to artefactual results caused by phenomena such as allele drop-out, amplification failure, preferential amplification, and contamination by extraneous DNA. In the late 1990s a number of key groups and scientists, including Dagan Wells, Pierre Ray, Karen Sermon, Jamie Grifo, and Charles Strom and their colleagues developed a variety of strategies to make single-cell PCR more reliable. Karen Sermon established that fluorescent PCR followed by fragment analysis on a DNA sequencer was highly sensitive and, in the late 1990s, highly polymorphic microsatellite markers were incorporated into the fluorescent PCR protocol (Sermon et al., 1998). This enabled simultaneous PCR analysis of the mutation and multiple sites around the mutation. For each individual case of monogenic PGD, markers for which the couple was polymorphic were chosen, effectively forming a DNA fingerprint around the mutation. This was a significant step forward because it enabled scientists to confirm the mutation result in a "belt and braces" approach as well as identifying artefactual results, particularly from contamination. This provided significantly more certainty and quickly became the gold standard adopted by most PGD labs throughout the world to provide PGD for families affected with autosomal recessive, dominant, and X-linked single gene diseases.

In my view, little changed in monogenic PCR over the next 10 or so years. Certainly there was a rapid increase in the number of different conditions that could be detected in a single blastomere and the published literature is full of such reports. But in the overwhelming majority of cases, the methodological approach was very similar. That is, monogenic PGD tests were developed for individual couples using fluorescent PCR for detection of the mutation with incorporated microsatellite markers to identify contamination and artefacts.

There was, however, an expansion of the use of PGD to perform HLA testing for tissue compatibility to an existing sick sibling. This was pioneered by Yuri Verlinsky and Svetlana Rechitsky who published their first paper on the topic in 2001 (Verlinsky et al., 2001). The rationale was to achieve the birth of a child not only free of the at-risk genetic disease, but one who could also provide matched hematopoietic stem cells to cure an affected sibling. This applied to conditions including Fanconi's anemia, thalassemia, and Wiscott–Aldrich syndrome. This was coined "savior sibling" PGD and was ethically controversial as healthy embryos were being discarded because they were not of the desired HLA type. Subsequently PGD with HLA matching was used for conditions that were not heritable, like leukemias, and couples were having IVF and PGD to select embryos purely on their HLA type to provide stem cells for the treatment of another family member. This was even more controversial, and in the State of Victoria was largely prohibited as IVF was only accessible as a treatment for infertility.

Karyomapping

In most PGD labs in the world, testing for monogenic disease has run alongside chromosome testing for translocation and infertility patients. Over the years, chromosome testing evolved from 2–3 chromosomes to 8–10 chromosomes using FISH, and then to a full molecular karyotype of all 24 chromosomes using some sort of array testing. It was a long-term frustration of mine that monogenic testing barely progressed for so many years, particularly because we could not simultaneously diagnose the chromosomal aneuploidies which we knew affected so many embryos. Too often for monogenic patients the joy of a pregnancy, unaffected with the disease that afflicted the family, was crushed when it was discovered that the fetus had a lethal aneuploidy that could not be detected during PGD. So I was very excited when, in 2010, Alan Handyside published a new method of universal genome analysis which he called karyomapping (Handyside et al., 2010). This was based on bioinformatic analysis of SNP array data where informative loci were grouped into haploblocks that enabled the parental and grandparental origin of short segments of chromosomes to be determined. The haploblock pattern close to the mutation of interest effectively provided a linkage analysis and the genotype of the DNA could be predicted. Importantly, karyomapping worked on just a few cells and for monogenic PGD patients it meant that there was an almost universal test that could be used to detect most mutations. It was no longer necessary to spend weeks or months developing an individualized monogenic PGD test for each couple, which resulted in substantial time and cost savings for patients. At Melbourne IVF, I set Sharyn Stock-Myer on the task of establishing karyomapping in our lab, and we paired with Illumina Inc., who were commercializing the system, to participate in the beta testing of karyomapping. Most significantly, karyomapping could simultaneously provide information on the chromosomal ploidy of embryos. Theoretically it could detect all monosomies and most meiotic trisomies, but it would be unlikely to detect post-zygotic trisomies. So although not quite the holy grail of simultaneous mutation and aneuploidy detection, in my experience karyomapping was the biggest game-changer in monogenic PGD in many, many years. It enabled us to double our throughput of monogenic PGD cases and provided a significant amount of information about aneuploidy. Importantly, it was faster and cheaper for patients.

What Next?

NGS is being used more extensively as a diagnostic tool in PGD and it is not unreasonable that protocols will be developed that will allow simultaneous detection of mutations and aneuploidy. The innovations in single-cell diagnosis since the inception of PGD in the 1980s have been striking and impressive. However, it has long been a disappointment of mine that there has been little change in embryo biopsy and cell sampling techniques, which effectively are the same as when they were first developed some 30 years ago (Wilton, 2009). The embryo biopsy process is laborious and time consuming and a bottleneck in the diagnostic work-flow. I would be delighted to see the process become simplified and perhaps automated.

With recent innovations in genome editing techniques, like CRISPR, it has been suggested that PGD may become redundant and, instead, mutations in embryos from couples who carry a genetic disease could be repaired. But it must be remembered that not all embryos from such couples would be affected by the condition and so one would still need to know which embryos needed mutation repair. So I think there is a place in clinical medicine for PGD for some time yet.

References

Gianaroli L, Magli MC, Ferraretti AP, et al. 1997. Preimplantation genetic diagnosis increases the implantation rate in human in vitro fertilization by avoiding the transfer of chromosomally abnormal embryos. *Fertil Steril* 72: 837–844.

Griffin DK, Wilton LJ, Handyside AH, Winston RML, Delhanty JDA. 1992. Dual fluorescent in situ hybridisation for simultaneous detection of X and Y chromosome-specific probes for the sexing of human preimplantation embryonic nuclei. *Human Genetics* 89: 18–22.

Griffin D, Wilton L, Handyside A, Winston R, Delhanty J. 1993. Pregnancies following the diagnosis of sex in preimplantation embryos by fluorescent in situ hybridisation. *Br. Med J.* 306: 1382–1383.

Handyside AH, Kontogianni EH, Hardy K, Winston RM. 1990. Pregnancies from biopsied human preimplantation embryos sexed by Y-specific DNA amplification. *Nature* 344(6268): 768–770.

Handyside AH, Lesko JG, Tarín JJ, Winston RM, Hughes MR. 1992. Birth of a normal girl after in vitro fertilization and preimplantation diagnostic testing for cystic fibrosis. *N Engl J Med.* 327(13): 905–909.

Handyside AH, Harton GL, Mariani B, et al. 2010. Karyomapping: a universal method for genome wide analysis of genetic disease based on mapping crossovers between parental haplotypes. *J Med Genet.* 47(10): 651–658.

Harper, J (2009) Introduction to preimplantation genetic diagnosis. In: *Preimplantation Genetic Diagnosis*, Harper J (ed.), Cambridge University Press, pp 1–47.

Kola I, Wilton LJ. 1991. Preimplantation embryo biopsy: detection of trisomy in a single cell biopsied from a four cell mouse embryo. *Mol Reprod Dev.* 29: 16–21.

Le Caignec C, Spits C, Sermon K, et al. 2006. Single-cell chromosomal imbalances detection by array CGH. *Nucleic Acids Res.* 12;34(9):e68.

Monk M, Handyside A, Hardy K, Whittingham D. 1987. Preimplantation diagnosis of deficiency for hypoxanthine phosphoribosyl transferase in a mouse model for Lesch–Nyhan syndrome. *Lancet* 2: 423–425.

Munné S, Weier HU, Grifo J, Cohen J. 1994. Chromosome mosaicism in human embryos. *Biol Reprod* 51: 373–379.

Munné S, Magli C, Bahçe M, et al. 1998. Preimplantation diagnosis of the aneuploidies most commonly found in spontaneous abortions and live births: XY, 13, 14, 15, 16, 18, 21, 22. *Prenat Diagn* 18: 1459–1466.

Sermon K, De Vos A, Van de Velde H, et al. 1998. Fluorescent PCR and automated fragment analysis for the clinical application of preimplantation genetic diagnosis of myotonic dystrophy (Steinert's disease). *Mol Hum Reprod* 4(8): 791–796.

Verlinsky Y, Cieslak J, Freidine M, et al. 1995. Pregnancies following pre-conception diagnosis of common aneuploidies by fluorescent in-situ hybridization. *Hum Reprod* 10: 1923–1927.

Verlinsky Y, Rechitsky S, Schoolcraft W, Strom C, Kuliev A. 2001. Preimplantation diagnosis for Fanconi anemia combined with HLA matching. *JAMA* 285(24): 3130–3133.

Voullaire L, Slater H, Williamson R, Wilton L. 2000. Chromosome analysis of blastomeres from human embryos using comparative genomic hybridization. *Human Genetics* 106: 210–217.

Wilton L. 2009. Preimplantation genetic diagnosis: the future. In: *Preimplantation Genetic Diagnosis*, Harper J (ed.), Cambridge University Press, pp. 274–285.

Wilton LJ, Trounson AO. 1986. Viability of mouse embryos and blastomeres following biopsy of a single cell. Proc. 18th Ann Conf Aust Soc Reprod Biol, Brisbane, Australia.

1989. Biopsy of preimplantation mouse embryos: Development of micromanipulated embryos and proliferation of single blastomeres in culture. *Biol Reprod* 40: 145–152.

Wilton L, Wells D. 2014. Use of comparative genomic hybridisation (CGH) and microarray-CGH for preimplantation genetic screening. In: *Human Gametes and Preimplantation Embryos: Assessment and Diagnosis*, Gardner DK (ed.), Springer Science.

Wilton L, Williamson R, McBain J, Edgar D, Voullaire L. 2001. Birth of a healthy infant after preimplantation confirmation of euploidy by comparative genomic hybridisation. *New Engl J Med*. 345: 1537–1541.

The Development of Embryo, Oocyte, and Ovarian Tissue Cryopreservation

Debra A. Gook and David H. Edgar

Introduction

Turning the clock back to the middle of the last century, the idea of potential human life being kept for long periods in cold storage would, for most people, have been restricted to the pages of science fiction novels. Today, however, the important role that cryopreservation of reproductive potential has played in the evolution of assisted reproductive technology (ART) cannot be understated. Although the factors that can be manipulated to allow biological material to be stored at very low temperatures in a viable state had been elucidated by a generation of notable cryobiologists, the specific application of these principles to human embryos, oocytes, and ovarian tissue has opened the door to significant alterations in clinical approaches to the treatment of infertility by IVF and offered new hope to those women who face imminent and abrupt loss of fertility when undergoing cytotoxic therapies, mainly for malignant disease. This chapter will retrace the evolution of "fertility cryopreservation" over the past three to four decades, in many cases in response to the need for potential solutions to specific clinical problems. For a more in depth review of the theoretical and methodological developments a list of suggested reading is included at the end of the chapter. Although there is inevitably some overlap, embryos, oocytes, and ovarian tissue will be dealt with individually in the interests of clarity. To list all the contributors and contributions to the development of cryopreservation of human reproductive material is an almost impossible task and well beyond the scope of this chapter, as is any attempt to analyze the theoretical and practical details of the methodology.

The Development of Human Embryo Cryopreservation

Slow Freezing of Cleavage Stage Embryos

In the early 1980s, it quickly became widely accepted that ovarian stimulation was necessary to achieve more consistent outcomes when collecting eggs for IVF. As a consequence, doctors were routinely faced with situations where multiple cleavage stage embryos were available for transfer. Multiple embryo transfer was normal practice at this time, partly to increase the probability of at least one implantation event but also because disposal of any non-transferred embryos would have been seen as lost potential when no other alternative was available. There was, however, growing concern over the frequency of multiple pregnancies. Restricting the number of embryos transferred would have been more acceptable if the remaining embryos could be made available in a potentially viable state following a period of storage after cryopreservation.

David Whittingham, together with Stanley Leibo and Peter Mazur (all notable cryobiologists), had demonstrated in the 1970s that this was possible with mouse embryos at similar developmental stages using a technique that employed the chemical dimethylsulfoxide (DMSO) to act as a permeating cryoprotectant in association with slow freezing and rapid thawing. There was no theoretical reason to suspect that this technique would not be successful with human embryos and, before the mid-1980s, the first human pregnancies and births using this approach were reported by Alan Trounson and Linda Mohr in Australia and by Zeilmaker and colleagues in The Netherlands. Application of this technique, however, was to be short-lived and the demonstration in the mid 1980s, by Lassalle and colleagues in France, of more consistent slow freezing results using the permeating cryoprotectant 1,2-propanediol (PROH) together with the non-permeating cryoprotectant sucrose led to this becoming the predominant method of choice for cleavage stage embryos for more than 20 years. As an aside, not all laboratories were able to achieve the same success as the French group in the early days and some sought hints by visiting Lassalle. It was rumored that, after such a visit, Bob Edwards commented that the only difference he could identify in the Lassalle lab was the distinct aroma of Gitanes in the atmosphere!

The widespread adoption of the PROH/sucrose method over this extended period was, in no small measure, assisted by the availability of commercial programmable freezing machines and a range of commercially available versions of the solutions required for freezing and thawing. While this ensured a measure of consistency in methodology between laboratories, it could be argued that it also inhibited the introduction of further improvements in slow freezing. Improvements were clearly desirable since the prevailing approach still left a significant proportion of thawed embryos that had suffered loss of cells as a consequence of the freeze/thaw process. So, while 80–90% of the thawed embryos may have had sufficient surviving cells to justify transfer, only around half would have been fully intact and have, therefore, retained their full pre-freeze potential for pregnancy. It was not until 2009 that our own work, prompted by our development of methodology for oocytes, resulted in a significant increase in the proportion of fully intact embryos (to 80%) by using a more rapid dehydration regime that employed an elevated concentration of sucrose. However, the embryo cryopreservation landscape had, at this point, undergone a marked transformation as a result of the growing move towards transferring embryos at the blastocyst stages and also the advent of vitrification.

Cryopreservation of Blastocysts

Although considered by many to be a recent concept, the potential advantage of selecting embryos for transfer after extended culture to the blastocyst stage was recognized in the early days of IVF. Pregnancies from both fresh and cryopreserved blastocysts were reported by Jacques Cohen and colleagues working at Bourn Hall in the early to mid 1980s. In this case, cryopreservation was by a slow freezing method using glycerol, a more slowly permeating cryoprotectant. However, mainly because of the inadequacy of the culture systems of the day, blastocyst transfer would have a significant wait before being accepted on a widespread basis.

Early in the 1990s, Yves Menezo in France and others began to explore the possibility of using co-culture systems in which the embryo in vitro was supported by a monolayer of somatic cells in order to enhance development to the blastocyst stage. This showed some initial promise and Menezo also published a method for slow freezing of co-cultured blastocysts, using both glycerol and sucrose, that resulted in a series of pregnancies. Again, however, this approach failed to gain widespread acceptance, in part owing to concerns over the use of somatic (predominantly Vero) cells.

It was the advent of defined sequential culture media permitting reliable extended development in vitro, as first described by David Gardner and Michelle Lane in the latter half of the 1990s, that finally resulted in blastocyst transfer becoming mainstream in IVF clinics worldwide. Optimization of cryopreservation for these highly selected embryos now became imperative. The more complex structure of the blastocyst, with populations of cells of different sizes and a fluid-filled blastocoelic cavity, posed a new challenge to cryopreservation methodology. The slow freezing methods previously mentioned, and some modifications of those, had been applied with varying degrees of success by many clinics but there was a pervading feeling that reproducibly high levels of survival were still not being achieved by many. As such, a number of clinics still resisted the advantages of blastocyst transfer or continued to transfer multiple blastocysts until they could be convinced of the reliability of the cryopreservation methodology. It was at this point that the technique of vitrification began to have an impact that was to revolutionize more than one area of fertility cryopreservation.

Vitrification of Embryos

As with culturing embryos to the blastocyst stage, the concept of ice-free cryopreservation by vitrification is not, as thought by many, a recent development. Studies on achieving the vitreous state go back as far as the work of Father Basile J. Luyet in the 1930s, and the notable cryobiologists Bill Rall and Greg Fahy reported successful vitrification of mouse embryos in 1985. It was the search for improved methods for cryopreserving mainly blastocysts and oocytes that led to a resurgence in interest in vitrification. One of the most significant (but rarely cited) studies that underpinned much of today's vitrification technology was that of Ali in 1993. This work assessed survival and pregnancy using various combinations of cryoprotectants, including sucrose, for blastocyst vitrification. The subsequent introduction of carriers such as the pulled straw (by Vajta) and cryoloop (by Mukaida and Lane) facilitated ultra-rapid rates of cooling and warming at a critical turning point for the clinical introduction of vitrification. The uptake of vitrification as the method of choice for blastocyst cryopreservation was rapid, spearheaded by Vajta, Kuwayama, Liebermann, Tucker, and Vanderzwalmen. The methodology being established could be shown, with relatively minor differences, to result in high survival rates of both cleavage stage embryos and blastocysts that implanted at equivalent rates to their fresh counterparts. These impressive results were being obtained with the use of a new generation of microcarriers that allowed embryos to be suspended in minute volumes of cryoprotectant solution prior to vitrification.

Embryo cryopreservation in the first decade of the new millennium had now reached a stage where its reproducibly high efficiency (often greater than 90% survival) was leading some to question whether its role in ART may be expanded in order to further improve clinical outcomes.

Clinical Outcomes From Cryopreserved Versus Fresh Embryos

Despite early reservations about the widespread introduction of embryo cryopreservation expressed by some, notably Professor (now Lord) Winston, the huge amount of data available on clinical outcomes from embryo cryopreservation has been reassuring and even suggests that birth outcomes may be improved, possibly as a consequence of allowing the cryopreserved embryo to be transferred in a more natural menstrual cycle. The application of embryo cryopreservation has now reached a stage where there are even advocates for the freezing of all viable embryos, with subsequent thaw and transfer into an unstimulated endometrium, as a strategy for achieving optimal outcomes.

Development of Human Oocyte Cryopreservation

While human embryo cryopreservation was developed mainly as a solution to the dilemmas associated with the availability of multiple embryos following ovarian stimulation and IVF, the development of technology for cryopreservation of the female gamete was driven initially in response to issues relating to a need for fertility preservation in young women undergoing cytotoxic therapies for malignant disease. The unique nature of the mature (metaphase II) oocyte was to pose the greatest challenge of all reproductive material for the cryobiologists. History will show us that overcoming this challenge has opened the door to potential

solutions to clinical, ethical, and logistic problems in human assisted reproduction.

Pre 1990s

It was the application of the DMSO-based method developed for embryos by David Whittingham in 1977 that led to the first report of mouse cryopreserved oocytes surviving, undergoing fertilization, and developing to term, and this success was soon replicated in other mammalian species. In the 1980s, although two live births were reported from human oocytes slow frozen with the DMSO method (by Chen in 1986, and van Uem and co-workers in 1987), these results could not be reproduced. This failure, combined with the concerns over abnormalities, particularly invoking the meiotic spindle and subsequent risks of aneuploidy, essentially resulted in the development of clinical oocyte cryopreservation being abandoned.

The 1990s

Data demonstrating the temperature sensitivity of the meiotic spindle and studies showing that cryoprotectant-like chemicals could induce the release of cortical granules in a phenomenon referred to as "zona hardening," indicated that, even if oocytes survived cryopreservation, the subsequent probability of fertilization would be very low and the risk of aneuploidy would be very high.

By this time, the PROH/0.1M sucrose slow freezing method was well established for cleavage stage embryos, so it seemed reasonable to us that we should at least explore it as a possibility. We found that the procedure was detrimental to mouse unfertilized oocytes but immediate post-fertilisation (pronuclear) stages survived well and went on to form blastocysts in vitro. At this point we were keen to explore the method with human oocytes and we are eternally grateful to many of our patients who were prepared to donate their precious oocytes to our work. To our initial surprise, some of these metaphase II oocytes survived and our subsequent studies showed that PROH had actually stabilized the spindle and not resulted in cortical granule release (Figure 24.1).

Although these experiments had proved difficult to perform, it was proving even more difficult to have the work accepted for publication, since it flew in the face of accepted dogma. During a chance meeting with Bob Edwards at a conference, I (DG) stressed that I believed that these results needed to be published in

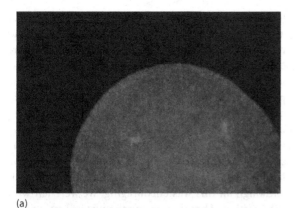

(a)

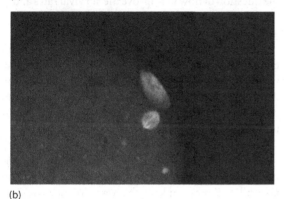

(b)

Figure 24.1 (a) A frozen thawed human oocyte stained to detect cortical granules. (b) The meiotic spindle within a frozen thawed human oocyte.

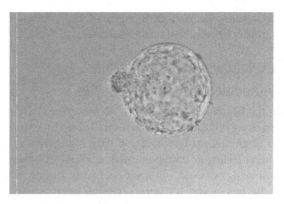

Figure 24.2 A hatching blastocyst which had developed from a frozen thawed human oocyte following ICSI.

order that they be confirmed or refuted and the paper subsequently appeared in *Human Reproduction*, which was under Bob's editorship at that time.

We now needed to see whether these oocytes were capable of fertilization and, if so, to examine them for subsequent aneuploidy. After much debate and discussion with our Victoria State regulatory body, we were able to assess the fertilization of thawed oocytes but only up to the point of pronuclear formation. This meant sleeping in the lab overnight in order to assess for pronuclei every two hours. We were able to establish that the fertilization rate of the frozen oocytes was similar to that of fresh oocytes using conventional IVF, a clear demonstration that, contrary to the prevailing dogma, zona hardening was not an issue. This fact continues to be overlooked in today's literature where it is often stated that sperm injection (ICSI) is necessary to achieve fertilization of cryopreserved oocytes.

Of course, the next question related to subsequent development, but the state legislation in Victoria,

Australia, prohibited this work, forcing us to carry it out in Sydney and in California. In Sydney, frozen/thawed oocytes were inseminated and one blastocyst developed, whereas in California two hatched blastocysts were obtained from oocytes injected using the new technique of ICSI, performed by two novices in the form of myself (DG) and Mitch Schiewe, guided only by the information in the literature (Figure 24.2).

It also has to be remembered that this was a time when only relatively simple culture media were available and culture of human embryos beyond day 3 was still extremely rare. The excitement of seeing hatching blastocysts was shared with a number of junior doctors in the unit, one of whom, Andrea Borini, would go on to champion clinical oocyte cryopreservation in Italy. In 1995, we published the evidence of development to the blastocyst stage of embryos generated from oocytes frozen with the PROH/sucrose method.

On the basis of this work, we had established the world's first frozen egg bank at the Royal Women's Hospital in Melbourne in 1994 as a resource for young women requiring fertility preservation prior to treatment for malignant disease. While this was an important initiative, it was clear that we would have to wait a considerable time before these stored oocytes were likely to be used and provide information on clinical outcomes following thawing. We were, however, aware that imminent changes to the legislation in Italy would preclude embryo cryopreservation and force clinics to consider freezing oocytes as an alternative and so began collaboration with a group in Bologna, Italy. Following a visit to establish their oocyte freezing program, the first birth from oocytes frozen using the PROH/sucrose method was reported by Eleanora

195

Porcu and colleagues in Bologna in 1997, followed soon after by reports of further successes.

Development of Slow Freezing Methodology for Human Oocytes

By the beginning of the 2000s, oocyte cryopreservation using PROH/sucrose had been adopted by a number of groups, predominantly in Italy, but there was a general feeling of disappointment at the level of survival being achieved – in most cases only around half of the frozen oocytes were surviving after thawing. Previously I (DG) had suggested that increasing the level of the non-permeating cryoprotectant, sucrose, and thereby increasing dehydration should result in a higher proportion of oocytes surviving cryopreservation. Raffaella Fabbri and her colleagues in Bologna were able to demonstrate that this approach could, in fact, increase the proportion of surviving oocytes after thawing and that raising the pre-freeze sucrose concentration threefold (to 0.3M) appeared to achieve higher survival than doubling it to 0.2M. Not surprisingly, with proclamation of the Italian law prohibiting embryo cryopreservation imminent and with low survival being the main concern being expressed with respect to the prevailing methodology, many groups were quick to adopt a modified approach using PROH and 0.3M sucrose. This move was further facilitated by the rapid appearance of commercial kits consisting of freezing and thawing solutions based on the findings. However, increasing the proportion of surviving eggs was not to be achieved without cost. A few years into the 2000s it started to become apparent that the implantation potential of embryos derived from oocytes frozen in PROH with 0.3M sucrose was compromised, and this was highlighted in our review published in 2007. Soon it was apparent from a number of studies that all was not well in terms of the early development of these embryos, with the demonstration of retarded early cleavage patterns, a likely consequence of perturbations of the cytoplasm and lysis of mitochondria within the oocytes.

Interestingly, as had been overlooked when raising the pre-freeze concentration to 0.3M, this alteration also had implications for the post-thaw levels of sucrose used to buffer the rehydration of oocytes, which had not been addressed in the method. While most groups active in oocyte cryopreservation had been seduced by the prospect of improved survival rates using 0.3M sucrose, we had taken a more stepwise approach by limiting the pre-freeze concentration to 0.2M while conducting all steps of the procedures at 37 °C to facilitate more complete dehydration and rehydration. The Borini group showed that this more conservative approach of dehydration in 0.2M sucrose, together with incorporating modifications to the post-thaw sucrose levels, could result in oocytes that generated embryos with similar developmental and implantation potential to those from fresh oocytes. We were also able to demonstrate this although, due to the small numbers of patients using their frozen oocytes in our unit, we did not publish our findings until 2011. Although all this was encouraging, we were left with the question of how to improve the survival rates above the approximately 70% ceiling that seemed to exist with this methodology.

It was an interesting time with many colorful and extremely passionate characters working in the area, both clinically and scientifically. This sparked heated debates at numerous ESHRE and ASRM meetings and it was always a challenge for the chairperson to maintain control.

As egg freezing became more common, interesting cases would occasionally arise in the literature, claiming to be the first report of some hitherto uncovered possibility. An example of this was a report from our clinic of a birth from a frozen embryo that had originally been created by injecting a frozen sperm into a frozen egg. Following the publication, a cartoon appeared in the *Melbourne Age* newspaper depicting a perplexed mother wondering why her child was continually trying to climb into the household refrigerator.

Concurrent alternative approaches had also been explored throughout the early 2000s, including direct injection of trehalose into the oocyte by Thomas Toth and substituting choline for sodium in the media used for cryopreservation by James Stachecki. These choline-based solutions were applied clinically with pregnancies reported in the USA and South America, but no firm conclusions could be drawn from the limited clinical data. However, before any improvements in slow freezing methodology for oocytes could be firmly established, the introduction of vitrification-based technology was to have a profound impact on clinical practice, as it did in the area of embryo cryopreservation.

Vitrification of Unfertilized Oocytes

While the slow freezing of oocytes was evolving during the late 1990s and early 2000s, parallel attempts to apply vitrification methodology to human oocytes were underway. This resulted in sporadic reports of success but no clear consensus was emerging on the optimal cryoprotectant composition or other critical parameters. An additional important restriction was the lack of availability of appropriate carriers (microtools) that would allow a broad range of users to consistently achieve the extremely rapid cooling and warming rates required for oocytes.

In 1999 the first birth with vitrification of human oocytes was reported by Kuleshova using brief exposure to an extremely high concentration (7.1M) of ethylene glycol (EG) and sucrose (0.6M) at 37 °C. Subsequent reports of births started to appear in the literature from the Cha group in Korea using what was thought, at that time, to be a more conservative concentration of 5.5M EG with 1.0M sucrose, but survival was low. The first development to significantly change the face of oocyte vitrification came in 2000 from a group in Taiwan, who showed that, by using a similar concentration to that used in slow freezing for initial dehydration followed by a short exposure to a high concentration of EG, survival jumped to over 90%. To this point, these reports had either been using copper EM grids, open pulled straws or conventional straws, all of which were relatively difficult to use and the next development came with introduction of a microtool or carrier; the cryotop. The cryotop had originated from work carried out in Japan by Katayama, Kuwayama, and co-workers including Gabor Vajta, Ed Stehlik and Stanley Liebo, the latter a reminder of the enduring debt to the early pioneers of cryobiology. Simultaneously, this group of eminent cryobiologists introduced the next development, based on the original philosophy of Rall and Fahy; the use of a combination of cryoprotectants which would reduce individual toxicity. This cocktail consisted of approximately equal concentrations of the permeating cryoprotectants EG and DMSO in combination with the non-permeating sucrose. It was the use of this approach in conjunction with the recently introduced carrier, the cryotop, that was to result in oocyte cryopreservation finally starting to gain traction.

However, there were still concerns regarding the toxicity of the cryoprotectants at these concentrations, and only a handful of pregnancies had been reported. In the mid to late 2000s the transition from case reports with oocyte vitrification to clinical series with autologous and donor oocytes began to emerge and oocyte vitrification started to gain momentum. In 2006, Antinori and co-workers, applying oocyte cryopreservation in the context of the Italian legislative framework,

reported survival of vitrified/warmed oocytes of well over 90% and equivalent fertilization, in-vitro development to day 3 and implantation rates comparable to fresh oocytes in a study involving over a hundred vitrified oocytes and 250 controls. It was unfortunate at this time that Antinori had been discredited for other reasons and these data were essentially ignored. However, the findings were reinforced in 2008 by Ana Cobo and her colleagues in Spain who reported survival rates greater than 90% and similar fertilization and development to the blastocyst stage in over 200 vitrified oocytes and a similar number of controls.

At this point it is interesting to reflect on the clinical context in which oocyte vitrification was occurring in Ana Cobo's laboratories. Up to that point in time, oocyte cryopreservation had been seen as essential in tackling the clinical situations presenting with imminent loss of fertility in women undergoing cytotoxic therapies. Also, although somewhat differently, in situations when the law precluded the option to cryopreserve embryos, but developments had been slow due to low numbers of patients returning to use the cryopreserved oocytes. In the Cobo study, the oocytes were obtained from donors (mean age of 27 years) in a large oocyte donation program. The obvious benefit in terms of advancing oocyte vitrification was that data on outcomes with high quality oocytes were generated quickly. It was clear that oocyte cryopreservation in this context, in contrast to synchronization of donor and recipient cycles, which was necessary for treatment using fresh oocytes, could offer significant logistic advantages. The encouraging results described above led to the Spanish group extending the use of vitrification in their donor oocyte programme and reporting, in their landmark study in 2010, the clinical results from over 3000 vitrified oocytes and a similar number of controls. The results were impressive, partly because of the average age of the oocyte donors (again 27 years) and the associated high quality of the gametes being used, but mainly because the clinical outcomes from the vitrified and fresh oocytes were almost identical and survival of the vitrified oocytes was again over 90%. Similar reports from other groups soon followed in the literature and oocyte cryopreservation had finally come of age.

Finally, the only outstanding criticism of vitrification, whether for oocytes or embryos, was the risk of potential contamination associated with all previously used open microtools, which has now been eliminated with the introduction of a closed microtool (Rapid-i). We have shown that the speeds required for successful vitrification can be achieved with a closed system without a requirement to increase cryoprotectant concentrations, and this has been reinforced by work from Ed Stehlik in mouse showing that the speed of vitrification is not as critical as speed of warming.

Reflecting again on the evolution of the technology and its role, we can see that "egg banking" has gone from being offered only in critical medical situations, where no alternative exists, to being a solution to legally imposed restrictions to becoming a valuable tool in large oocyte donation programmes. The story will not end there for oocyte cryopreservation; while a small number of patients may choose to access this (now well-proven) technology to avoid ethical issues associated with stored embryos, it is more likely that the next chapter will be dominated by a growing demand for "social egg freezing." So we are likely to see young women choosing to defer conception until their circumstances make them more comfortable with that choice, while at the same time having access to the biological vigor of their young gametes that have been suspended in time. How would the pioneers of cryobiology have viewed that prospect?

Development of Human Ovarian Tissue Cryopreservation

As discussed in the previous section, the dramatic improvements achieved with oocyte cryopreservation have broadened the scope of its application within and beyond its originally envisaged role in preserving female fertility prior to cytotoxic treatments. However, the urgent need to commence these treatments often leaves little time to complete one or more cycles of oocyte collection and storage, leaving this group of patients unable to benefit from these scientific advances. In such cases, the option of cryopreserving and storing ovarian tissue has been explored on the basis that the human ovary, at least in younger women, is likely to contain a large reservoir of oocytes, albeit predominantly in very immature (primordial) stage follicles.

Animal Studies

Evidence that ovarian tissue, frozen using glycerol, could function after thawing and grafting had been reported in rodents as early as the 1950s but follicle preservation was very inefficient, pregnancy was rare, and litter size was reduced. It was the work of Roger Gosden, working with David Baird and others in Edinburgh, that rekindled interest in this as a clinical possibility. Using

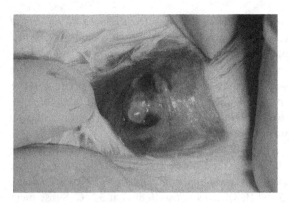

Figure 24.3 Antral follicle developed from frozen human ovarian tissue xenografted under the kidney capsule in an immunodeficient mouse.

DMSO as a cryoprotectant for freezing strips of ovarian cortex from sheep, in 1994 they reported restoration of fertility following grafting of thawed tissue. This was of particular interest given the similarity in follicle distribution in sheep and human ovaries.

Cryopreservation of Human Ovarian Tissue

Although we had established an oocyte cryopreservation program with the aim of offering it to young women who were about to start cytotoxic therapy, we quickly became aware that very few of this group had sufficient time available to undergo a cycle (or cycles) of ovarian stimulation, and so we began investigating cryopreservation of ovarian tissue. Our preliminary experiments showed the method for oocyte cryopreservation could be adapted to ovarian tissue and in 1995, due to urgent demand but with no real knowledge of whether the tissue had potential, we began clinical cryopreservation of ovarian tissue. It is interesting to note that tissue cryopreserved at that time has subsequently been transplanted back to a patient who has now been cycling regularly for over 11 years. At the same time visiting clinicians working in Gosden's laboratory, including Outi Hovatta, Kutluk Oktay, and Dror Meirow, were subsequently able to demonstrate that human primordial follicles in ovarian cortical tissue could survive cryopreservation and that this could be achieved using DMSO, EG, or PROH as the cryoprotectant during slow freezing. Of course, this and our own evidence was largely based on histological examination but functional survival was soon confirmed when follicle development up to antral stages was reported in thawed ovarian tissue that had been grafted into immunodeficient mice (Figure 24.3).

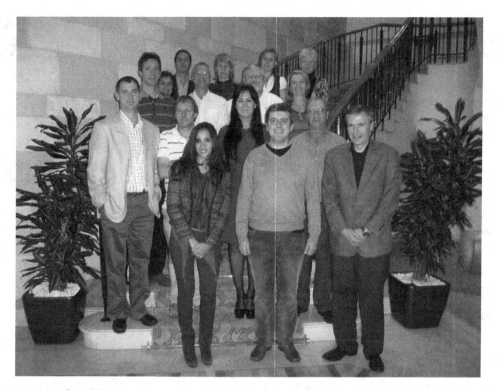

Figure 24.4 Members of the Alpha consortium.

While vitrification has not been ignored in the context of ovarian tissue cryopreservation, the specific issues associated with using this approach for pieces of cortex that are vastly different from embryos or oocytes has restricted development in this area. The Japanese group of Nao Suzuki has developed tools and cryoprotectant solutions suitable for ovarian tissue vitrification and recently reported three births from transplanted cryopreserved ovarian tissue. Although technically challenging this may be a way forward for the future, as may cryopreservation of isolated follicles.

While successful preservation was being described by many groups, it would be fair to say that there was no systematic attempt to optimize the methodological variables associated with success in rigorous comparative studies. This can be partly attributed to the availability of material, but also to the fact that the assessment of tissue survival is much more complex than the clearly defined endpoints associated with embryo and oocyte cryopreservation.

As the prospect of survival following cytotoxic therapies was improving, it was inevitable that some patients whose ovarian function and/or fertility had not returned would be keen to use tissue that had been cryopreserved and stored. The ultimate evidence of successful cryopreservation would, of course, only be available when the tissue could be shown to have resulted in pregnancy and birth after thawing and grafting it back to the patient on whose behalf it had been stored.

Clinical use of Cryopreserved Ovarian Tissue

Grafting of frozen/thawed ovarian tissue can be either to the original ovarian site (orthotopic) or a non-ovarian site (heterotopic). Understandably, orthotopic grafting has, in general, been the approach of choice given the relative simplicity of the procedure and the fact that it allows the possibility of natural conception, at least in cases where the Fallopian tubes are intact. After demonstrations of resumption of ovarian function, the first birth following orthotopic grafting of thawed tissue was reported by Jacques Donnez and colleagues in Brussels. To date, around 80 births have been reported from this approach by a number of groups around the world, notably those from Belgium, Denmark, Israel, and Germany. However, at least from a theoretical standpoint, unequivocal evidence of the birth originating from gametes in the transplanted tissue would only be obtained if the oocytes had been aspirated from the transplanted tissue.

In 2004, Kutluk Oktay had first reported fertilization and embryo development in oocytes aspirated from tissue grafted at a heterotopic site (forearm). This tissue had been frozen using DMSO as cryoprotectant. Unequivocal evidence of birth from cryopreserved (PROH) ovarian tissue following heterotopic transplantation (abdominal wall), follicle aspiration, and embryo transfer was reported by our group in 2013 and subsequently repeated in our clinic. Confirmatory evidence has also been reported by Donnez's group and that of Claus Andersen in Copenhagen using tissue cryopreserved with DMSO and EG respectively.

Reflections on the Development of Cryopreservation in Reproductive Medicine

It is difficult to imagine how the history of assisted reproductive treatment (ART) might have looked if it had not been possible to cryopreserve and store human embryos and eggs. Having to consider the pros and cons of either transferring multiple embryos or disposing of potential life is, thankfully, not a situation that we have to face in current practice. Successful outcomes from cryopreserved embryos are now an expectation but success was variable and never taken for granted in the early days. Similarly, the comparable current success of oocyte cryopreservation has evolved from a situation when it was being offered more in hope than expectation. Current expectations are reflected by the publication of international benchmarks by the Alpha Scientists in Reproductive Medicine expert group that included many who had contributed to today's success (Figure 24.4).

While ovarian tissue cryopreservation can, to some extent still be viewed as being in its infancy, we look forward to the possibility of technology that allows the primitive oocytes in this tissue to be matured in vitro and used for IVF procedures, thereby overcoming the problems associated with tissue transplantation.

Wherever the future takes us, it serves us well to constantly remind ourselves of the massive debt we owe to the pioneers of cryobiology who took us from the realms of science fiction into a world of previously unthinkable possibilities (Figure 24.5).

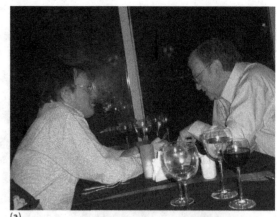

(a)

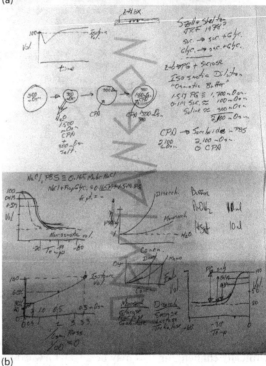

(b)

Figure 24.5 (a) Pierre Vanderzwalmen and Stanley Liebo discussing cryopreservation. (b) Diagrams of cryopreservation principles drawn by Stan Liebo.

Select Bibliography

Ali J, Shelton JN. (1993) Design of vitrification solutions for the cryopreservation of embryos. *J Reprod Fertil* 99(2), 471–477.

Balaban B, et al. (2012) The Alpha consensus meeting on cryopreservation key performance indicators and benchmarks: proceedings of an expert meeting. *Reprod Biomed Online* 25, 146–167.

Cobo A, Meseguer M, Remohi J, Pellicer A. (2010) Use of cryo-banked oocytes in an ovum donation programme: a prospective, randomized, controlled, clinical trial. *Hum Reprod* 25, 2239–2246.

Cobo A, de los Santos MJ, Castello D, et al. (2012) Outcomes of vitrified early cleavage-stage and blastocyst-stage embryos in a cryopreservation program: evaluation of 3,150 warming cycles. *Fertil Steril* 98, 1138–1146.

Donnez J, Dolmans MM, Demylle D, et al. (2004) Livebirth after orthotopic transplantation of cryopreserved ovarian tissue. *Lancet* 364, 1405–1410.

Edgar DH, Gook DA. (2012) A critical appraisal of cryopreservation (slow freezing versus vitrification) of human oocytes and embryos. *Human Reproduction Update* 18, 536–554.

Gook DA. (2011) History of oocyte cryopreservation. *Reprod Biomed Online* 23, 281–289.

Gook DA, Edgar DH. (2007) Human oocyte cryopreservation. *Human Reproduction Update* 13, 591–605.

Gook DA, Edgar DH. (2011) Ovarian tissue cryopreservation. In: *Principles and Practice of Fertility Preservation*, eds. Donnez J and Kim SS, Cambridge University Press, pp. 345–359.

Gook DA, Schiewe MC, Osborn SM, et al. (1995) Intracytoplasmic sperm injection and embryo development of human oocytes cryopreserved using 1,2-propanediol. *Hum Reprod* 10, 2637–2641.

Gosden RG, Baird DT, Wade JC, et al. (1994) Restoration of fertility to oophorectomized sheep by ovarian autografts stored at –196 °C. *Hum Reprod* 9, 597–603.

Kuwayama M. (2007) Highly efficient vitrification for cryopreservation of human oocytes and embryos: the Cryotop method. *Theriogenology* 67, 73–80.

Kuwayama M, Vajta G, Kato O, Leibo SP. (2005) Highly efficient vitrification method for cryopreservation of human oocytes. *Reprod Biomed Online* 11, 300–308.

Lassalle B, Testart J, Renard JP. (1985) Human embryo features that influence the success of cryopreservation with the use of 1,2 propanediol. *Fertil Steril* 44, 645–651.

Leibo SP. (2004) Cryopreservation of mammalian oocytes. In: *Preservation of Fertility*, eds. Tulandi T and Gosden R, Taylor & Francis: London.

Oktay K, Buyuk E, Veeck L, et al. (2004) Embryo development after heterotopic transplantation of cryopreserved ovarian tissue. *Lancet* 363, 837–840.

Porcu E, Fabbri R, Seracchioli R, et al. (1997) Birth of a healthy female after intracytoplasmic sperm injection of cryopreserved human oocytes. *Fertil Steril* 68, 724–726.

Rall WF, Fahy GM. (1985) Ice-free cryopreservation of mouse embryos at –196 °C by vitrification. *Nature* 313, 573–575.

Rall WF, Wood MJ, Kirby C, Whittingham DG. (1987) Development of mouse embryos cryopreserved by vitrification. *J Reprod Fertil* 80, 499–504.

Stern CJ, Gook D, Hale LG, et al. (2013) First reported clinical pregnancy following heterotopic grafting of cryopreserved ovarian tissue in a woman after a bilateral oophorectomy. *Hum Reprod* 28, 2996–2999.

Trounson A, Mohr L. (1983) Human pregnancy following cryopreservation, thawing and transfer of an eight-cell embryo. *Nature* 305, 707–709.

Vajta G, Nagy ZP. (2006) Are programmable freezers still needed in the embryo laboratory? Review on vitrification. *Reprod Biomed Online* 12, 779–796.

Whittingham DG. (1977) Fertilization in vitro and development to term of unfertilized mouse oocytes previously stored at –196 °C. *J Reprod Fertil* 49, 89–94.

Whittingham DG, Leibo SP, Mazur P. (1972) Survival of mouse embryos frozen to –196 degrees and –269 degrees C. *Science* 178, 411–414.

Zeilmaker GH, Alberda AT, van Gent I, Rijkmans CM, Drogendijk AC. (1984) Two pregnancies following transfer of intact frozen-thawed embryos. *Fertil Steril* 42, 293–296.

The Development of Ovarian Stimulation for In-Vitro Fertilization

Colin M. Howles

Introduction

Prior to the start of in-vitro fertilization (IVF), pharmaceutical preparations containing biologically active gonadotropins had been in use for about 75

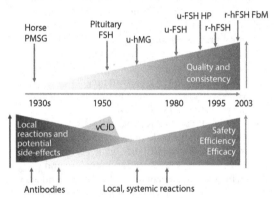

FbM, filled by mass; PMSG, pregnant mare serum gonadotrophin; u-hMG, urine-derived hMG; vCJD, variant Creutzfeldt–Jakob disease

Figure 25.1 Increased quality and consistency of gonadotrophin preparations for clinical use.

The evolution of novel gonadotrophin purification technologies was driven by the need to eliminate extraneous molecules from the final product. This mirrored the development of products in other therapeutic areas, such as insulin and pituitary hormone.

In the early 1960s, the purity of human menopausal gonadotrophin (hMG) was only 5%, the activity was low and it contained significant amounts of other proteins. As a result, problems – including poor fertilization rates, lower viability and allergic reactions – were common.

In 1983, advances in purification technology led to the production of u-FSH, which contains only small amounts of LH. Nevertheless, the purity of this product was still only 5%, with 95% of the protein remaining unwanted.

By the late-1980s, affinity purification processes were used to produce u-FSH HP, which has a purity of up to 95%.

Even higher purities of 99% were achieved when r-hFSH products entered the market in the 1990s. These r-hFSH products also have greater specific activities than the earlier generations of gonadotrophins.

Donini P, Montezemolo R. Rassegna di Clinica, Terapia e Scienze Afini. A publication of the Biologic Laboratories of the Instituto Serono 1949;48:3–28

Mazer. Diagnosis and treatment of menstrual disorders and sterility. New York: Paul B Hoeber Inc., 1946

years. As reviewed by Lunenfeld (2004) and Howles (2006) (Figure 25.1), major advances in technology have brought the field of gonadotropin therapy a very long way since the era of animal – human pituitary (whose use from 1958 for ovulation induction, led 20 years later, to a number of cases of iatrogenic Creutzfeld–Jakob disease (CJD) in material prepared by national agencies from France, Australia and UK) – and urinary-derived hormones. For almost 30 years, human menopausal gonadotropin (hMG) had been the main gonadotropin available for clinical use. Table 25.1 lists the characteristics of FSH preparations that have been commercially available. The FSH and LH content of hMG (or menotropin) are equal in terms of biological activity (75 IU of FSH and 75 IU of LH) as measured by animal derived bioassays. The use of the term IU's and FSH quantities in multiples of 75 IUs is still used today even in the era of recombinant gonadotrophins.

The early years (1980–1995) of ovarian stimulation protocols for assisted reproduction were shaped firstly from pioneering work in animal models (see review by Edwards (1996)) and then through the use of urinary-derived gonadotrophins, in particular menotrophin (human menopausal gonadotrophin; HMG) and human chorionic gonadotrophin (hCG), which were first scientifically described for use together in an IVF ovarian stimulation protocol by Steptoe and Edwards in their landmark 1970 *Lancet* paper (Steptoe and Edwards, 1970). Following the replacement of human embryos in 77 cases without a pregnancy and an ectopic occurring after the use of 900 IU HMG followed by hCG (Steptoe and Edwards, 1976), the pioneering team decided to change tack. Bob Edwards and Patrick Steptoe abandoned HMG use, and the first IVF births (two from UK and one from Australia) were all after natural cycle IVF. A wide range of stimulation protocols were then investigated (Edwards et al., 1980); however, HMG was reintroduced in particular by the US Norfolk IVF program (Jones et al., 1982). In 1983, the Bourn Hall

Table 25.1 Characteristics of gonadotrophin preparations commercially available

	Purity (FSH content)	Mean specific FSH activity (IU/ mg protein)	Injected protein per 75 IU (mcg)
hMG	< 5%	~100	~750
u-FSH	< 5%	~150	370–750
hMG HP	< 70%	2000–2500	~18
u-FSH HP	> 95%	~9000 (highly variable)	6–11
r-hFSH			
Follitropin beta	–	7000–10,000	8.1
Follitropin alfa	> 99%	13,645	6.1

Early urine-derived products have minimal purity. This purity has improved over the years as advances were made in gonadotrophin purification methods. r-hFSH contains over 99% FSH and has a greater purity than even u-FSH HP. Furthermore, r-hFSH is not contaminated with other human proteins; this may reduce the risk of antigenic reactions.

The specific activity of these products ranges from approximately 100 IU/mg to over 13,000 IU/mg of protein, with r-hFSH showing the highest specific activity and the lowest variability.

Because r-hFSH is so pure, only 6.1 mcg of protein needs to be injected to give a 75 IU dose of FSH. In contrast, as much as 750 mcg of the first-generation urine-derived gonadotrophins needs to be injected to deliver the same dose of FSH.

Loumaye *et al*. Hum Reprod 1996;11:95–107 (hMG)

van de Weijer *et al*. Reprod Biomed Online 2003;7:547–557 (hMG HP)

Howles *et al*. Hum Reprod 1996;2:172–191 (u-FSH/u-FSH HP, amount of protein injected per 75 IU)

Le Cotonnec *et al*. Hum Reprod 1993;8:1604–1611 (u-FSH/u-FSH HP, specific activities)

Giudice *et al*. Hum Reprod 1994;9:2291–2299 (u-FSH HP)

Bassett *et al*. Reprod Biomed Online 2005;10:169–177 (follitropin alfa and beta)

Giudice *et al*. J Clin Res 2001;4:27–33 (hMG, specific activity)

team reported detailed results describing the treatment of 1200 patients, in cycles that produced a maximum of four oocytes per retrieval (mean of 2.1–2.6 oocytes) and fertilization rates of 88–92%, depending on the type of stimulation used (Edwards and Steptoe, 1983).

Bob Edwards was particularly concerned about the endocrinology of the HMG/HCG protocol, which was associated with a shortened luteal phase. It was then combined with clomiphene citrate (CC), which had initially been successfully used by the Melbourne groups (Trounson et al., 1981). The CC/HMG/HCG protocol was utilized at Bourn Hall Clinic in the early 1980s and proved more successful than CC alone (Edwards et al., 1984; Fishel et al., 1985). For a comprehensive review

of the early pioneering years of ovarian stimulation for IVF see Hillier (2013).

The CC/HMG/hCG protocol was the backbone of the stimulation armamentarium when I entered the then novel world of IVF back in 1984. With a fully tuned embryological department, staffed by future lab innovators such as Jacques Cohen and Simon Fishel, intensive endocrine monitoring (requiring the collection of patient's urine around the clock), highly experienced medical staff (including John Webster, Jon Hewitt, and Tom Matthews), it was the norm to have three positive plasma hCG tests out of every ten patients with an embryo transfer. Each patient's progress during the ovarian stimulation phase was discussed daily at the lunchtime meeting by members of the clinical and scientific teams. Bob Edwards and Patrick Steptoe were generally in attendance and strongly contributed to the decision-making process.

It was clear though that change was required. One of the problems associated with the use of CC in combination with gonadotrophins was that up to 20% of patients underwent an endogenous LH surge (Macnamee et al., 1988) prior to the clinical decision to administer human chorionic gonadotrophin (hCG). Ovarian stimulation didn't inhibit the surge (Glasier et al., 1988), but often caused it to be attenuated (Messinis et al., 1985) and hence difficult to detect. The outcome of the attenuated LH surge, which was not detected, led to one of two scenarios. Firstly, depending upon the severity of attenuation, all of the events normally associated with ovulation; re-initiation of meiosis, luteinization, and follicular rupture, did not always occur. Thus, "premature" oocyte maturation, which is very sensitive to rising LH levels, was probably a relatively common event following superovulation therapy with CC/HMG.

Secondly, the attenuated LH surge led to ovulation and hence the appropriate time of oocyte recovery was mistimed. The occurrence of LH surges also posed a problem in the organization of clinics, as patients had to undergo oocyte recovery 24–28 h after the surge had been first detected in plasma to avoid excessive follicular rupture and lost oocytes. Thus, it was essential to know when the LH surge commenced so that oocyte recovery was performed at the correct time.

It is not surprising, therefore, that many early IVF programs that did not have an adequate monitoring system experienced variable oocyte quality. As described above, poor oocyte quality was probably due to the occurrence of a highly attenuated LH surge that

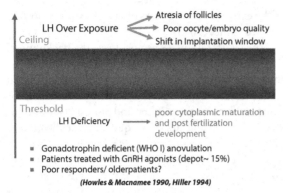

Figure 25.2 Laying the foundation for the "LH therapeutic window."

had not been detected, thus leading to mistiming of oocyte recovery.

Howles and colleagues working in the late 1980s (Howles et al., 1986, 1987), hypothesized that these elevated levels of LH indicative of attenuated LH surges arising from the use of clomiphene citrate and HMG in IVF patients was associated with poor embryo viability. Later, based on this work, Howles and MacNamee (1990) suggested that there was an LH window for normal follicle growth; if levels exceeded this window then follicular atresia and premature oocyte maturation would ensue.

Hillier further expanded upon this concept from in-vitro studies, and suggested that a high LH level led to follicular atresia, especially of the smaller follicles, leading to what he termed the "ceiling" level of LH (Hillier, 1994)(Figure 25.2).

Coming back to the challenges associated with mistimed oocyte recovery, when I arrived at Bourn Hall the main tool to monitor urinary LH was a modified hemagluttination assay (Fishel et al., 1983) which relied upon the sedimentation of erythrocytes coated with LH antibody, called Hi-Gonavis from Mochida Pharmaceuticals, Japan. The presence of LH in a urine sample modified the form of sedimentation. This assay was, at the best of times, a bit like making predictions through the reading of tea leaves spread around the bottom of a teacup. We tried other alternatives such as ovulation (LH) test sticks, but the sensitivity was not sufficient to detect subtle changes indicative of an attenuated LH surge.

Working with a Finnish company, we modified their DELFIA Immunofluorometric assay to detect low levels of LH in urine (Howles et al., 1986; 1987). It was a major step forward and facilitated a more precise

timing of oocyte retrieval. It also allowed us to closely document 24-hourly LH output and to correlate with outcome.

There still remained, however, the logistical challenge of carrying out oocyte recoveries at the whim of LH, leading to patients being taken into theater at any time between 7 am to 11 pm at night. There were some early reports of the use of a GnRH analog with agonistic properties (Fleming et al., 1982) in ovulation induction patients and then used in IVF patients. We started to explore this use first in PCOS type patients. It was not though a simple transition and we had to work on the right dosing schedule and the dose injected or given intranasally. After some fine tuning with regard to the daily agonist dose used, we virtually changed all stimulation protocols over to the luteal phase GnRH agonist protocol coupled with HMG or u-FSH with hCG trigger. The clinical utility of the GnRH agonist drugs is based on their ability to reversibly block pituitary gonadotropin secretion, thereby preventing a premature surge of luteinizing hormone (LH), which causes luteinization and disruption of normal follicle and oocyte development, a situation that was observed frequently with CC/HMG or HMG only stimulation protocols. Although a single dose of GnRH agonist stimulates the release of gonadotrophins, the administration of multiple doses causes a reversible blockade of pituitary function after an initial stimulatory phase (the so-called "flare-up" effect).

Thus in the mid-1980s a revolution in stimulation practices occurred following the introduction of the GnRH agonist into the IVF clinic. The luteal start GnRH agonist protocols are still used today and based upon the early experiences (Porter et al., 1984). The use of the GnRH agonist "long protocol" to block gonadotrophin release from the pituitary (Fleming et al., 1982; Howles et al., 1986) led to a major step forward in the clinical management of IVF patients; eliminating the incidence of an attenuated LH surge (Macnamee et al., 1987), reduction in hormone monitoring (no need for 24 h urine collections) and ultrasound scans, ability to program patients start of FSH stimulation, development of a more homogenous follicle cohort, allowing improved timing of hCG administration and the scheduling of oocyte retrieval, but at the same time increasing the period of drug treatment and number of injections (GnRH agonist pre-treatment and stimulation period), as well as increasing FSH consumption. However, the most important advantage was improved pregnancy rates across IVF centers. A host of other

GnRH agonist regimens appeared (short or flare for "poor responders", microdose or ultrashort; Howles et al., 1987), mostly used in poor responders. The GnRH long agonist regimen still reigns worldwide (≈60% cycles) as the preferred adjunct therapy and this is in spite of the fact that even today it is not registered in all markets (e.g. USA) for use in IVF. Its popularity is probably partly due to convenience for the clinic in terms of cycle scheduling. However, the GnRH agonist is now being seriously challenged by the GnRH antagonist protocol. Serono launched the first GnRH antagonist in 1999 to a tremendous fanfare (shorter treatment period, less FSH required), but it took almost 10 years to find its place in the stimulation armamentaria. The early years of the GnRH antagonist were difficult; clinics had to learn a completely new way of ovarian stimulation and monitoring, as well as losing some of the advantages of the GnRH agonist protocol such as cycle programming as well as a tendency to recruit, on average, one less oocyte and with reports of lower clinical pregnancy rates. However, with time and experience and fueled by its ability to be coupled with GnRH agonist as the "trigger" for timing oocyte retrieval (Kol et al., 2005; Humaidan et al., 2005), leading to the promise of an "OHSS free IVF clinic" (Devroey et al., 2011), the GnRH antagonist protocol continues to be more widely used.

Soon after the general introduction of the GnRH agonist into IVF stimulation protocols, I left Bourn Hall and joined Serono Pharmaceuticals, who were a major manufacturer of urinary gonadotrophins and were themselves starting on a journey to replace the urinary gonadotrophins with those manufactured using recombinant DNA technology.

Following the introduction of recombinant human insulin in 1982, drugs produced through the use of recombinant DNA techniques became a welcome alternative source of complex biological proteins across medical practice. The fact that r-hFSH preparations have a fully controlled production process from bulk to finished product, full traceability from the starting material (cell line) to the final product, unlimited supply with batch-to-batch consistency, free from urinary protein contaminants, is considered as advantageous (Howles, 1996; Loumaye et al., 1996). The conclusion has, thus, been reached that r-hFSH, indeed, is less immunogenic than the older urinary-derived medications and, at least from this point of view and overall safety, is preferable. However, the question whether recombinant derived FSH products are beneficial from the clinical perspective, has long been debated in the literature. This is in sharp contrast with other recombinant biotech drugs used in other therapeutic areas such as diabetes or growth deficiency; the widespread use of these products was not motivated by clinical superiority over biological/organic derived products but replacement was driven just on the basis of their potentially better safety profile. This argument has never really taken hold in reproductive medicine.

I was a member of the team that introduced in 1996 the first r-hFSH (follitropin alfa) (see Figure 25.2). This heralded the start of the recombinant era in reproductive medicine with the follow-up launch by the end of the decade of both r-hLH and r-hCG. In 2010 a recombinant fusion molecule (FSH coupled to the CTP of hCG, the development of which was initiated by Organon; see review by Fauser et al., 2009) with a longer FSH action was registered in EU, followed in 2014 by the launch in EU of the first biosimilar FSH (Rettenbacher et al., 2015). In 2017 another FSH (follitropin delta) with different pharmacokinetic properties compared to existing FSH products will enter the EU market (Nyboe Andersen et al., 2017). There is also a recent report of another modified FSH (follitropin epsilon) with different phamacodynamic properties from follitropin alfa, which has undergone Phase I and Phase II trials. Overall, the advances in available gonadotrophin preparations have brought improved product consistency and methods of injection delivery. However, urinary derived gonadotrophins are still prevalent in many countries and look likely to continue being part of the stimulation armament in years to come.

In IVF studies comparing gonadotropins, the most feasible primary efficacy endpoint is the number of oocytes retrieved from aspirated hCG or "LH surge" primed follicles. This is the endpoint recognized by, for example, the European Medicines Agency as pharmacologically the human FSH receptor, is only located in the female, on the granulosa cell. FSH stimulation of the granulosa cell leads to repeated cell division leading to follicle growth and cell differentiation. Whilst pregnancy and live birth are the desired outcomes for all stakeholders, implantation and pregnancy rates are influenced by a number of variables unrelated to gonadotrophin stimulation of the ovaries, such as laboratory conditions and the embryo transfer technique. Pregnancy rates can vary widely between clinics within a country and also across international borders for the same patient population (Boostanfar et al., 2012). Over the years, the measurement of gonadotrophin "efficacy" has been a subject of a multitude of generally underpowered studies, which were then combined into numerous meta analyses, yielding no major meaningful clinical difference.

Today, as a result of the availability of a combination of established as well as new techniques we are beginning to witness a total re-evaluation of how ovarian stimulation is carried out. These are the use of GnRH antagonist pituitary blockade with GnRH agonist trigger, optimized COS using biomarkers such as AMH/AFC, vitrification, new generation sequencing for PGS, and a move to segmented ART ("freeze only" cycles).

Thus, following careful, highly controlled laboratory culture and analysis using time-lapse technologies and/or preimplantation genetic screening (PGS), ideally one high-quality embryo can be transferred to the uterus, thus bringing closer to reality the mantra "one embryo one baby."

Supernumerary oocytes and/or embryos can now be more reliably cryopreserved for future use. Vitrification is a rapid freezing technique for embryos and oocytes. Vitrified, warmed embryos have very good survival rates and the technique is becoming increasingly more widely used (Cobo et al., 2015). The success of this technique in terms of both oocyte and embryo survival rates has facilitated an increased focus on documenting the cumulative live birth rate following a combination of these strategies.

While COS is aimed at maximizing the beneficial effects of treatment, the potential risks associated with ovarian hyperstimulation syndrome (OHSS) and multiple pregnancy must be taken into account (Fauser et al., 2008). OHSS is the most serious complication of COS and is triggered or exacerbated by human chorionic gonadotropin (hCG) and results in increased capillary permeability, hemoconcentration, and hypovolemia (Aboulghar and Mansour 2003). In order to minimize the incidence of OHSS, there has been an increased use of GnRH antagonist protocols coupled with a GnRH agonist (Humaidan et al., 2005) to induce final follicular maturation and to time oocyte recovery (Dosouto et al., 2017). This in itself has caused consternation with regard to the integrity of the subsequent luteal phase and its ability to support implantation, leading to a lengthy debate on how best to avoid OHSS (Devroey et al., 2011) and also how to support the luteal phase (Humaidan et al., 2015) after fresh embryo transfer.

Summary and Concluding Remarks

The use of gonadotrophins for controlled ovarian stimulation will continue to be a cornerstone of a successful ART treatment cycle. The use of segmented ART protocols will gain ground due to the need to reduce the risk of OHSS and also because of concerns about the integrity of the stimulated endometrium to allow implantation. Additionally, vitrification as well as techniques to identify a healthy embryo are facilitating a "one at a time" embryo replacement policy and a focus on cumulative live birth rates from a single course of ovarian stimulation.

References

Aboulghar MA, Mansour RT. Ovarian hyperstimulation syndrome: classifications and critical analysis of preventive measures. *Hum Reprod Update* 2003;9: 275–289.

Boostanfar R, Mannaerts B, Pang S, et al. A comparison of live birth rates and cumulative ongoing pregnancy rates between Europe and North America after ovarian stimulation with corifollitropin alfa or recombinant follicle-stimulating hormone. *Fertil Steril* 2012;97: 1351–1358.

Cobo A, Garrido N, Pellicer A, Remohí J. Six years' experience in ovum donation using vitrified oocytes: report of cumulative outcomes, impact of storage time, and development of a predictive model for oocyte survival rate. *Fertil Steril* 2015;104: 1426–1434.

Devroey P, Polyzos NP, Blockeel C. An OHSS-Free Clinic by segmentation of IVF treatment. *Hum Reprod* 2011;26: 2593–2597.

Dosouto C, Haahr T, Humaidan P. Gonadotropin-releasing hormone agonist (GnRHa) trigger – State of the art. *Reprod Biol* 2017;17: 1–8.

Edwards RG. The history of assisted human conception with especial reference to endocrinology. *Exp Clin Endocrinol Diabetes* 1996;104: 183–204.

Edwards RG, Steptoe PC. Current status of in-vitro fertilisation and implantation of human embryos. *Lancet* 1983 (Dec. 3);2(8362): 1265–1269.

Edwards RG, Steptoe PC, Purdy JM. Establishing full-term human pregnancies using cleaving embryos grown in vitro. *Br J Obstet Gynaecol* 1980; 87: 737–756.

Edwards RG, Fishel SB, Cohen J, et al. Factors influencing the success of in vitro fertilization for alleviating human infertility. *J In Vitro Fert Embryo Transf* 1984;1: 3–23.

Fauser BC, Diedrich K, Devroey P. Predictors of ovarian response: progress towards individualized treatment in ovulation induction and ovarian stimulation. *Hum Reprod Update* 2008;14: 1–14.

Fauser BC, Mannaerts BM, Devroey P, et al. Advances in recombinant DNA technology: corifollitropin alfa, a hybrid molecule with sustained follicle-stimulating activity and reduced injection frequency. *Hum Reprod Update* 2009;15: 309–321.

Fishel SB, Edwards RG, Walters DE. Follicular steroids as a prognosticator of successful fertilization of human oocytes in vitro. *J Endocrinol* 1983 (Nov);99(2): 335–344.

Fishel SB, Edwards RG, Purdy JM, et al. Implantation, abortion, and birth after in vitro fertilization using the natural menstrual cycle or follicular stimulation with clomiphene citrate and human menopausal gonadotropin. *J In Vitro Fert Embryo Transf* 1985;2: 123–131.

Fleming R, Adam AH, Barlow DH, et al. A new systematic treatment for infertile women with abnormal hormone profiles. *Br J Obstet Gynaecol* 1982;89: 80–83.

Glasier A, Thatcher SS, Wickings EJ, et al. Superovulation with exogenous gonadotrophins does not inhibit the luteinizing hormone surge. *Fertil Steril* 1988; 49: 81.

Hillier SG. Current concepts of the roles of follicle stimulating hormone and luteinizing hormone in folliculogenesis. *Hum Reprod* 1994;9: 188–191.

Hillier SG. IVF endocrinology: the Edwards era. *Mol Hum Reprod* 2013 (Dec.);19(12): 799–808.

Howles CM. Genetic engineering of human FSH (Gonal-F). *Hum Reprod Update* 1996;2: 172–191. Recombinant gonadotrophins in reproductive medicine: the gold standard of today. *Reprod Biomed Online* 2006;12: 11–13.

Howles CM, Macnamee MC. The endocrinology of stimulated cycles and influence on outcome. In: Mashiach S et al. (eds.) *Advances in Assisted Reproductive Technologies*. New York Plenum Press, 1990, p. 311.

Howles CM, Macnamee MC, Edwards RG, Goswamy R, Steptoe PC. Effect of high tonic levels of luteinising hormone on outcome of in-vitro fertilisation. *Lancet* 1986;2(8505): 521–522.

Howles CM, Macnamee MC, Edwards RG. Follicular development and early luteal function of conception and non conceptional cycles after human in vitro fertilisation: endocrine correlates. *Hum Reprod* 1987; 2: 17.

Short term use of an LHRH agonist to treat poor responders entering an in-vitro fertilization programme. *Hum Reprod* 1987 (Nov);2(8): 655–656.

Humaidan P, Bredkjaer HE, Bungum L, et al. GnRH agonist (buserelin) or hCG for ovulation induction in GnRH antagonist IVF/ICSI cycles: a prospective randomized study. *Hum Reprod* 2005;20: 1213–1220.

Humaidan P, Engmann L, Benadiva C. Luteal phase supplementation after gonadotropin-releasing

hormone agonist trigger in fresh embryo transfer: the American versus European approaches. *Fertil Steril* 2015;103: 879–885.

Jones WJ Jr., Jones GS, Andrews MC, et al. The program for in vitro fertilization at Norfolk. *Fertil Steril* 1982;38:14–21.

Kol S, Muchtar M. Recombinant gonadotrophin-based, ovarian hyperstimulation syndrome-free stimulation of the high responder: suggested protocol for further research. *Reprod Biomed Online* 2005;10: 575–577.

Loumaye E, Martineau I, Piazzi A, et al. Clinical assessment of human gonadotrophins produced by recombinant DNA technology. *Hum Reprod* 1996;11 Suppl. 1: 95–107.

Lunenfeld B. Historical perspectives in gonadotrophin therapy. *Hum Reprod Update* 2004;10: 453–467.

Macnamee MC, Edwards RG, Howles CM. The influence of stimulation regimens and luteal phase support on the outcome of IVF. *Hum Reprod* 1988;3 (suppl. 2): 43.

Macnamee MC, Howles CM, Edwards RG. Pregnancies after IVF when high tonic LH is reduced by long-term treatment with GnRH agonists. *Hum Reprod* 1987 (Oct.);2(7): 569–571.

Messinis IE, Templeton AA, Baird DT. Endogenous LH surge during superovulation induction with sequential use of cc and pulsatile HMG. *J Clin Endocrinol Metab* 1985;61: 1076.

Nyboe Andersen A, Nelson SM, Fauser BC, et al. ESTHER-1 study group. Individualized versus conventional ovarian stimulation for in vitro fertilization: a multicenter, randomized, controlled, assessor-blinded, phase 3 noninferiority trial. *Fertil Steril* 2017;107: 387–396.

Porter RN, Smith W, Craft IL, Abdulwahid NA, Jacobs HS. Induction of ovulation for in-vitro fertilisation using buserelin and gonadotropins. *Lancet* 1984;2(8414):1284–1285.

Rettenbacher M, Andersen AN, Garcia-Velasco JA, et al. A multi-centre phase 3 study comparing efficacy and safety of Bemfola(®) versus Gonal-f(®) in women undergoing ovarian stimulation for IVF. *Reprod Biomed Online* 2015;30: 504–513.

Steptoe PC, Edwards RG. Laparoscopic recovery of preovulatory human oocytes after priming of ovaries with gonadotrophins. *Lancet* 1970 ;1(7649): 683–689.

Reimplantation of a human embryo with subsequent tubal pregnancy. *Lancet* 1976;1(7965): 880–882.

Trounson AO, Leeton JF, Wood C, Webb J, Wood J. Pregnancies in humans by fertilization in vitro and embryo transfer in the controlled ovulatory cycle. *Science* 1981;212: 681–682.

Chapter 26

The Development of Microsurgery for Male and Female Infertility

Sherman J. Silber

My 47-year history of developing what was once considered an innovative technique of microsurgery began in 1970 when I was a urology resident at the University of Michigan in Ann Arbor, not at all interested in infertility. My goal was to understand compensatory renal hypertrophy, i.e. why when you remove one kidney, the other kidney compensates by getting bigger, and renal function of the remaining kidney is almost doubled. So I decided to transplant extra kidneys into animals, to see if the reverse would occur, i.e. would the kidneys "hypotrophy?" I did not want the experiment to be hampered by rejection, and the largest animal inbred enough to avoid rejection was the rat. So I developed in my earliest papers the original microvascular surgery which created the three and four kidney rat model (Silber and Crudop, 1973). With the help of a brilliant janitor at the University of Michigan animal lab, Jimmy Crudop, I transplanted extra kidneys from one Lewis rat into another Lewis rat using donor renal artery and vein anastomosis to the recipient aorta and vena cava. I developed my microsurgical skills by developing the technique of renal transplantation in rats using an operating microscope. We also developed what is even now a modern approach to preventing allograft rejection using prior properly timed injection of donor antigens (Silber, 1974). Thus when I left Ann Arbor, Michigan, and Melbourne, Australia, I was known as a kidney transplanter and microvascular surgeon. But I had no idea I would ever be an infertility doctor. In fact I hated the smell of semen.

While in Melbourne, I worked with Bob Fowler and Douglas Stephens, who were very unhappy with their popular "Fowler–Stephens" operation for intra-abdominal cryptorchid testis, because of ischemic testis atrophy. So I developed the microvascular testis autotransplant procedure, using the same microvascular technique on human spermatic artery and vein that Jimmy Crudop and I had developed for renal artery and vein in rats (Silber and Kelly, 1976). We divided the spermatid artery and vein of these young boys, which

was at that time always avoided (thus in the past keeping the testis tethered up high), and we re-anastomosed them to the inferior epigastric artery and vein. This amazingly allowed the intra-abdominal testis, otherwise high up near the kidney, to be safely brought down to the scrotum. This had never been done before. These boys then did not suffer testis atrophy after these procedures, and grew up to be fertile young men. Fowler and Stephens adopted this procedure and indeed gave me credit for it. But urologists who were not microvascular surgeons continued to use only the more destructive Fowler–Stephens operation.

Before leaving Melbourne in 1975, I worked with the famed plastic surgeon Ian Taylor, to perform the first human free microvascular skin graft. I had taught Ian Taylor how to do microvascular anastomoses in rats in Peter Morris's lab in Melbourne, and Ian had worked out the anatomy of the skin of the groin. So together we performed the world's first free huge vascularized skin flap, which revolutionized reconstructive plastic surgery (Figure 26.1).

In 1978, using these same microsurgery techniques we performed the first human testis transplant, from an identical twin with two normal testes to his brother with anorchia (born with no testes) (Silber, 1978b). These testis transplants worked perfectly, and resulted in five healthy babies from spontaneous pregnancies. This achievement was hailed as a great newsworthy advancement at the AUA (American Urological Association) meeting that year and was praised by the great Dr. Willard Goodwin of UCLA urology fame.

But I never dreamed my greatest reputation would come from vasectomy reversal. In fact I considered that to be just an insignificant fun thing to do, but not very important. I honestly thought that no one who had a vasectomy would ever want it reversed. So the original papers I wrote on microsurgery to reverse vasectomy seemed to me to be trivial.

So finally came microsurgery for vasectomy reversal and vasoepididymostomy after presentation of a

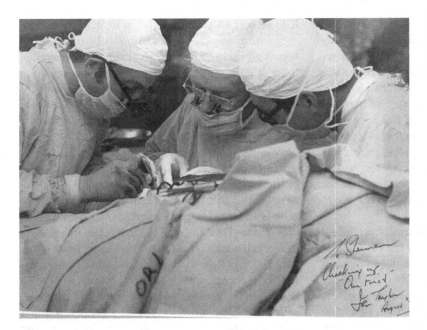

Figure 26.1 The author and Dr. Ian Taylor in 1975 performing the world's first free microvascularized groin and bone flap, using techniques honed in the rat lab.

live telecast to 20,000 surgeons on closed-circuit TV at the American College of Surgeons meeting in San Francisco in October of 1975. It was immediately the main story on the front page of the *New York Times* (Brody, 1975). This was in 1975, three years before IVF. It was shocking to the world that we could get such high pregnancy rates in otherwise azoospermic men by simply doing a better microsurgical anastomosis (Brody, 1975). It had been thought erroneously before this that the consistent failure of vasectomy reversal was due to sperm antibodies, which has subsequently been completely disproven. The cause of the consistent failure of vasectomy reversal was not some obscure autoimmunity, but rather just mechanical failure to re-establish accurate continuity. This news made the front page of almost every newspaper in the world. There was no internet or web then, but it hit the AP wire service and the news spread everywhere.

There was, however, great controversy. Some called vasectomy reversal "immoral." They would actually argue at urology meetings, "If a man has had a vasectomy, it is unethical to reverse it." Others said, "You don't need a microscope," and some even apocryphally claimed they already were doing this (although only Earl Owen of Sydney began to do this around the same time that I did). No one could believe we actually performed a two-layer anastomosis of this tiny structure. We used 10-0 nylon interrupted stitches for the inner mucosa, and 9-0 for the outer muscle. Most urologists

had no idea what a 10-0 nylon suture was. Some who resisted using a microscope claimed that two layers were not necessary. But eventually everyone finally accepted that microsurgical two layer anastomosis was the proper procedure for vasovasostomy. Nonetheless, I suffered extreme criticism either because of professional jealousy or fear of a future they could not grasp. Only Bruce Stewart of the Cleveland Clinic and Earl Owen of Sydney supported me. But eventually all urologists in the world reluctantly adopted my procedure.

However, we noted in my 1977 papers that if there was no sperm in the vas fluid at the time of vasovasostomy, the operation always failed, despite a perfect anastomosis. Furthermore the testis biopsy, despite no sperm in the vas fluid, always showed normal spermatogenesis. Also if there was a sperm granuloma at the vasectomy site, there was always sperm in the vas fluid, and virtually all vasovasostomies in that case were successful (Silber, 1977). In fact, we recommended "open-ended" vasectomy to ensure the formation of sperm granuloma as early as 1978. We were promptly ridiculed for this suggestion, but we were, and still are, correct.

Because of this observation, we explored the epididymis in men with no sperm in the vas fluid (remember, spermatogenesis is always normal in these men), and found pressure induced secondary epididymal extravasation and blowouts, and thus, secondary epididymal obstruction was found in all of these

209

cases with no sperm in the vas fluid (Silber, 1979). We found that there was always increased pressure buildup after vasectomy. At that time we found that the longer the duration of time since vasectomy the greater was the incidence of epdidymal blowouts, due to a longer interval of increased pressure. Poor results were not caused by damage to the testis owing to a long duration of obstruction, although to this day patients are erroneously being told this. We actually wrote the original papers that showed success rates for vasovasostomy were better if the vasectomy was less than ten years before the reversal. However, this was not due to testicular damage.

In 1978 we developed a microsurgical procedure for anastomosing the inner mucosa of the vas deferens to the very delicate specific tubule of the epididymis proximal to the site of obstruction (Silber, 1978a). The results were, astoundingly, as good as with vasovasostomy when there was sperm in the vas fluid. This again was at first greeted with disbelief and initially disdain. Most urologists shy away from this approach even today, but our success rate of over 95% argues in favor of it. Nonetheless, the epididymal tubule is so tiny and fragile that very few urologists even today attempt this procedure. But this procedure revolutionized the surgery for obstructive azoospermia.

However, there were cases of obstructive azoospermia where there was no vas (congenital absence of vas, CBVAD), for which we developed the microepidymal sperm aspiration (MESA) procedure first with IVF in 1986, and then with intracytoplasmic sperm injection (ICSI) in 1992 (Devroy et al., 1994). Again, remarkably, pregnancy and live baby rates were no different from couples with normal sperm counts in their ejaculate.

Then even more remarkably, in Brussels, when there was no epididymis at all, we reported in 1993 that testicular non-motile sperm with ICSI resulted in normal pregnancy and live baby rates (Devroy et al., 1995). We termed that procedure TESE (testicular sperm extraction). We still have the original napkin from the surgeon's lounge in Brussels where Paul Devroey wrote this down when we coined the eponym "TESE" (Silber et al., 1995). We also changed the basic science concept of epididymal function. It had been thought that the most motile sperm would be the most distal, that had transversed through most of the epididymis, but we discovered the opposite was true in cases of obstruction, and found good motility only in the most proximal sperm. This discovery revolutionized IVF and

ICSI success with MESA. Then, in 1994, we found that even with azoospermic men without obstruction (and seemingly no spermatogenesis at all), there were often (over 50%) a very tiny number of rare spermatazoa in the testis, which were adequate for successful ICSI with normal pregnancies (Silber et al., 1996). This was based on our original papers on quantitative histologic examination of testis biopsies in the 1970s.

We then used these early pioneering micro TESE patients to map and sequence the Y chromosome, beginning in 1995 in the Page Lab at MIT, and we were the first to discover genes that control spermatogenesis and are deleted in infertile men. This was the now famous DAZ (deleted in azoospermia) gene – we in fact coined the term DAZ. From there again at the Page Lab, we (Reijo et al., 1995) discovered autosomal DAZL on chromosome 3. As it now turns out DAZL is the major ancestral universal gene that "licenses" early embryonic stem cells to become germ cells, either sperm or in fact eggs. This discovery, in 1995, turns out to be the central most common key to spermatogenesis and oogenesis in most animals going far back in the phylogenetic tree (Silber, 2011).

With our development of microsurgical TESE, we discovered the simplest way to avoid adhesions, which applies obviously to tubal microsurgery as well. Whenever we had to re-operate on these men with non-obstructive azoospermia, to retrieve more sperm, there were never any adhesions in the tunica albuginea space. It was as though there had never been any previous surgery in his scrotum. We realized that this was an affirmation, within the scrotum, of the principles of minimal tissue trauma, perfect hemostasis, and pulsatile irrigation with heparinized saline promulgated by Gomel and Winston. There was no commercial adhesion prevention product that could compare with just keeping the tissue constantly wet with heparinized saline, and using micro-bipolar forces for hemostasis with no tissue damage.

As important as prevention of adhesions we learned from our 30-year history with TESE, was how to avoid testis tissue damage with microsurgery, despite total exploration of the testis to find the rare sperm in an azoospermic male that had appeared to be making no sperm. We avoided intra-testicular swelling and subsequent testis atrophy by stopping all bleeding with microbipolar forceps and closing the tunica albuginea (which has no elasticity) with 9-0 nylon interrupted sutures, rather than the prevailing running stitch with 4-0 vicryl. This prevents a purse string reduction in testis volume and subsequent pressure atrophy. Furthermore we studied the location of spermatogenic stem cells (SSCs) and realized that the surgeon does not have to "dig into" the testis to find the rare sperm. That procedure, called "microdissection," actually destroys testis tissue and creates ischemic atrophy by interruption of testis "end-arteries." One can stay on the periphery of the seminiferous tubules and sample nonetheless every anatomic lobule. If there is a spermatogenic stem cell (SSC) anywhere within the testis, you will find sperm at the periphery of the tubule where it loops around. Thus you avoid any internal testis damage (as occurs usually with the so-called "microdissection" technique).

Varicocoelectomy has been a very popular operation for infertile men since 1952, for well over half a century. I am no longer an advocate of that procedure, even though for many urologists it is still very popular. However, I did make it a much safer procedure in 1979 by being the first to introduce a microsurgical approach, thus sparing damage to the tiny spermatic artery (Silber, 1979). Prior to that, there was a 5% incidence of painful hydrocele, and often testicular atrophy or a reduction (rather than increase) in spermatogenesis because of spermatic artery damage. In addition, recurrence of the varicocoele, because of failure to ligate every spermatic vein, was common. Although before 1979 no one used a microsurgical approach to varicocoelectomy, now everyone does.

Despite my popularization of the microsurgical approach to varicocoelectomy, I realized in the mid 1980s and early 1990s that varicocoelectomy results were no better than controls who never underwent varicocoelectomy. In well-performed studies, (most notable Baker et al. in Melbourne, Australia, and Neischlag et al. in Germany) it was clearly shown that varicocoelectomy was a worthless procedure for improving male infertility. My papers and talks on this subject have severely angered, and still anger, most urologists, despite the fact that the vast majority of infertility doctors, who are not urologists, completely agree with me. In fact, when men undergo this pointless procedure, waiting for the sperm count to improve, the wife's eggs are simply getting older. So going through this varicocoelectomy approach is actually detrimental to the couple's chances for having a baby. My views on this have severely alienated urologists who desperately cling to this operation.

Most recently, we have turned our attention to culturing and freezing spermatogonial stem cells (SSCs) in order to transplant them back after sterilizing chemotherapy in pre-pubertal boys with cancer. We have analyzed, with single cell analysis of gene transcription, the entire genomics of spermatogenesis, and identified the heretofore-elusive human SSCs. We can easily freeze a TESE specimen from a pre-pubertal boy, and then when he is an adult, culture and amplify the number of SSCs, and then transplant them later into his azoospermic testis. Such spectacular progress in Andrology was made possible by dispensing with hopeless treatments such as varicocoelectomy and hormonal stimulation, and focusing instead on microsurgical TESE, genetics, and cell culture.

Our microsurgery for male infertility also now has great application to females. Tubal microsurgery was first introduced in England by Winston (Winston, 1977) and in Canada by Gomel (Gomel, 1977) in the mid 1970s. However we were among the first to perform successful tubal microsurgery (to reverse tubal ligation) in the United States, bringing to America the techniques of Winston and Gomel (Silber and Cohen, 1984). Then in 2004 we performed the first fresh human ovary transplant in the world between identical twins using microsurgery (Silber et al., 2005) (Figure 26.2) – just like the world's first testis transplants we performed in 1976 and 1978. We later performed the first successful frozen ovary transplant in the United States, following those of Donnez in Belgium and Meirow in Israel (Silber, 2016). We now (at the time of writing in 2017) have a series from our center alone of 23 healthy babies from these procedures in women who had been menopausal for more than five years, either from premature ovarian failure (POF) or from cancer treatments (Silber, 2016).

We are the only center in the United States with such success with fresh or frozen ovary transplants. Finally, as a result of our scientific study of this remarkable series of human ovary transplants, we have deciphered the duration of time in the human between primordial follicle recruitment and ovulation, as well as the heretofore mysterious control of that recruitment (Silber et al., 2015) Furthermore, currently, by studying the development of human oocytes from the skin cells of our identical twins discordant for premature ovarian failure we are determining at what embryonic stage primordial germ cell (PGC) specification occurs in the human embryo.

So it has been a long, almost half a century, journey from my first microsurgical experiments in rats to remarkable advances in the understanding and

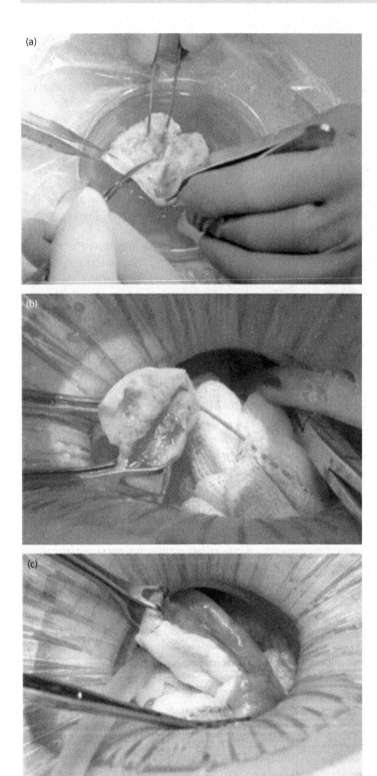

Figure 26.2 Picture of first successful human ovary transplant.

treatment of human infertility, both in the male and the female. In fact our results with vasectomy reversal, tubal reversal, and vasoepidymostomy are still stunning, despite the great ease now of microsurgery for MESA, TESE, and IVF, which evolved from those original studies in the early 1970s in rats. The future for male infertility now is testis freezing and SSC transplantation, as well as deciphering the entire genetic transcriptome of spermatogenesis. In the female, it is ovary freezing, transplantation and creation of stem cells (IPS) and oocytes from skin.

References

Brody, EJ. (1975, October 8). *New York Times*, p. 1. Retrieved from http://www.nytimes.com/1975/10/08/archives/microsurgery-successful-in-vasectomy-reversals-vasectomy-test.html?mcubz=0

Devroey P, Liu J, Nagy Z, et al. Normal fertilization of human oocytes after testicular sperm extraction and intracytoplasmic sperm injection. *Fertil Steril* 1994;62:639–641.

Pregnancies after testicular sperm extraction and intracytoplasmic sperm injection in non-obstructive azoospermia. *Hum Reprod* 1995;10:1457–1460.

Gomel V. Tubal reanastomosis by microsurgery. *Fertil Steril* 1977 Jan.;28(1):59–65.

Reijo R, Lee TY, Salo P, et al. Diverse spermatogenic defects in humans caused by Y chromosome deletions encompassing a novel RNA-binding protein gene. *Nat Genet* 1995;10:383–393.

Silber SJ. The prevention of acute tubular necrosis in renal transplantation by chronic salt loading of the recipient. *Aust N Z J Surg* 1974;44:410–412.

Silber SJ. Sperm granuloma and reversibility of vasectomy. *Lancet* 1977;2:588–589.

Silber SJ. Microscopic vasoepididymostomy: specific microanastomosis to the epididymal tubule. *Fertil Steril* 1978a;30:565–571.

Transplantation of a human testis for anorchia. *Fertil Steril* 1978b;30:181–187.

Microsurgical aspects of varicocele. *Fertil Steril* 1979;31:230–232.

Silber SJ. The Y chromosome in the era of intracytoplasmic sperm injection: a personal review. *Fertil Steril* 2011;95:2439–2448, e1–5.

Unifying theory of adult resting follicle recruitment and fetal oocyte arrest. *Reprod Biomed Online* 2015;31:472–475.

Silber S. Ovarian tissue cryopreservation and transplantation: scientific implications. *J Assist Reprod Genet* 2016;33:1595–1603.

Silber SJ, Crudop J. Kidney transplantation in inbred rats. *Am J Surg* 1973;125:551–553.

Silber SJ, Cohen R. Microsurgical reversal of tubal sterilization: factors affecting pregnancy rate, with long-term follow-up. *Obstet Gynecol* 1984;64:679–682.

Silber SJ, Kelly J. Successful autotransplantation of an intraabdominal testis to the scrotum by microvascular technique. *J Urol* 1976;115:452.

Silber SJ, Van Steirteghem AC, Liu J, et al. High fertilization and pregnancy rate after intracytoplasmic sperm injection with spermatozoa obtained from testicle biopsy. *Hum Reprod* 1995;10:148–152.

Silber SJ, van Steirteghem A, Nagy Z, et al. Normal pregnancies resulting from testicular sperm extraction and intracytoplasmic sperm injection for azoospermia due to maturation arrest. *Fertil Steril* 1996;66:110–117.

Silber SJ, Lenahan KM, Levine DJ, et al. Ovarian transplantation between monozygotic twins discordant for premature ovarian failure. *N Engl J Med* 2005;353:58–63.

Silber S, Pineda J, Lenahan K, DeRosa M, Melnick J. Fresh and cryopreserved ovary transplantation and resting follicle recruitment. *Reprod Biomed Online* 2015;30:643–650.

Winston RM. Microsurgical tubocornual anastomosis for reversal of sterilisation. *Lancet* 1977;1(8006):284–285.

Chapter 27

Embryonic Stem Cells, Medicine's New Frontier

Ariff Bongso

In-Vivo Fertilization and Early Human Embryonic Development

Clinical embryologists see fertilization as a complex series of events between two highly specialized cell types, one as small as 3–5 μm (head of spermatozoon) and the other the largest cell in the human body, approximately 100–120 μm (oocyte). Very little was known visually during fertilization in vivo until it was possible to fertilize oocytes with sperm in a laboratory dish. Although a human male can produce as many as 100 million sperm in his ejaculate, only 20 million are required to be deposited at the cervix during intercourse to bring about a pregnancy. Approximately 2000 actively motile sperm finally reach the ampullary region of the Fallopian tube to allow one spermatozoon to fertilize the oocyte. Once the sperm enters the oocyte, the first four days of conception (fertilization to the mulberry-shaped morula stage) occur within the Fallopian tube after which the five-day-old embryo (an early blastocyst) enters the uterus to find its site of implantation in the endometrium to establish a pregnancy around days 7–9. Confirmation that the blastocyst enters the uterus at the early cavitating stage and then undergoes cleavage to expanded and hatching blastocysts was established from lavaged flushings of the uterus after hysterectomies. More than one blastocyst was found in the uterus, suggesting that there is a high degree of reproductive wastage in the human.

Following implantation, cells migrate within the expanded blastocyst to lay down two distinct cell layers, a peripheral layer of trophectoderm (TE) destined to become the placenta, and a cluster of cells (the inner cell mass, ICM) that protrude from the inner wall of the blastocyst and are destined to become the fetus. The ICM later develops into the hypoblast and epiblast. The hypoblast produces the yolk sac, which eventually degenerates, while the epiblast gives rise to the three germ layers (ectoderm, mesoderm, and endoderm) from which the various organs are produced. The

umbilical cord (UC) is physiologically and genetically part of the fetus and contains part of the yolk sac and allantois. It forms during the fifth week of development, replacing the yolk sac as the source of nutrients, and carries within it the three umbilical blood vessels (two arteries and a vein) that then begin to shuttle nutrients between mother and fetus (Bongso and Fong, 2013).

In-Vitro Fertilization

The possibility of transferring embryos from the reproductive tract of one mammal to another with the production of viable offspring that are fostered by a surrogate mother goes as far back as 1890 in some elegant experiments in the rabbit. Later, in the 1940s, this idea was practised in farm animals where the ovaries of genetically superior females (cows with high lactation yields) were stimulated with hormones to produce many oocytes and then artificially inseminated with the sperm of genetically superior males (bulls with a genetic history of producing offspring with high lactation yields). The resulting embryos at the blastocyst stage were flushed out of the uteri non-surgically and then transferred to "ordinary" genetically inferior surrogates to produce offspring with the highest genetic merit for milk production. From a single donor, at least 5–10 blastocysts could be obtained. Today, the procedure of multiple ovulation–embryo transfer is routinely used in the farm animal industry to produce increased yields of protein for human consumption. The average "take-home offspring rate" using this method is about 60%.

This protocol was later modified to the human, where oocytes generated from stimulated ovaries of subfertile women were aspirated and fertilized in a laboratory dish (in-vitro fertilization, IVF). The more detailed events occurring during human fertilization and early embryonic growth could then be recorded. Fertilization rates of over 80% could be obtained by exposing an optimal number of washed motile sperm to a single oocyte. Ovarian stimulation protocols that produced mature oocytes that yielded high fertilization rates and embryos that had a high chance of implantation were then optimized. For men with suboptimal sperm parameters, a single sperm could be microinjected into an oocyte to produce an embryo for transfer (intracytoplasmic sperm injection, ICSI). In the early years of IVF up to three day-2 embryos (two- to four-cell stage) were replaced with take-home baby rates of 10–15%.

The ability to visualize early embryonic events under the microscope led to very accurate recordings of important cleavage events in the human. Successful fertilization was recognized in vitro when two pronuclei were formed in the oocyte approximately 18–22 h after insemination. Male and female pronuclei could be distinguished from size, the larger being the female, and fusion of the two pronuclei leads to syngamy with the disappearance of the pronuclei. Thereafter, the pronuclei fuse and cleavage is initiated with the formation of two equal-sized blastomeres that cleave to four equal-sized blastomeres (day-2, four-cell stage) about 46 h post-insemination. After 72 h post-insemination, the four-cell stage embryo cleaves to the eight-cell stage on day 3.

Cryopreservation of Human Embryos

In order to increase the cumulative pregnancy rate and for reasons that required the delay of transfer of embryos, it became necessary to develop freezing protocols to store such human embryos at various embryonic stages. The first successful cryopreservation procedure of high thaw-survival rates of four- and eight-cell human embryos followed by the establishment of a pregnancy after the transfer of one frozen-thawed eight-cell embryo was reported in 1983 (Trounson and Mohr, 1983). Later, cryopreservation studies on 97 day-2 and day-3 human embryos showed that thaw-survival was possible using different cryoprotectants and freezing procedures. These included programmed slow-cooling methods and dimethyl sulfoxide (DMSO) as a cryoprotectant. Today, these methods are used routinely in the freezing of early stage embryos in IVF programs (Mohr and Trounson, 1985). After the development of blastocyst culture, slow freezing methods with glycerol as cryprotectant and faster snap-freezing (vitrification) methods with ethylene glycol as cryoprotectant were successfully developed for the storage of blastocyst-stage embryos (Yokota et al., 2001).

Blastocyst Culture Sets the Stage for the Isolation of Embryonic Stem Cells

It has been claimed that the transfer of embryos on day-2 into the uterus results in suboptimal pregnancy and delivery rates. Discordance between the stage of embryo replaced and the receptivity of the uterus significantly limits the "take-home" success rate because physiologically it is a blastocyst that reaches the uterus for implantation. The replacement of blastocysts was previously impossible because only 15–20% of human embryos actually reach the blastocyst stage under conventional culture conditions with simple culture media, because of an "in-vitro embryonic block" between day 2 and day 3 in the human when transcription events were being handed over from mother to embryo.

To enable blastocyst development in vitro, it was necessary to mimic the conditions of the Fallopian tubal environment. This was accomplished by growing human embryos on a feeder layer of Fallopian tubal epithelial cells harvested from the inner lining of the Fallopian tubes of women undergoing hysterectomy. Called the co-culture technique, the tubal cells provided the nutrients to not only improve the quality of four- and eight-cell stage embryos but also to extend their growth to blastocysts with cleavage rates of as high as 68%. The replacement of co-cultured blastocysts into the uterus produced increased pregnancy rates of nearly 42% in patients aged 35 years or older who had experienced two previous IVF failures (Bongso et al., 1999). Embryos grown on such cell monolayers showed less fragmentation, had expanded blastomeres and cleaved faster at rates close to in-vivo conditions. In the human Fallopian tubal in-vitro environment, expanded blastocysts of improved viability were produced on day 5 and hatching commenced on day 6. A grading system for blastocyst quality became available and it was possible to observe the behavior of such human embryos during co-culture for up to six or seven days. The mechanism of the co-culture system was via the secretion of embryotrophic factors that enhanced embryo growth and/or the cells removing toxic or unwanted metabolites from the medium. Some of the embryotrophic factors that were identified included insulin-like growth factor-1, platelet-derived growth factor, transforming growth factor and glycoproteins. During the negative conditioning process there were alterations in the energy substrates or stabilization of the oxygen and carbon dioxide tensions in the medium (Bongso et al., 1999). The tubal cells were later replaced with cell-free sequential culture media where pronuclear embryos were grown in the first medium up to day 2 and then switched to a second more complex culture medium on day 2 to generate blastocysts (Gardner et al., 2002). Blastocyst transfer, with high birth rates, is practised today in some IVF centers.

From IVF to Blastocysts to Embryonic Stem Cells

Nature has provided remarkable regenerative abilities for animals and this has fascinated man for a long time. In some animals when tissues are lost, the remaining tissues organize themselves to form the missing body part. Amongst the invertebrates, planarian flatworms and hydra regenerate their tissues with great speed. Some vertebrates such as the salamanders regenerate their lost body parts through the dedifferentiation of specialized cells into new precursor cells. Most of the higher chordates do not have the capabilities of whole-organ regeneration but possess the machinery to generate new tissues during embryonic development (Bongso and Richards, 2004). Most mammals have lost their regenerative abilities but have been rewarded with efficient wound healing capabilities as a trade-off. The complete replacement of antlers during the rutting (mating) season in elks is the most significant form of regeneration known in mammals, while liver regeneration after partial hepatectomy is the only form of natural regeneration known in the human. It has been claimed that tissue repair in mammals are dedifferentiation-independent events that result from the activation of pre-existing stem or progenitor cells lying within the tissues. The stem cell is the common denominator for nearly all types of regeneration which are either already pre-existing or created during the process of dedifferentiation. Stem cells are buzzwords today and we read about them in almost every journal across various disciplines. At the same time, there is also a lot of hype as to how stem cells can treat every imaginable disease and even prolong the life span of the human being. Furthermore, embryonic stem cell research has often been unjustly associated with reproductive cloning (Bongso and Richards, 2004).

Bone marrow stem cell transplantation has been the traditional form of stem cell therapy for malignant hematopoietic diseases and has been the source of inspiration to explore for other sources of stem cells with wider plasticity that could help treat a wider spectrum of diseases. The concepts of co-culture and blastocyst culture in IVF set the stage for the isolation and development of human embryonic stem cells (hESCs). Without the advent of blastocyst culture to improve IVF pregnancy rates, hESC research would have never evolved, since blastocysts with a recognisable ICM were required to isolate hESCs. The use of feeder layers (co-culture) to prolong the growth of human embryos beyond day 7 was also an important milestone that assisted the derivation of hESCs. This is because the initial derivation of hESCs from ICMs could not be successfully achieved under feeder-free conditions even with the best of culture media.

With the development of blastocyst culture, it became clear that the cells of the ICM were omnipotent and that nature had her own recipe of differentiation factors to program differentiation of the ICM cells into all the respective tissues of the human being via the three primordial germ layers. In 1994, our group was the first to recognize and report the isolation and culture of human embryonic stem cell-like cells from the ICMs of blastocysts (Bongso et al., 1994). Patients enrolled in our IVF program donated their surplus embryos which were co-cultured on human Fallopian tubal ampullary epithelial feeders to generate blastocysts. Once cavitating blastocysts were formed, the medium was changed to Chang's medium supplemented with human serum and human recombinant leukaemia inhibitory factor (hLIF), which was a differentiation inhibitor. The blastocysts were left undisturbed for 48 h to allow hatching, attachment and continued non-differentiated growth of the ICM and TE in the presence of hLIF on the feeder layer. The ICM grew as a piled-up lump on the monolayer and large trophoblast cells began to spread out from the peripheral regions of each lump on days 8 and 9. The ICM lumps were then mechanically separated, disaggregated into clusters of cells using trypsin-EDTA, and re-cultured on fresh Fallopian tubal ampullary feeder layers bathed in Chang's medium containing hLIF. The nest-like ICM colonies of cells took on the typical morphological characteristics of hESCs (circular small cells with high nuclear-cytoplasmic ratios and prominent nucleoli), which were non-committed cells that had the potential to enter a full range of developmental pathways. These hESCs were grown for up to two passages without differentiation (Bongso et al., 1994). Four years later, the

216

ICMs of human blastocysts were isolated by immuno-surgery, grown on irradiated mouse embryonic fibro-blasts as feeders, and the first hESC line established (Thomson et al., 1998). Following these two seminal papers, hESC lines were then readily derived by other groups (Reubinoff et al., 2000; Cowan et al., 2004).

Characterization and Differentiation of Human Embryonic Stem Cells

The stemness properties of hESCs can be character-ized using a battery of assays. These include biochemi-cal and gene expression markers (SSEA-4, TRA-1-81, alkaline phosphatase, TERT, OCT4, SOX2, NANOG), confirmation of pluripotency by the production of tera-tomas in immunodeficient mice, stability of a normal karyotype in serial culture, telomerase production, and the ability to differentiate into tissues originat-ing from all three primordial germ layers (ectoderm, mesoderm, and endoderm) (Gokhale and Andrews, 2013).

The hESCs are social cells that love their neigh-bors. If disassociated, they would differentiate into undesirable cell types. The challenge therefore is to keep them undifferentiated and then take control of their differentiation into a specific desired lineage. The first report of differentiation of hESCs was into neural progenitor cells (Reubinoff et al., 2000). After prolonged cultivation of hESCs to high density (four to seven weeks), vesicular structures appeared above the plane of the feeder layer and among these struc-tures were clusters of cells with elongated processes that extended out from their cell bodies forming net-works as they contacted other cells. The cells and the processes of these neural derivatives stained positively with antibodies against neurofilament proteins and the neural cell adhesion molecules. These cell areas were isolated and re-plated in serum-free medium after which they formed spherical structures within 24 h. Cells in these neurospheres initially expressed markers of primitive neuroectoderm (polysialylated N-CAM, the intermediate filament proteins nestin, vimentin and transcription factor Pax-6). Later, these differentiated cells began to display the morphology and expression of structural markers characteristic of mature neuronal differentiation (160 and 200 kDa neurofilament proteins, b-tubulin, Map2a, b, and syn-aptophysin) (Reubinoff et al., 2000). Today, a variety of differentiation protocols have been developed to differentiate hESCs into almost any lineage of choice,

the most notable being for the differentiation of pan-creatic islet cells that secrete insulin (Millman et al., 2016).

Clinical Grade Human Embryonic Stem Cells

Reliance on xeno-support systems such as murine embryonic feeder fibroblasts introduces considerable disadvantages with respect to exploiting the therapeu-tic potential of hESCs. A major drawback is the risk of transmitting pathogens from the animal feeder cells or culture medium to the hESCs. A protocol for the deri-vation of the first xeno-free hESC line was reported in 2002 (Richards et al., 2002). The hESCs were derived and propagated from a human embryo on mitomycin-C-treated human fetal muscle feeders in the absence of hLIF and in the presence of human-based ingre-dients. There was no exposure to animal feeders, matrices, or animal-based products in the in-vitro system. The same authors also showed that a variety of human feeder cell types could support the propaga-tion of hESCs such as human fetal muscle and human fetal and adult skin from in-house derived and com-mercial sources. It was thus possible to collect a skin biopsy from the IVF patient donating an embryo for hESC derivation to act as an autologous feeder layer to derive and propagate hESCs. These feeders would be disease-free as the patient would have been previ-ously screened for HIV and hepatitis B before entering the IVF program, thus eliminating the risk of cross-contamination of the hESCs with pathogens from the human feeders (Richards et al., 2002). The production of such a xeno-free culture system set the stage for the later development of clinical grade hESC lines for cell-based therapies (Crook et al., 2007).

Hurdles in Taking hESCs to the Clinic

There are some hurdles that have to be overcome before hESC-derived tissue therapy becomes a routine proce-dure. Some of these challenges include their contro-versial nature as their source are human embryos, the risk of immunorejection as the tissues derived from them originate from donor embryos and the risk of tumorigenesis if they are accidently transplanted in an undifferentiated state. The problems of immuno-rejection and use of human embryos were overcome by reprogramming already differentiated adult skin cells to the embryonic state. Viral vectors carrying genes encoding for transcription factors (KLF4, OCT 3/4, SOX2, c-MYC; KOSM factors) were introduced into skin fibroblasts (transduction) to produce pluripotent cells with hESC characteristics (human induced pluripotent stem cells, hiPSCs) that could then be differentiated to produce personalized tissues for the patient from whom the skin cells were taken for the reprogramming process thus preventing immunorejection (Takahashi et al., 2007).

Today, several reports have been published using lentiviral and adenoviral somatic cell reprogramming with fewer pluripotent genes. In addition to adult somatic cells a variety of fetal cell types have also been successfully reprogrammed using these methods. However, there are several disadvantages with viral-integrated reprogramming such as the low efficiency of hiPSC colony formation, faulty faithful reprogramming and the potential integration of the viral genome into the host genome raising concern with respect to the safety of the derived tissues from such hiPSCs for clinical application. The importance of using low-risk integration-free methods for reprogramming has therefore been stressed to eliminate the risks of integration of foreign genomic sequences. Non-viral integration-free methods for reprogramming have been recently successfully used to produce safer hiPSCs (mRNA and defined factors, peptides, proteins, nucleofection, episomal plasmid and minicircle vectors and piggyback transposition). To make reprogramming even safer some have suggested the use of other methods such as somatic cell nuclear transfer (SCNT) ("Dolly the sheep technology"), cell fusion, and human pluripotent cell extracts.

Basic research using hESCs and hiPSCs has progressed with much speed, but their use as a routine clinical procedure still faces some roadblocks. The risk of tumorigenesis still remains the major obstacle in moving hESC and hiPSC technology to the clinic. Such tumours (teratomas) originate from a few rogue undifferentiated hESCs or hiPSCs lying within the hESC/hiPSC-derived tissue population that have not completed the differentiation process. Small numbers of undifferentiated hESCs and hiPSCs can induce teratomas in immunodeficient mice. At doses of 1000 hESCs, 32–40% of mice develop teratomas and at 10,000 hESCs, 100% of mice develop teratomas. Some injection sites favor teratoma formation while others do not. The incidence of teratoma formation under the kidney capsule and in subcutaneous regions is greater than intratesticular and intramuscular regions and

hESCs injected into the liver generated huge tumors in 3–4 weeks while subcutaneous hESC implants produced slower-growing teratomas. It has been suggested that environmental cues affect such differences in stem cell behavior between graft sites. The production of teratomas is much more aggressive and formation is much earlier with hiPSCs compared to hESCs (Cunningham et al., 2012). All these studies are using animal models and it is not clear as yet whether such teratomas will be produced in the human after hESC and hiPSC-derived tissue therapy. After reviewing the features of such tumors from the animal models it was postulated that they most closely resembled spontaneous benign teratomas that occur early in mouse and human life (Cunningham et al., 2012).

Several studies are being undertaken to prevent tumorigenesis by trying to remove such renegade undifferentiated hESCs or hiPSCs from the differentiated cell population. These protocols include: (1) the search and destruction of undifferentiated hESCs or hiPSCs in their differentiated tissue populations using antibodies and specific agents, (2) separating the undifferentiated hESCs or hiPSCs from their differentiated cell populations using flow cytometry and other separation methods, and (3) extending the period of differentiation to provide time for the remaining undifferentiated hESCs or hiPSCs to differentiate further.

Clinical Trials Using hESC and hiPSC-Derived Tissues

Despite the challenges in taking hESC and hiPSC-derived tissues to the clinic, a few clinical trials have been approved to test specific hESC and hiPSC-derived tissues for the treatment of specific diseases. The Investigational New Drug (IND) review process for the clinical use of hESC and iPSC-derived tissues requires a high level of scrutiny because of their potential to form tumors. Cell-based therapies that are injected locally or contained within a device that controls their migration are easier to receive approval than treatments that are injected systemically. As such, the current approved testing is predominantly for eye diseases such as retinal macular degeneration and Stargardt's disease. The eye was approved for Phase I and I/II trials because the retina is considered an immuno-privileged site, it is an isolated environment and is accessible for local injection. Moreover, the patient can be monitored non-invasively and the trial suspended if there are any adverse effects. Currently, eight hESC-derived retinal pigmented epithelial (RPE) cell and one hiPSC-derived RPE cell-approved clinical trials are active, in the recruiting process or approved but not yet recruiting. The other approved clinical trials are one for hESC-derived cardiac progenitors for heart failure, one hESC-derived pancreatic endoderm for Type 1 diabetes and two for hESC-derived oligodendrocyte progenitors for spinal cord injury (Kimbrel and Lanza, 2015).

Other Beneficial Uses of hESCs and iPSCs

The hESCs and hiPSCs possess other advantages in that they are an ideal tool to understand the pathogenesis of diseases and to test and develop candidate drugs for specific organ systems as they are pluripotent and can be easily differentiated into a variety of tissues. Currently, animal cell lines, immortalized cancer cell lines, somatic cell explants, and live animal models are used for testing, discovering, and validating new drugs that are not reliable, reproducible, and physiologically not the same as human cell lines. The reprogramming of primitive fetal cells (such as those from the fetus, fetal membranes, or umbilical cord) into hiPSCs and then deriving tissues from them (which will be primarily of fetal origin) will serve as a useful and reliable model to understand the pathogenesis of congenital anomalies such as Down syndrome and help to evaluate the effects of teratogens and other toxic agents that affect the unborn child during pregnancy.

Stem Cells from Birth-Associated Tissues

Mesenchymal stem cells (MSCs) from fetal and adult organs and hematopoietic stem cells (HSCs) from the adult bone marrow are other sources of stem cells that have been studied in depth and have had clinical application for certain diseases. However, the disadvantages of adult MSCs are their limited cell numbers, retention of stemness properties for short times in vitro and ability to differentiate only into a few desirable lineages (multipotency). Fetal MSCs are controversial as they are derived from human abortuses. HSCs are unipotent and have the disadvantage of differentiation into blood lineages only. The various disadvantages of fetal and adult MSCs, HSCs, hESCs, and hiPSCs have prompted the search for other sources of stem cells.

Stem cells from birth-associated tissues such as the umbilical cord, placenta, and amnion have drawn tremendous interest recently. It is well known that as pregnancy advances and the fetus becomes an adult, stem cells begin to lose their pluripotent properties and their plasticity diminishes. Since birth-associated tissues lie mid-way on the human developmental map, the stem cells isolated from them would still remain primitive as they are not exposed to the insults of the external environment and may thus possess certain benefits. Of the birth-associated tissues, the umbilical cord (UC) has been the most popular because, in addition to HSCs from cord blood, pure homogeneous populations of stromal cells with unique stemness properties could be isolated from the other compartments of the cord. Stromal cell populations with stemness properties have been isolated from the umbilical blood vessel adventitia, endothelium and perivascular region, amnion, subamnion, and Wharton's jelly. Significant differences in stemness characteristics between the cells of these compartments have been reported (Subramanian et al., 2015). Utmost caution has therefore been emphasized to avoid simplistic derivations of stromal cells from entire pieces of UC using simple explant culture protocols as they would contain a heterogeneous mixture of cell populations from all compartments. Stromal cells derived directly from pure uncontaminated Wharton's jelly (hWJSCs) appear to have the greatest stemness properties and offer the best clinical utility compared to the other compartments. Cells in the Wharton's jelly comprise of small populations of CD40+ fibroblasts, macrophages, and CD24+ and CD108+ mesenchymal cells while the majority of the cells possess stemness properties similar to MSCs. The Wharton's jelly occupies the largest surface area within the UC from which it has been shown that nearly 4.61 ± 0.57 million fresh hWJSCs/cm of UC could be isolated without the need for in-vitro expansion compared to other compartments. The Wharton's jelly compartment also has significantly lesser CD40+ contaminants (26–27%) and show greater osteogenic and chondrogenic differentiation potential compared to cells from other compartments. Cells from the Wharton's jelly offer the best clinical utility as (i) they have less non-stem cell contaminants, (ii) can be generated in large numbers with minimal culture avoiding changes in phenotype, (iii) their derivation is quick and easy to standardize, (iv) they are rich in stemness characteristics, and (v) have high differentiation potential (Subramanian et al., 2015).

The hWJSCs appear to have several unique properties. They can be harvested painlessly in large numbers, they are proliferative, possess stemness properties that last more than 20 passages in vitro, are multipotent, hypo-immunogenic, and do not induce tumorigenesis in laboratory animals, primates, and in the human. Furthermore, their regenerative ability has been confirmed in xenograft animal models and human clinical trials. Using microarray transcriptome profiling it was shown that hWJSCs had several beneficial genes including tumor suppressor genes that were not seen in other types of stem cells. Interestingly, hWJSCs also possess tumoricidal properties, support HSC expansion ex vivo and inhibit keloid cell growth (Fong et al., 2014; Lin et al., 2014). They are thus attractive autologous or allogeneic "off-the-shelf" stem cell sources that can be stored as adjuncts to HSCs in cord blood banks for differentiation into non-hematopoietic lineages for cell based therapies.

Clinical Applications of Umbilical Cord Wharton's Jelly Stem Cells

There are many exciting applications of hWJSCs that are being developed. These include wound healing, alternative therapies for hematopoietic diseases, understanding the pathogenesis of gestational diabetes mellitus, and studying other fetal developmental defects induced by the ZIKA virus (ZIKV) and other teratogens during pregnancy.

Some patients suffer from hard-to-heal diabetic foot ulcers, bed-sores, and burns, while others are prone to abnormal wound healing leading to ugly scars called keloids which are a cosmetic nuisance and psychosocial burden. Also, some surgical interventions end up with severe adhesions that interfere with normal organ function. Current methods such as chemicals, dressings, and skin grafts aimed to correct these disorders have met with limited success. Wound dressing patches made up of nano-scaffold carriers impregnated with hWJSCs were shown to enhance the healing of surgical and diabetic wounds in laboratory scratch-wound assays and in animal models and hold tremendous promise in the treatment of hard-to-heal wounds in patients (Tam et al., 2014). Recent reports have suggested that a benign neoplastic stem cell-like phenotype in an altered cytokine microenvironment drives scar formation in wounds with uncontrolled cell proliferation, leading to the formation of keloids. Modification of the stem cell niches in the wounds of

such patients is an attractive approach to keloid prevention. It was shown that the conditioned medium of hWJSCs had putative anti-fibrotic factors that could inhibit keloid cell growth (Fong et al., 2014).

The hWJSCs have contributed to the understanding and management of diseases of reproductive importance such as gestational diabetes mellitus. Pregestational and gestational diabetes mellitus (GDM) affects about 20–25% of pregnancies and the offspring of such mothers are usually large and have a life-long increased risk of glucose intolerance, obesity, metabolic syndrome, hypertension, and cardiovascular disease. Maternal hyperglycemia leads to fetal hyperglycemia because glucose readily traverses the placenta. Thus, unchecked fetal hyperglycemia results in hypertrophy of fetal pancreatic islets and hyperinsulinemia. The diabetic environment also promotes vascular injury and it has been suggested that adult endothelial cardiovascular disease may have its origins during fetal development. Much of the attention has been on the management of the diabetic mother with limited information on the pathogenesis and treatment of the infant of the diabetic mother (IDM) (Fong et al., 2017). Since tissues from the IDM are inaccessible to study the effects of maternal hyperglycemia, hWJSC can help generate tissues that mimic those of the IDM. Thus far, it has not been possible to differentiate fetal hWJSCs directly into *bona fide* pancreatic beta islets that secrete insulin. However, the reprogramming of fetal hWJSCs from the umbilical cord of the IDM into hiPSCs and then differentiating such hiPSCs into pancreatic insulin-secreting islets, cardiac, or any other tissue, provides an unprecedented platform to study the effects of glucose on the organs of the IDM and develop novel approaches of managing GDM. Established protocols are now available to differentiate hiPSCs into pancreatic islets, cardiac derivatives, muscle, hepatocytes, and endothelial cells (Fong et al., 2017).

It was recently shown that ZIKV exposure readily infects forebrain-specific cortical neural progenitors derived from multiple lines of hiPSCs in monolayer cultures (Tang et al., 2016). Protocols have been established to differentiate adult skin-derived hiPSCs into neural lineages corresponding to different CNS regions both in monolayer cultures and as brain organoids, including forebrain, midbrain, hypothalamus, retina, and heterogeneous organoids of multiple brain regions (Qian et al., 2016). Instead of using adult skin as the parent cell for reprogramming to hiPSCs, fetal hWJSC-derived hiPSCs will mimic better and provide a more

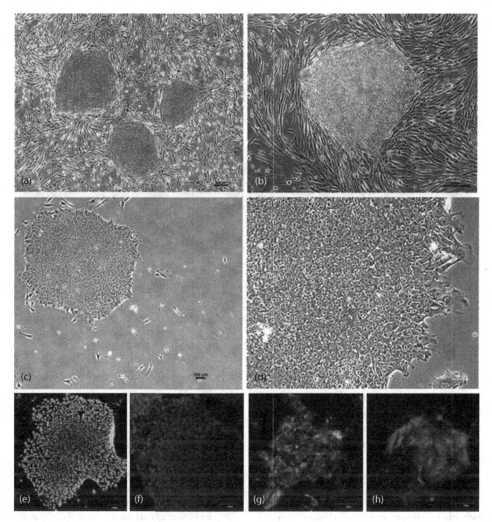

Figure 27.1 Morphology and characterization of hiPSCs reprogrammed from hWJSCs. (a) Low magnification phase contrast image of three rhomboid-shaped hWJSC-hiPSC colonies growing on murine embryonic fibroblasts. (b) High magnification phase contrast image of a hWJSC-reprogrammed hiPSC colony growing on murine embryonic fibroblasts. (c) High magnification phase contrast image of a hWJSC-hiPSC colony growing on matrigel without murine feeder cells (feeder-free). (d) High magnification of a hWJSC-hiPSC colony showing individual hWJSC-hiPSCs with high nuclear-cytoplasmic ratios and prominent nucleoli (dark dot in center of each cell) typical of embryonic stem cell morphology. (e)hWJSC-hiPSC colony staining positive for OCT4. (f) hWJSC-hiPSC colony staining positive for SOX2. (g) hWJSC-hiPSC colony staining positive for Tra-1-60. (h) hWJSC-hiPSC colony staining positive for Tra-1-81. (Figure courtesy of Selvarajoo V, Kong CM, Biswas A, Fong CY, Bongso A. (2017), unpublished data.)

reliable platform to produce brain organoids, neurospheres, and neural derivatives to study ZIKV-induced microcephaly and other developmental defects during pregnancy. The hWJSC-hiPSC-neural derivative platform will also be useful in screening novel anti-viral drugs against ZIKV (Figures 27.1 and 27.2).

The currently available treatment option of bone marrow HSC transplantation for the treatment of malignant hematopoietic diseases has its limitations. Cord blood HSC transplantation has advantages over bone marrow because of less stringent HLA matching, reduced GvHD, lack of donor attrition, and urgent and readily available HLA typed HSCs for those who find a match difficult. However, the number of HSCs available from a single umbilical cord is low, resulting in suboptimal engraftment and delays in hematopoietic reconstitution. There is thus an urgent need to increase the number of HSCs available and reduce engraftment failure rates. The hWJSCs possess remarkable tumoricidal properties against lymphomas and also provide

Brain organoids　　　　　**Neurospheres**

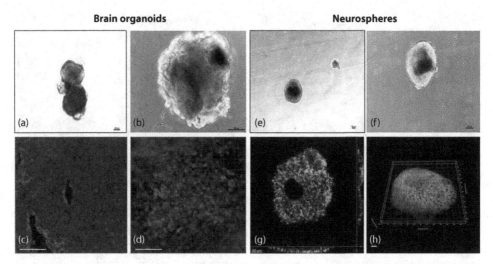

Figure 27.2 Differentiation and characterization of brain organoids and neurospheres differentiated from hWJSC-hiPSCs. (a) Low magnification of a brain organoid after 13 days of differentiation from hWJSC-hiPSCs. (b) High magnification of a brain organoid after 17 days of differentiation from hWJSC-hiPSCs. (c) Forebrain region of brain organoids staining positive for DAPI-FOXG1 (day- 32). (d)Neural stem cells in brain organoids staining positive for DAPI/PAX6 (day-32). (e) Low magnification of a neurosphere after 12 days of differentiation from hWJSC-hiPSCs. (f)High magnification of a neurosphere after 12 days of differentiation from hWJSC-hiPSCs. (g) Neurospheres staining positive for DAPI/Nestin-Type IV intermediate filament (neuroectodermal stem cell marker) (day-12). (h) Neurospheres staining positive for DAPI/Pax6 (neuroectoderm specification) (day-12). (Figure courtesy of Selvarajoo V, Fong CY, Biswas A, Bongso A. (2017), unpublished data.)

molecular cues for HSC expansion (Lin et al., 2014). Co-transplantation of hWJSCs (as a substitute for bone marrow MSCs) together with HSCs (expanded using hWJSC stromal support) would be an attractive alternative novel approach to the management of hematopoietic diseases.

References

Bongso A, Richards M. History and perspective of stem cell research. *Best Pract Res Clin Obstet Gynaecol* 2004; 18: 827–842.

Bongso A, Fong CY. The therapeutic potential, challenges and future clinical directions of stem cells from the Wharton's Jelly of the human umbilical cord. *Stem Cells Revs Reports* 2013; 9: 226–240.

Bongso A, Fong CY, Ng SC, Ratnam S. Isolation and culture of inner cell mass cells from human blastocysts. *Hum Reprod* 1994; 9: 2110–2117.

Bongso A, Fong CY, Matthew J, et al. Benefits to human in vitro fertilization of transferring embryos after in vitro embryonic block: Alternatives to day-2 transfers. *Assisted Reprod* 1999; 9 (2): 70–78.

Cowan CA, Klimanskaya I, McMahon J, et al. Derivation of embryonic stem-cell lines from human blastocysts. *The New England J Med* 2004; 350: 1353–1356.

Crook JM, Peura TT, Kravets L, et al. The generation of six clinical-grade human embryonic stem cell lines. *Cell Stem Cell* 2007; 1: 490–494.

Cunningham JJ, Ulbright TM, Pera MF, Looijenga LHJ. Lessons from human teratomas to guide development

of safe stem cell therapies *Nature Biotech* 2012; 30: 849–857.

Fong CY, Biswas A, Subramanian A, et al. Human keloid cell characterization and inhibition of growth with human Wharton's jelly stem cell extracts. *J Cellular Biochem* 2014; 115: 826–838.

Fong CY, Biswas A, Stunkel W, Chong YS, Bongso A. Tissues derived from reprogrammed Wharton's jelly stem cells of the umbilical cord provide an ideal platform to study the effects of glucose, Zika virus, and other agents on the fetus. *J Cellular Biochem* 2017; 118 : 437–441.

Gardner D, Lane M, Stevens J, Terry Schlenker T, Schoolcraft WB. Blastocyst score affects implantation and pregnancy outcome: towards a single blastocyst transfer. *Fertil Steril* 2002; 73: 1155–1158.

Gokhale PJ, Andrews PW. Characterization of human pluripotent stem cells. *Neuroreport* 2013; 24: 1031–1034.

Kimbrel EA, Lanza R. Current status of pluripotent stem cells: moving the first therapies to the clinic. *Nature Rev Drug Discovery* 2015; 14: 661–692.

Lin HD, Fong CY, Biswas A, Choolani M, Bongso A. Human Wharton's jelly stem cells, its conditioned medium and cell-free lysate inhibit the growth of human lymphoma cells. *Stem Cells Revs and Reports* 2014; 10:573–586.

Millman JR, Xie C, Van Dervort A, et al. Generation of stem cell-derived β-cells from patients with type 1 diabetes. *Nature Communications* 2016; 7: 11463.

Mohr LR, Trounson AO. Cryopreservation of human embryos. *Ann N Y Acad Sci* 1985; 442: 536–543.

Qian X, Nguyen HN, Song MM, et al. Brain-region-specific organoids using mini-bioreactors for modelling ZIKV exposure. *Cell* 2016; 165: 1238–1254.

Reubinoff B, Pera MF, Fong CY, Trounson A, Bongso A. Embryonic stem cell lines from human blastocysts: Somatic differentiation in vitro. *Nature Biotechnol* 2000; 18: 399–404.

Richards M, Fong CY, Chan WK, Wong PC, Bongso A. Human feeders support prolonged undifferentiated growth of human inner cell masses and embryonic stem cells. *Nature Biotechnol* 2002; 20:933–936.

Subramanian A, Fong CY, Biswas A, Bongso A. Comparative characterization of cells from the various compartments of the human umbilical cord shows that the Wharton's jelly compartment provides the best source of clinically utilizable mesenchymal stem cells. *PLOS ONE* 2015; 10: e0127992.

Takahashi K, Tanabe K, Ohnuki M, et al. Induction of pluripotent stem cells from adult human fibroblasts by defined factors. *Cell* 2007; 131: 861–872.

Tam K, Cheyyatraviendran S, Venugopal J, et al. A nanoscaffold impregnated with human Wharton's jelly stem cells or its secretions improves healing of wounds. *J Cellular Biochem* 2014; 115: 794–803.

Tang H, Hammack C, Ogden SC, et al. Zika virus infects human cortical neural progenitors and attenuates their growth. *Cell Stem Cell* 2016; 18: 587–590.

Thomson JA, Itskovitz-Eldor J, Shapiro SS, et al. Embryonic stem cell lines derived from human blastocysts. *Science* 1998; 282: 1145–1147.

Trounson AO, Mohr LR. Human pregnancy following cryopreservation, thawing and transfer of an eight-cell embryo. *Nature* 1983; 305: 707–709.

Yokota Y, Sato S, Yokota M, Yokota H, Araki Y. Birth of a healthy baby following vitrification of human blastocysts. *Fertil Steril* 2001; 75: 1027–1029.

28

The Regulation and Legislation of In-Vitro Fertilization

Louis Waller and Sandra Dill

Legislation of Assisted Reproduction – the Australian Experience – Louis Waller

In the Beginning

Candice Reed, the first Australian test-tube baby, as she was entitled then, was born in Melbourne on June 23, 1980. That was nearly two years after Louise Brown was born in Oldham in England, the first human being to enter our world whose life had begun in a Petri dish in a laboratory.

The arrival of Candice Reed, and several more in-vitro fertilization (IVF) babies in 1981, excited Australian interest in and controversies about the phenomenon. In January 1982 the Catholic Archbishop of Melbourne and the Anglican Archbishop of Sydney publicly expressed deep concerns about the "test-tube baby programme," especially about the fate of embryos used in experimental activities.

Side by side with critics and questioners were those who advocated for the many infertile couples and their families and friends, who saw IVF as a success story. Couples who had struggled to have a child and who had either decided that adoption was unacceptable or who were, for whatever reasons, marked as unsuitable adopters, were especially adamant.

In the decade that followed that first Australian IVF birth, several Australian states and several national bodies investigated, considered, debated, and framed legislation to manage the arrival of assisted reproduction. Victoria was in the forefront of this enterprise, in which religious organizations, medical and allied health professionals, the legal profession, and practitioners in social work all participated.

The Victorian IVF Committee

In 1982, the Victorian IVF Committee was convened. I was the Law Reform Commissioner of Victoria, and I

was appointed Chairman of the Committee. The eight other members included two professors of medicine, two clerics, and a barrister whose expertise was in family law. The Committee's terms of reference obliged it to deliver an Interim Report three months after its first meeting. In that Report the committee concluded that IVF in the most common situation, that is when a married couple who had been unable to achieve a pregnancy and whose gametes were used in the procedures, was acceptable in Victoria. The Committee then published two further reports, on the use of donor gametes in IVF, and on embryo storage, embryo experimentation, and on surrogacy in IVF. The first of these led the Victorian Government to decide that legislation would be introduced, in two Bills: the first to make the status of all children born from assisted reproduction, including donor insemination, as well as IVF where donor gametes were employed, was clear and unambiguous. Gamete donors were not to have any legal relationship with children born as a consequence. The second Bill would create a system for the licensing, monitoring, and regular reviews of IVF providers. The legislation was enacted in 1984. The IVF Committee's third Report was published after the Bills had been introduced, and some of its most significant recommendations were incorporated into the *Infertility (Medical Procedures) Act 1984*. This was a pioneering enactment in Australian legislation on IVF and related issues. It was probably the first statute of its kind in the common law world, and beyond. The Act created a Standing Review and Advisory Committee on Infertility, SRACI. I was its first Chairman. SRACI was linked to the Department of Health, and housed in its premises. It was replaced, in 1995, by the Infertility Treatment Authority. This body will be described later.

Other States and Territories

Committees or other bodies charged with the same tasks as the Victorian IVF Committee were established in several Australian jurisdictions. The most substantial, in terms of constitution, powers, and resources, was the New South Wales Law Reform Commission, which published several Reports on IVF.

There has been federal legislation on IVF issues. The pioneering *Family Law Act* 1975 was amended to declare that children born to a married woman (or one in a *de facto* relationship) were the children of that woman's husband or partner. Any child born to such women as a result of assisted reproductive technology is the child of that woman and her partner if there has been mutual consent to the ART procedure. A gamete donor is denied any parental status.

The *Prohibition of Human Cloning for Reproduction Act* 2002 makes it an offence to create an embryo outside the body of a woman for any purpose other than achieving a pregnancy in a woman. Research on human embryos is restricted to those created for reproductive purposes but untransferred, and only where that specific research is authorized by a licence and is conducted in an accredited ART clinic. The third federal enactment, the *Prohibition of Human Cloning for Reproduction Act* 2002, prohibits commercial trading of any kind in relation to the supply of any human gametes or embryos, or the import or export of any prohibited embryos.

The two federal bodies have published non-legislative guidelines on ART. The National Health and Medical Research Council's *Ethical Guidelines on the Use of Assisted Reproductive Guidelines in Clinical Research and Practice*, 2007, underpins the regulation of ART practice, especially in those states which have not enacted comprehensive legislation. The Reproductive Technology Accreditation Committee, established by the Fertility Society of Australia, has published a *Code of Practice for Reproductive Technology Units*, last revised in 2014, to which treatment providers must agree if they are to comply with legislation and guidelines in some Australian jurisdictions.

Three Australian States have followed Victoria's example of enacting legislation on ART. New South Wales has the *Assisted Reproductive Technology Act* 2007. In South Australia the *Assisted Reproductive Treatment Act* 1988, and the *Family Relationships Act* 1975, provide a comprehensive statutory regime, as does the *Human Productive Technology Act* 1991 and the *Artificial Conception Act* 1985 in Western Australia. Queensland, Tasmania, and the Australian Capital Territory and the Northern Territory had enacted legislation to effect parent and child status in ART

procedures, but have no regulatory enactments, except in relation to surrogacy, of which more later.

The Victorian Regulatory Experience

The Act of 1984 came into force in parts. The Standing Review and Advisory Committee was constituted by the Minister of Health in 1985. Its eight members included five who had been members of the IVF Committee. I was its first Chairman. The Committee gave advice to the Minister on several important issues, including freezing and storage of embryos, embryo experimentation, and novel methods of assisted reproduction, gamete intra-Fallopian transfer (GIFT), pronuclear surgical transfer (PROST), and zygote intra-Fallopian transfer (ZIFT). Amending legislation to bring these methods into the ambit of the 1984 legislative scheme of approval and regulation by the Minister was speedily affected by the *Infertility (Medical Procedures) Amendment Act* 1987. One of SRACI's most important recommendations was that "embryo" meant that entity where sperm had penetrated the ovum and the chromosomes released by each gamete were aligned on the mitotic spindle. This occurs about 22 or 23 hours after the spermatozoon penetrates the zona pellucida of the ovum. Cell division happens about 26–36 hours after penetration, and two daughter cells result. Though there was division of opinion in SRACI on this matter, ultimately the view that before syngamy penetrated ova might be the legitimate subjects of permitted experimentation was incorporated into the 1987 statutory amendment.

The establishment of a Central Register to contain and preserve comprehensive information on gamete donors whose donations resulted in births was one of the most important creations of the Act of 1984. The Register was opened in 1988, and its establishment underlines the absence of accurate comprehensive information before that date. A Voluntary Register was also created, but its value has depended on submissions of information by people or institutions motivated by the realization that children born from ART may want to know who their father or mother was, and that gamete donors and their offspring may want to know who their progeny or their siblings are. The Minister of Health asked SRACI to undertake a comprehensive review of the 1984 legislation, which resulted in three Reports, the last published in October 1991. This contained what was entitled a plain English version of The Infertility Treatment Bill. This major recommendation was the replacement of ministerial consideration, approval and oversight of ART providers, and of ART practitioners and counselors, by a system of licensing with penal provisions only as sanctions of last resort. After a change of government in October 1992, and extensive consultations, including several with SRACI, the Kennett Government introduced amending legislation in 1995. As happened with the pioneering legislation of 1984, the new Bill enjoyed both bipartisan and bicameral support, and received assent on June 27, 1995. It created an Independent statutory Infertility Treatment Authority (ITA) charged with the responsibility of administering the regulatory regime of ART in Victoria. I was appointed its first Chairman. Before the rest of the Act was proclaimed on January 1, 1998, the 1995 Act was amended to provide access to ART procedures to people in *de facto* relationships, that is, "where a man and a woman . . . are living together as husband and wife on a genuine domestic basis, though not married". The *Infertility Treatment (Amendment) Act 1997* also abolished SRACI.

As the twentieth century drew to its end, the Victorian Government charged the Victorian Law Reform Commission (VLRC) "to enquire into and report on the desirability and feasibility of changes to the Infertility Treatment Act 1984 to expand eligibility criteria in all or any forms of assisted reproduction and adoption . . . ." The VLRC published its Final report in February 2007. After comprehensive discussions and debates the *Assisted Reproductive Treatment Act 2008* received assent on December 11, 2008. Its purposes are to regulate ART and artificial insemination, and to establish a new entity, the Victorian Assisted Reproductive Treatment Authority, VARTA, and to repeal altogether the Act of 1995. The transition from the ITA to VARTA occurred in 2009, with the ITA delivering its Twelfth and Final Report to the Victorian Government in June 2009.

The Act of 2008 provides that any woman, regardless of sexuality or marital status, may access ART Services, provided that woman has satisfied she is unlikely to become pregnant, or able to carry a pregnancy, or is at risk of transmitting a genetic abnormality to a child.

The Act mandates consent by the woman and her partner, if any, to the ART treatment sought. An approved counsellor who has provided counselling to the woman, and her partner, must certify that she or he has sighted a criminal records check on the woman, and her partner, performed by a member of the police force. A child protection order in relation to an ART applicant must also be sighted. The Act creates a Patient Review Panel which may consider applications by any person who is denied access to ART because of an unfavorable criminal record check or child protection order. No other Australian jurisdiction prescribes this requirement.

The Act of 2008 has been substantially amended. First, the *Assisted Reproductive Treatment Amendment Act* 2013 provides a new comprehensive regime for the storage of embryos. Secondly, the *Assisted Reproductive Treatment Amendment Act* 2016 broadens the capacities of people born from donor treatment procedures using gametes donated before January 1, 1988, when the provisions in the Act of 1995 on collection and preservation and disclosure of donor procedures and their outcomes, came into effect.

Information and its Disclosure

In its Second Report, on Donor Gametes in IVF, published in August 1983, the Victorian IVF Committee wrote:

> Whether or not a person pursues her or his origins, it should be possible for everyone to discover them . . . There is . . . a substantial and growing view that the values of honesty and integrity are crucial to the creation of a happy family . . .

The specific recommendation to establish and maintain a Central Register of identifying information on donors of gametes and embryos whose donations resulted in births, to be the responsibility of the Health Commissioner (later the Department of Health) was embodied in the Act of 1984. The 1984 Register was inaugurated in 1988, and was incorporated into the 1995 Central Register. The original legislation enabled donor-conceived people who were 18 or older and donors to access non-identifying information about their origins or their outcomes, but identifying information was only available if the person to whom the information related consented.

The ITA established a Voluntary Register in 2001, to record information about ART procedures which took place before July 1, 1988. In its Final Report of 2007, the VLRC recorded that there were 101 donor registrations and 26 offspring registrations in the pre-1988 and post-1988 voluntary registrations.

The Act of 1995 contains provisions which enable people conceived with gametes donated on or after January 1, 1998 to obtain identifying information about the relevant donor or donors without obtaining their consent, provided the applicant is 18 years old. Applications for information on donor-conceived people under 18 must be made by their parents, and its release depends on the donor's consent.

In 2006 the ITA launched its *Time to Tell* campaign, specifically to provide accurate information and support to families with children born as a result of donor ART procedures. Many would be turning 18 in 2006, since over 4400 had been born in Victoria since the pioneering Act of 1984 was implemented in 1988. The campaign received extensive media publicity and the ITA and its successor, VARTA, have continued the campaign. As I write this, I have a copy of VARTA's invitation to its recent *Time to Tell* Seminar, held on September 9, 2017, where "tips to parents on how, when and what to say to their donor-conceived children" will be the focus of the assembly. As well, I have a copy of VARTA's request for information on donor sperm or egg practices and medical and health records in Victoria July 1988. "We need your help to fill the gaps."

Surrogacy

Surrogacy arrangements may be effected without recourse to ART procedures. It is an arrangement where a woman is, or will become pregnant, and hand over the child she bears to another, surrendering all her parental rights. She may enter into this arrangement with another woman or two women or with a married or *de facto* couple, or with a man, or two men. The much-publicized cases in the 1980s in the USA and the United Kingdom resulted in the citation of biblical examples of the practice, where the matriarchs Sarah and Rachel, struck by infertility, recruited second wives or concubines for their husbands, so that they might be "builded up through her."

The regulation of surrogacy and its parentage and status consequences has resulted in both Commonwealth and state and territory legislation. The presumptions of parenthood in the *Family Law Act* 1975, described above, may affect surrogacy arrangements. An amendment to that Act provides that if a court makes an order under a prescribed law of a State or Territory to the effect that the parentage of a child is transferred from a surrogate mother and her married or *de facto* partner to the couple who intend to be that child's parents, they will be presumed to be the parents under the Commonwealth Act. So far relevant legislation in New South Wales, Victoria, Queensland,

Western Australia, South Australia, and the ACT have been so prescribed.

There has been sustained opposition to what is described as commercial surrogacy since the first arrangements came to light in the context of the IVF developments in the 1980s. Every state and the ACT have enacted specific surrogacy legislation. Commercial surrogacy, sometimes described as the selling and the buying of babies, has been prohibited, and in several, advertising for surrogacy, even altruistic surrogacy, is also a criminal offence. The Northern Territory is the only jurisdiction which does not prohibit the practice. Altruistic surrogacy arrangements may be permissible, but generally any altruistic surrogacy agreements are unenforceable. In New South Wales, Queensland, and the ACT, it is a criminal offence to enter into an overseas commercial surrogacy agreement.

In Victoria and Western Australia an altruistic surrogacy arrangement requires the approval of the relevant statutory authority. In Victoria that is the Patient Review Panel, created under the ART legislation and in Western Australia it is the Reproductive Technology Council. Approval depends on the intending parents' fertility, risk of pregnancy, or likelihood of transmitting a genetic disorder. Most State statutes prescribe age requirements for the surrogate mother, and prescribe legal advice and specific counselling. Whilst material benefits or advantages may not be received by the surrogate, reasonable medical expenses, costs of legal advice, and travel costs may be paid.

The Future

There is little doubt that issues of the use, and misuse, of ART procedures will arise in Australia in the decades ahead. The most pressing is the international regulation of a growing commerce in overseas surrogacy arrangements. Episodes in Asia involving Australian would-be parents have attracted persistent media attention and comment. Proscription of such arrangements in some countries has resulted in the selection of others, where surrogacy arrangements may be effected, with large payments exchanged for the transfer of the child involved. Australian citizens have travelled to the USA, Canada, and some European countries to enter into such arrangements.

A plebiscite to decide whether same-sex marriage legislation should be permitted in Australia has recently been held. After overwhelming support, same-sex marriage has been legislated, as has now happened in many jurisdictions. This will clearly result in some LGBTI couples who are currently ineligible to access ART programs seeking access to them. New ways of family formation are no longer imagined. They are clearly contemplated and many have been established.

The growth in the information accessible by donor-conceived children and by gamete donors may also continue, at a faster pace. There are important consequences which may flow, in terms of the discovery of formerly unknown genetic connexions, and of specific genetic conditions. The continuing exploration of the human genome will also have its consequences in this connexion.

The continuing unravelling of the human genome will undoubtedly foster the attempts of some would-be parents to use ART procedures and preimplantation genetic manipulation to bear "designer babies." Preimplantation diagnoses have been effectively used legitimately to avoid catastrophic genetic conditions being transmitted. For some couples, gender selection is the result they, sometimes desperately, seek. Current legislation in Australia clearly prohibits such selection.

Conclusion

It is now clear that the recommendation of the Victorian IVF Committee, in its Second Report in 1983, that legislation enacted by the parliament should be the method adopted for the regulation and monitoring of the novel ART procedures already employed, and those that followed as research and clinical practice developed, has been the best course to follow in today's Australia. In 1981, Sir Ninian Stephen, then a Justice of the High Court of Australia and later the Governor-General, put it so in his Southey Memorial Lecture in the University of Melbourne in 1981:

> An elected legislature as the identified and visible maker of laws can be seen to be responsive to legitimate pressures, and to the strongly held views of the community. Courts, on the other hand, confer no democratic legitimacy upon the law they make and their judgments are neither responsive to nor afford any relief for, the pressures of community concern which bear so strongly upon an elected legislature which must periodically go to the people.

What he wrote about courts, even final courts of appeal, applies also to administrative bodies, or professional associations, no matter how eminent.

How will those who come after us regard the efforts which have resulted in the statutory enactments and their implementation in the regulation of ART in Australia? One swift comment is that in a country where, despite distance, the same considerations, questions, and difficulties exist in each of its jurisdictions, a national legislative scheme should be developed. It is a goal our posterity should thoughtfully and sensitively pursue.

The Effect of Regulation on Infertile Couples – Government at the Bedroom Door – Sandra Dill

Infertility is an extremely isolating experience. This is exacerbated because infertility and the death of a child are taboo subjects. Society has difficulty dealing with these sad experiences. Infertile people need medical and social choices to help them deal with infertility. Assisted reproductive technology (ART) has provided IVF and related treatments as another way of overcoming infertility and childlessness.

However, in order to access medical treatment, those who need it have government at the bedroom door deciding if they can have legal and affordable access to ART and we are mindful that there is "very little distance between policy and politics" (Shenfield, 1997).

The United Nations Declaration of Human Rights recognizes that, "Men and women of full age, without any limitation due to race, nationality or religion, have the right to marry and found a family" (UN Convention). This is supported by the European Convention on Human Rights which guarantees respect for family life and the right to found a family (EU Convention). It can be argued that these provisions create a positive right to access ART to achieve this goal, one taken for granted by fertile people in the community. For between 13% and 24% of couples who need medical assistance to form their families, infertility causes immense suffering. For those who finally remain without a child, infertility can have lifelong implications (Greenhall and Vessey, 1990).

The Limited Recognition of Infertility as a Disease or Medical Condition

Governments worldwide have been reluctant to acknowledge that infertility is a disability or medical condition. In most countries infertility treatment is viewed as an elective procedure and therefore not worthy of reimbursement. For example, in Bangladesh, infertility is considered a curse that brings couples bad luck and the possibility of treatment is unknown to the majority.

The need to have access to health care is balanced against the need for governments to responsibly manage scarce resources and to distribute them justly and equitably for the good of the whole community. The challenge for consumers of infertility services is to persuade governments that infertility is a medical disability that causes suffering and as such is worthy of inclusion in their national health plan. This is one of the objectives of the International Consumer Support for Infertility (iCSi), which brings patient leaders together to discuss common interests. In addition, national patient associations in many countries provide support for infertile people and advocate for access to affordable infertility treatment.

In 2011, the patient association FINE in Japan met with government Ministers to discuss expansion of reimbursement, then sent a petition to the Cabinet.

The World Health Organization has recommended that "Infertility should be recognized as a public health issue worldwide, including developing countries" (WHO, 2001).

Conversely, the government in Uganda ignored this when they told the patient association JOYCE that, with one of the highest fertility rates in Africa, they would not support infertility treatment which would result in more births. This failed to recognize that identifying ways to reduce the number of births from fertile women would be more effective than restricting access to ART for infertile people.

In 2013 in Argentina, after the patient association Concebir had lobbied the government for several years, a national law was approved by Congress. There is no age limit for women and access is permitted for single mothers and lesbian couples. Treatment is free. For low complexity ART (insemination), free access is provided for four cycles each year. Three cycles are free for IVF or ICSI. Gametes for the couple or donor insemination are permitted for all ART. In 2015 a new Civil Code recognized the right of people born through ART with gamete donation to have access to clinical and identifying information about the donor. The national donor registry will be controlled by the Ministry of Health.

The Impact of Legislation – Government Sneaking into the Bedroom

Governments internationally have enacted restrictive legislation, which in some cases has compromised safe health care and the wellbeing of infertile people and their families. The legislative changes in Italy in recent years have provided a sobering example. In this ultra conservative climate it is crucial that infertile people and their health care professionals work in partnership to ensure that governments understand the suffering that infertility causes and the need to provide equity of access to safe, effective health care to overcome infertility.

In 2004, Italy passed Law 40 which:

a. permitted only three eggs to be inseminated and obligated doctors to transfer simultaneously all embryos obtained. This assumed that doctors could control the number of embryos created but if not then all created had to be transferred;

b. prohibited embryo freezing, which meant that no excess embryos could be saved;

c. prohibited preimplantation genetic diagnosis (PGD) and donor (use of donor sperm or eggs) ART.

In 2009, after many efforts made by patient associations supported by pro bono lawyers who lodged 22 appeals to the First Level Court and Constitutional Court, the law partially changed. Parts (a) and (b) above were removed, allowing for the possibility of embryo cryopreservation.

Many criteria are used in deciding which patient will receive health care. It has been argued, as in New Zealand, that determining an initial eligible pool of patients based on substantive standards and procedural rules is preferable to the decision making process being left to the final selection of an individual for a particular procedure (Beauchamp and Childress, 1989)

Governments continue to intrude into the lives of infertile people. This is inconsistent with existing legal choices for women in relation to human reproduction which respect individual autonomy. These include contraception, abortion, where it is permitted (in many countries the father has no say), female sterilization and tubal reversals.

In 1993, the Canadian Royal Commission claimed as paramount, "good government power . . . immediate intervention and concerted leadership are required . . . citizens in provinces with insufficient regulation may suffer harm" (Proceed With Care, 1993).

Rushed legislative responses to some emerging technologies have resulted in strange anomalies, such as:

- allowing sperm donation but not in an IVF cycle (Norway and Sweden) or
- allowing sperm donation but not oocyte donation (Denmark and Germany) or
- recommending that the use of a woman's frozen embryo (created with her husband) be disallowed if her husband dies, but allowing that same woman to receive donor sperm (United Kingdom, France, Germany, and Canada).

The power of government to destroy the reproductive futures of individuals was evident in 1996 (Edwards and Beard, 1997). To avoid prosecution, UK IVF clinics were forced by the Human Fertilisation Embryology Authority to destroy more than 3000 embryos that had reached their five-year statutory limit (Deech, 1997). This was despite many couples not being able to be contacted, and who found out about the destruction after the event.

In 2008, The Victorian Government in Australia passed the Assisted Reproductive Technology Bill which permitted access to ART to lesbian women. A late amendment required anyone seeking ART treatment to undergo a police and child protection check beforehand. The Attorney General admitted to two directors of the patient association ACCESS that this was a ruse to capture lesbian women, who some members of the Cabinet considered likely to abuse children. To single them out would have been in breach of the Commonwealth Sex Discrimination Act, so they applied it to everyone. They offered no supporting evidence to support their claim. Douglas has argued that instituting a "fitness to parent" code is "difficult enough to apply in cases concerning children who are in existence, let alone those who are only a twinkle in the doctors' eye and it is open to many different assessments, depending on the person making the judgement" (Douglas, 1994).

For couples with the disability of infertility, the bedroom has become a nostalgic metaphor for lost privacy (Jansen and Dill, 2009). The evidence is that government intrusion is set to increase.

These examples raise questions of how, and on what basis and authority, elected members of parliament legislate for ethically laden matters such as IVF in which a diversity of opinions will be found. This is not the same as how a group within society, such as a church or major faith, makes decisions that they will regard as binding on members. While society may impinge on our lives in many ways, we question whether the rights of a government will outweigh the rights of potential parents.

Consumers of ART services seek politicians with integrity who have the courage to act fairly rather than expediently. More than five million children have been born through ART. Many of them have reached voting age and show great interest in how their elected officials value their existence.

C. Everett Koop, former US Surgeon General, introduced sex education in schools to slow the progress of the AIDS epidemic. Responding to criticism from his conservative Christian community, he argued that personal moral beliefs should not automatically be enacted in laws enforced by the State (Yancey, 2001).

Consumers as Partners not Passive Participants

A significant factor in the success of negotiations with government in relation to regulation and reimbursement in Australia has been the commitment of consumers and providers to work in partnership to achieve common goals. This coalition of the committed has provided a model for other countries. This paradigm shift from consumers as passive participants to partners has been difficult for IVF clinicians in some countries but the political benefits for consumers and providers can be significant. These partnerships are also appropriate as they recognize that consumers of ART services must live with the consequences of policy and treatment decisions (Dill, 2006).

Real Costs of Infertility: Emotional, Social, Societal

Governments have argued that the costs of providing reimbursement for infertility treatment are too high but it can be argued that the financial costs are less significant than the real costs of infertility.

The Royal College of Obstetricians and Gynaecologists and the British Infertility Counselling Association found, based on papers by infertility specialists and interviews with medical, scientific, and psychological experts, that infertility costs the nation in absenteeism, poor productivity, and wasted resources (Kon, 1993).

There are also social costs to consider such as marital relationships, taking time off work, refusing promotions, strained family relationships, exclusion from inheritances or family mementos, and isolation from friends. The quality of life for some infertile people can become marginal when they have difficulty coping with a friend's pregnancy, seeing babies and young children, or watching television advertisements featuring babies. For infertile couples, events such as Christmas, Mother's Day, and Father's Day can be painful reminders of other people's fertility and success and are times to be endured.

In 1993, the London newspaper, the *Daily Mail*, reported on the 15th birthday of "Bubbly Louise" (Brown), the world's first baby born through IVF (*Daily Mail*, 1993a). A few pages away appeared a story headlined "Tragic teacher who longed for a baby": Gillian Martine, a 34 year old primary school teacher from Southampton and her husband, Michael, after trying to conceive for some years, had been told by their doctors the heartbreaking news that they would never have a child. Depressed and discouraged, she committed suicide (*Daily Mail*, 1993b). On the same day, the joy of assisted parenthood and the desperation and despair of infertility were graphically contrasted.

The question is not whether infertile people have a right to infertility treatment reimbursement, but rather why they should be discriminated against in being denied access to appropriate health care services. The international family of patient associations will continue to bring the needs of infertile people to governments. We will not rest until all those we represent are treated with the dignity enjoyed by others in our communities. As citizens and taxpayers, we assert our right to equity of access to affordable quality, health care services for the medical condition of infertility.

Bibliography

Annual Reports of SRACI, the ITA and VARTA, 1986 to date.

Assisted Reproductive Treatment Bill 2008.

Beauchamp T and Childress J. *Principles of Biomedical Ethics*, 1989, ch. 6, p. 292.

Daily Mail, 27/3/1993a, 9.

Daily Mail, 27/3/1993b, 15.

Deech R. A reply from the chairman of the HFEA. *Hum Reprod* 1997; 12: 5–6.

Dill S, International treatment differences: Policy, politics, partnerships and ART. In: Valverde JL (Ed.) *2050: A Changing Europe. Demographic Crisis and Baby Friend Policies, Pharmaceuticals Policy and Law*, Vol. 9, 2007.

Douglas G, Law, fertility and reproduction, 1991, pp. 119–122, in *Medical Law*; 2nd edn, Kennedy & Grubb, Butterworths, London, 1994.

Edwards RG and Beard HK. UK law dictated the destruction of 3000 cryopreserved human embryos. *Hum Reprod* 1997; 12: 3–5.

European Convention on Human Rights and its Five Protocols, Articles 8 & 12.

Greenhall E and Vessey M. The prevalence of subfertility. *Fertility Sterility* 1990; 54(6): 978–983.

Jansen R and Dill S. When and how to welcome government to the bedroom. *Medical Journal of Australia* 2009; 190(5).

Keane Loanne in video link from the USA at the annual scientific meeting of the Fertility Society of Australia, December 1997.

Kon A. *Infertility: The Real Costs, ISSUE, CHILD for National Fertility Week*, 1993.

Medical, Ethical and Social Aspects of Assisted Reproduction (2001: Geneva, Switzerland) Current practices and controversies in assisted reproduction: report of a WHO meeting / editors, Effy Vayena, Patrick J. Rowe and P. David Griffin.

Nicol M. *Loss of a Baby, Understanding Maternal Grief, Transworld, Moorebank, NSW*, 1989, 4.

Page H. Estimation of the prevalence and incidence of infertility in a population: A pilot study. *Fertility Sterility* 1989; 51(4): 571–577.

Proceed with Care. *Final Report of the Royal Commission on New Reproductive Technologies, Canada Communications Group*, Ottawa, 1993, 19.

Reports of the Victorian IVF Committee, 1982, 1983 and 1984.

Shenfield F. "Justice and access to fertility treatments". In: *Ethical Dilemmas in Assisted Reproduction*, Shenfield F, Sureau C (Eds.), Parthenon Publishing Group, London, 1997.

Skene L. *Law and Medical practice: Rights, Duties Claims and Defences*, 3rd ed., 2008.

Universal Declaration of Human Rights, Article 16.1, United Nations, 1948.

Vayena, E., Rowe, P. J., and Griffin, D. P., Current Practices and Controversies in Assisted Reproduction; Report of a meeting on "Medical, Ethical and Social Aspects of Assisted Reproduction", WHO, 2001.

Victorian Law Reform Commission: Assisted Reproductive Technology & Adoption, Final Report 2007.

Waller L. Australia: the law and infertility – the Victorian Experience. In McLean SAM (Ed.), *Law Reform and Human Reproduction*, 1992.

Yancey P. *Soul Survivor, How My Faith Survived the Church*, Hodder & Stoughton, London, 2001.

Chapter 29

Research on Assisted Reproduction Families: A Historical Perspective

Susan Golombok

I first met Bob Edwards in Paris in 1991. I was giving a paper on psychological aspects of in-vitro fertilization (IVF) at the Second International Conference of IVF Nurse Co-ordinators and Support Personnel. Bob was in the audience and, with his irrepressible enthusiasm, strongly and publically supported the fledgling research that my team had initiated on the psychological consequences for children of being born by IVF. Back then, clinicians and embryologists were focused on achieving pregnancies and the birth of healthy babies. The longer-term psychological outcomes for the children conceived through their pioneering reproductive technologies was of little interest. But that was not the case with Bob. He was interested in the children right from the start. He was not only a vocal advocate of our research but also made sure that it was discussed by ethics committees and at conferences on the social and ethical aspects of assisted reproduction. It was just like Bob to turn up at a conference for nurses and support personnel. Indeed, he was the driving force behind them. For Bob, the contribution of nurses, counselors, and other support staff was every bit as important as that of scientists and doctors. Luckily for me, he also believed that social science research was central to the overall endeavor of creating healthy families through IVF. Caught up by his boundless energy, I found myself attending meetings on ethics and law; meetings that were well out of my comfort zone as a developmental psychologist. In fact, he wouldn't take no for an answer. In 2004, I was preparing to go on sabbatical to Columbia University in New York when he held a conference on the Ethics, Science, and Moral Philosophy of Assisted Reproduction at the Royal Society. I agreed to speak on the basis that I would not have to produce a written paper. "Don't worry," said Bob. "I shall have your talk recorded and transcribed. All you will need to

do is look it over." What he didn't say was that the transcriber he had in mind for the job was Czechoslovakian and could hardly speak English. I spent the first week of my sabbatical cursing Bob and trying to undo the mess. But you couldn't be angry with Bob for long. He was the warmest, kindest person you could ever hope to know. He was the first person to invite me to lunch when I moved to Cambridge in 2005, and one of the first to arrive at my housewarming party. He went out of his way to welcome a newcomer and I think that says it all.

IVF and ICSI Families

It's hard to imagine it now, but when the first IVF children were born they were treated with suspicion and sometimes outright hostility. I met women at that time who told me stories of being shunned in the street, or shouted at, because of their "test-tube" babies. Even close relatives were wary of the new addition to their family. As one of the first IVF mothers said to me, "I think my mother-in-law thought he was going to come out with two heads . . . . She does love him, I'm sure she does, but there's always been that little something . . . even when she came to the hospital after he was born, she didn't pick him up."

Although the concerns of the medical profession focused on the possible risks of IVF for the health and physical development of the children, concerns were expressed more broadly about the potentially adverse psychological effects. Owing to the stressful nature of infertility and its treatment, it was thought that parenting difficulties might arise when a long-awaited baby would eventually be born. It was argued that parents who had had difficulty conceiving may be over-protective of their children, or have unrealistic expectations of them or of themselves, as parents.

Do mothers and fathers who become parents through IVF behave differently towards their children than do mothers and fathers of naturally conceived children? A number of studies have been carried out to address this question, focusing on parents of children of different ages. Research on infants aged 4 months and 1 year has been conducted in Australia. In Belgium, IVF families were investigated when the children were aged 2 years, again when they were aged 8–9 years, and finally at age 15–16 years. The European Study of Assisted Reproduction Families, conducted in the United Kingdom, the Netherlands, Spain, and Italy, assessed IVF families when the children were aged around 6 years, again at age 12 years, and, in the UK only, as they became adults at age 18. In the first study to be conducted in a non-Western culture, IVF families with preschool and early school age children were investigated in Taiwan.

So, is it the case that the mothers and fathers of children born through IVF experience difficulties in parenting their long-awaited children? It seems that IVF mothers may be less confident in the children's early months of infancy than are mothers who have not undergone fertility treatment. However, this difference seems short-lived. In children's preschool and early school years, IVF mothers and fathers appear to show more positive parenting than do natural conception parents, although there may be a tendency towards over-involvement and over-protection among a minority of mothers. By the time children reach adolescence, IVF mothers and fathers seem very similar to those who have conceived their children naturally in both their approach to parenting and in the quality of their relationships with their children. In general, mothers and fathers whose children have been conceived through IVF appear to be highly committed and involved parents – a finding that is perhaps not surprising given the obstacles they faced in their quest for a child.

What about the children? Do IVF children experience psychological difficulties associated with the method of their conception? The Australian study found some evidence of elevated levels of behavioral difficulties in IVF infants, compared with naturally conceived infants. However, there was no difference at age one year old in the proportion of IVF and natural conception infants classified as securely attached to their mothers. In the European Study of Assisted Reproduction Families, the IVF children did not differ from the comparison group of naturally conceived children in terms of psychological adjustment as rated by parents or the children's teachers. The same was true of the Belgian study and of other studies of the psychological adjustment of IVF children. The age 18 follow up of the UK sample in the European Study of Assisted Reproduction Families provided the first opportunity to ask young people directly how they felt about the unusual nature of their conception. Not one was distressed about having been conceived by IVF. Indeed, many commented that they had forgotten all about it until the researchers turned up!

So, contrary to the fears voiced in the early days of IVF, children conceived in this way do not appear to be at risk for emotional and behavioral difficulties. Although there is some evidence of temperamental problems in infancy, this may reflect the perceptions of anxious mothers, rather than the difficulties of their infants. IVF children are just as likely as their naturally conceived counterparts to be securely attached to their mothers. No studies found raised levels of psychological problems in IVF children. As some investigations also administered questionnaires to teachers in order to obtain independent reports, greater confidence can be placed in the findings than would otherwise be possible had the questionnaires been completed by parents, alone. It seems, therefore, that the tendency towards over-protection by IVF mothers does not result in psychological problems for children. Neither does the greater quality of parenting shown by IVF parents result in even more positive child adjustment.

Although concerns about ICSI families have centered on the effects on children rather than on parents, the same concerns regarding parenting that have been expressed in relation to IVF parents, such as the possibility of their over-protecting their children, also apply to ICSI parents. For this reason, researchers have examined parenting in ICSI families. A large-scale, study conducted in Belgium, Denmark, Greece, Sweden, and the United Kingdom identified few differences in parenting between ICSI, IVF, and natural conception families, and there were no differences in children's feelings towards, or involvement with, their mothers or fathers. Similar findings were reported from a study in the Netherlands. It appears, therefore, that parents of ICSI children are similar to parents of IVF children, in that they are highly committed to parenting and have positive relationships with their children.

Whereas initial anxieties about IVF families arose largely from speculation and fear of the unknown, ICSI raised more tangible concerns due to the direct manipulation of eggs and sperm in the fertilization process. As a result, a number of studies have examined the psychological development of ICSI children. No differences in emotional or behavioral problems have been found between ICSI children and comparison groups of either IVF or natural conception children. Attention has also focused on the cognitive development of ICSI children. A variety of samples of ICSI children of different ages have been studied in comparison with IVF and natural conception children by researchers in Belgium, Australia, Denmark, Greece, Sweden, the United Kingdom, and the Netherlands. Although there has been some variability in the findings, there is little evidence to suggest that ICSI results in cognitive impairment in children.

Despite the positive outcomes for families created by IVF or ICSI, the experience can be extremely difficult. As one father described it, "I think for anyone going through it it's hard, the ups and downs, you know the little victories when the injections start reacting and working and then you're counting the embryos and then you see the little picture of the two cell or four cell embryos; and they are highs. And then the lows when it doesn't work. And knowing you've got to wait and go through it all again. It's really hard." Some parents commented on the lack of understanding of others which they found difficult; "I don't think my mother-in-law realises quite how much we went through to have children. It's all very well saying 'Oh yeah we underwent IVF' – if only it was that simple." However, those whose treatment was successful generally felt that it was all worthwhile. One mother told us, "They're miracles. They are absolute miracles. She came out of the freezer and he was fresh." And another mother summed it up like this, "I tell her that she's very special but then, you know, all children are, but personally I think IVF babies are a little bit, little bit more."

Gamete Donation Families

Although IVF has attracted much publicity, assisted reproduction involving the donation of sperm, eggs, or embryos has had a more fundamental impact on the family owing to the absence of a genetic connection between one or both parents and the child. It has been suggested that parents may be more distant from, or hostile towards, a non-genetic child. It has also been argued that keeping the child's genetic origins secret may be psychologically harmful to the child. Concerns about secrecy have arisen from research on adoption, the family therapy literature, and the personal accounts of those who found out about their donor conception later in life.

Until recently, the majority of parents who gave birth to donor-conceived children did not tell their children about their genetic origins. Even in Sweden, where legislation giving donor offspring the right to obtain information about the donor's identity came into force in 1985, more than a decade later, only 11% of parents were found to have informed their children of their donor conception. When asked about their reasons for secrecy, parents of children born through egg, sperm, and embryo donation have said they were worried that their children would be upset, shocked, and confused by the knowledge that they were not genetically related to one parent (or both parents). The parents were also concerned about jeopardizing the positive relationship that existed between the non-genetic parent(s) and the child, fearing that their child would no longer love the non-genetic parent(s) if they were to find out.

In recent years, there has been a rise in the number of parents intending to tell their children that they were born through donated gametes. However, in spite of these intentions, many parents do not actually disclose this information. In the UK Longitudinal Study of Assisted Reproduction Families, a longitudinal study of children born through gamete donation initiated at the millennium, 46% of parents of infants conceived by donor insemination and 56% of parents of infants conceived by egg donation planned to tell their children about their donor conception. However, only 28% of donor insemination parents and 41% of egg donation parents actually did so by the time their children were seven years old, the age by which most adopted children are told about their adoption. Moreover, some parents who reported that they had told their children had discussed the use of fertility treatment, but not the more fundamental issue of the use of donated eggs or sperm. Many parents of children conceived by embryo donation have been found to similarly give only partial information about the nature of the conception to their children.

There is anecdotal evidence that the removal of donor anonymity in some countries has resulted in an increase in the proportion of parents who tell their children about their donor conception. However, there is little systematic data on the removal of donor anonymity on disclosure rates. A Swedish study of both egg and sperm recipients published in 2011 found that 90% were in favor of disclosure, which suggests a shift towards greater openness; nonetheless, only 16% of parents had begun the process of disclosure by the time their children were four years old. In New

Zealand, where disclosure has been encouraged since 1985 and legislated since 2004, a study found that only 35% of young adults who had been conceived by donor insemination had been told about the nature of their conception. However, an investigation of New Zealand families with younger children found that one-third of the parents had told their children about their donor conception, and, of the parents who had not told, three-quarters intended to do so. In the only systematic study of disclosure since the removal of donor anonymity in the United Kingdom, only around one-third of part-nered mothers had told their 4–8-year-old children about their donor conception. It seems that social and legislative changes may have resulted in parents' greater openness with their donor-conceived children about their biological origins, but it remains the case that a substantial proportion of parents still choose not to tell.

Whether or not parents should tell their children about their donor conception is still a live issue. In 2013, the Nuffield Council on Bioethics published a report on donor conception concluding that it was best for children to be told about their genetic origins at an early age. However, in 2017, Guido Pennings published a controversial letter in the journal Human Reproduction arguing that there was no need to tell. This prompted an animated response not only by coun-selors and social scientists who disagreed, but also by donor-conceived people themselves. My own reading of the research literature leads me to the conclusion that openness is generally in the best interests of the child.

Parents who talk to their young children about their donor conception generally begin to do so by the time they are four years old. These parents tend to tell their children stories about needing help to have a baby, rather than giving detailed explanations of the reproductive process. Contrary to parents' concerns, it appears that children who are told about their donor conception in their preschool years respond neutrally, or with curiosity, rather than distress. However, chil-dren appear to have little understanding of egg or sperm donation by age seven, the age by which most adopted children understand what it means to be adopted. It is not until age 10 that most donor-conceived children are able to give clear accounts of the nature of their con-ception. In a study in the United States of the thoughts and feelings of adolescents who had grown up with the knowledge that they were donor conceived, the major-ity reported feeling comfortable about their donor conception and felt that learning about their donor conception had not had a negative impact on their relationships with their parents. It is noteworthy that parents do not appear to regret telling their children about their donor conception.

The experience of those who are told or find out about their donor conception in adolescence or adult-hood, as opposed to early childhood, can be strik-ingly different. Participants in qualitative studies have reported that secrecy about the nature of their con-ception caused them psychological harm, and many have reported feeling deceived by their parents and angry towards them. Moreover, in a survey of donor-conceived adolescents and adults who were members of the Donor Sibling Registry, a website that helps donor-conceived persons search for their donor and donor siblings (see below for further details of this study), those who had found out about their donor conception in adolescence or beyond were more likely to report feeling upset, angry, shocked, and confused than were those who had been told in childhood. It is important to point out that the participants in these studies had either joined a support group for donor conceived offspring or had joined the Donor Sibling Registry, and thus the extent to which they were rep-resentative of individuals aware of their donor con-ception is not known. Also, all had been conceived by donor insemination; no data are yet available on the feelings and experiences of adolescents and young adults conceived by egg or embryo donation.

A key aim of the UK Longitudinal Study of Assisted Reproduction Families was to investigate the psycho-logical consequences of openness with children about their donor conception. So far, the families have been assessed when the children were aged one, two, three, seven, ten, and 14 years. In the preschool years, the differences identified between family types pointed to more positive parent–child relationships in families cre-ated by gamete donation than in the comparison group of natural conception families, with no differences in the quality of family relationships according to whether the children lacked a genetic connection to their father (in the case of donor insemination) or mother (in the case of egg donation). The donor-conceived children were found to be functioning well, but, in spite of their parents' highly involved parenting, did not show higher levels of adjustment than their counterparts from natural conception families. These findings repli-cated those obtained in the European Study of Assisted Reproduction Families conducted 15 years earlier.

In contrast to the more positive outcomes for the donor conception families in the preschool years, greater difficulties emerged when the children were seven years old, the age by which children show a greater understanding of biological inheritance and the meaning and implications of the absence of a biological connection to parents. The gamete donation mothers who had kept their children's origins secret showed higher levels of emotional distress than did those who had been open with their children about their origins. With respect to the relationship between parents and children, interview and observational assessments of mother–child interaction revealed less positive interaction in the donor-conceived families in which parents had not disclosed the method of conception to the children than in the natural conception families. There were no differences for fathers, apart from higher negativity shown by donor-insemination children during an observational assessment of interaction with their fathers. It is important to note that the differences identified when the children were aged seven were not indicative of dysfunctional family relationships, but, instead, reflected variation within the normal range. Moreover, these differences do not necessarily mean that non-disclosure caused the less positive outcomes for families who did not tell their children about their origins; the non-disclosing families may have been less communicative generally. When the children reached adolescence, the quality of mother–child relationships remained good. However, less positive relationships were found between mothers and adolescents in egg donation families than in donor insemination families, suggesting that the absence of a genetic link between mothers and their children is associated with less positive mother–adolescent relationships than is the absence of a genetic link between the father and the child. In addition, parents who had been open with their children about their origins from an early age had more positive relationships with them at adolescence. This finding came from data obtained independently from both mothers and adolescents which gives greater weight to the finding than had the data come from the mother alone.

In terms of child adjustment, the absence of a genetic connection to either the mother or the father was not associated with emotional or behavioral problems when the children were aged three, seven or 10 years, unless the mother herself was experiencing emotional problems, in which case the children showed higher levels of difficulties at age seven. At age 10, the children were interviewed about their relationships with their parents; those who were aware of their origins were asked about their feelings about having been donor-conceived. The large majority in all three family types perceived their relationships with their mothers and fathers as warm and involved; the absence of genetic relationships did not appear to affect children's feelings of closeness to their parents. Most had positive feelings about their donor conception. However, they tended not to discuss this with friends and family, and some reported feeling embarrassed when talking about the subject. At adolescence, there were no differences in psychological well-being between adolescents in the different family types.

In the only study of parenting and child development in families formed through embryo donation, families were found to be functioning well when the children were of preschool age and in middle childhood. The parents differed from comparison groups of adoptive and IVF parents only in terms of greater emotional over-involvement with their children. However, the children were not found to be at increased risk of psychological problems either in their preschool or their early school years.

As mentioned above, it has been suggested that research on adoption can provide valuable insight into how donor-conceived offspring may feel about searching for and contacting their genetic relations. The main reason given by adopted individuals for searching for birth relatives is to gain a more complete understanding of their family history in order to enhance their own sense of identity. There is growing evidence that similar processes are at play for children born through gamete donation, although, so far, the available data come from studies of those who have been conceived through donated sperm, rather than donated eggs or embryos. In 2000, the Donor Sibling Registry – an internet site designed to facilitate the search for donor relations – was established in the United States by a donor-conceived teenage boy and his mother. Since that time, more than 40,000 people have registered with this website and more than 10,000 matches between donor offspring, donors, and donor siblings have been made. Thus, it appears that knowledge of biological origins is important for the identity formation of some donor-conceived persons, just as it is for some adopted persons. Nevertheless, the proportion of donor-conceived people who search for their donor and donor siblings remains unknown.

Surveys of Donor Sibling Registry members have been carried out to examine why people seek out their donor relatives and what happens when they are found.

The mothers' main reasons for searching were curiosity and for their children to have a better understanding of who they were. Although many of the offspring wished to meet their donor, no one gave the desire to form a relationship with him as their main reason for searching. A striking finding was of just how many donor siblings were found. Donor siblings are genetic half-siblings who have been born from the same donor but raised in different families. In the first survey, half of the families found at least five donor siblings, with many finding more than 10 and one sibling constellation numbering 55! Since that time, even larger donor sibling networks have been identified through the Donor Sibling Registry. Unexpectedly, it was found that families with a child born from the same donor often experienced a strong emotional bond when they met, and they often viewed each other not as new acquaintances, but as family. The families were more interested in forming relationships with the donor siblings than with the donor. They wanted to meet the donor to find out what he was like, but it was the siblings with whom they particularly wanted to stay in touch. Few had met the donor. Nevertheless, those who had made contact with him generally reported these meetings, and the ensuing relationship between the donor and the child, to be positive. Some children were also in touch with the donor's family, including the donor's children and parents, who were effectively their half-siblings and grandparents.

Studies that have included lesbian and single-mother families have found that children are more likely to have been told about their donor conception – and to have been told at an earlier age – than their counterparts from two-parent heterosexual families. This is not surprising, given that the mothers in these families have to address their children's questions about their father. In addition, the majority of parents who search for donor relations are lesbian couples or single mothers, which suggests that these families may be more interested in searching for their children's donor relatives than are heterosexual two-parent families. A much higher proportion of donor-conceived offspring from lesbian mother families tell their non-biological mothers that they are searching for their donors than donor-conceived offspring from two-parent heterosexual families tell their fathers. This suggests that children in heterosexual parent families wish to avoid upsetting their fathers.

So what have we learned about the family relationships and psychological wellbeing of donor-conceived children? It appears that children whose parents begin

to talk to them about their donor conception from an early age seem to integrate this information into their developing sense of identity, whereas some donor offspring who find out about their donor conception in adolescence or adulthood report enduring psychological distress. Moreover, evidence is emerging from longitudinal research of more positive functioning in families in which parents have disclosed the child's donor conception. Thus, it appears that disclosure to children in the preschool years is optimal in terms of the emotional well-being of donor offspring. Those who are aware of their donor conception may search for their donor and donor siblings, generally because they are curious and wish to find out about their ancestral background in order to incorporate this information into their life story. Whilst most donor offspring who search for their donor do not wish to form a parental relationship with him, some do wish to form a fraternal relationship with their donor siblings. It seems that a new phenomenon is taking place – family relationships based on genetic connections between children who were not previously aware of each other's existence are being created across multiple family units. The generally positive functioning of families with children born through egg, sperm, or embryo donation suggests that the absence of a genetic link to one or both parents does not, in itself, have an adverse effect on parenting quality or the psychological well-being of the child.

Surrogacy Families

In spite of the contentious nature of surrogacy and the adverse publicity it has attracted, surprisingly little empirical research has been conducted to determine its impact on parents and children. In the only in-depth investigation, a group of families created by surrogacy was included in the UK Longitudinal Study of Assisted Reproduction Families. Contrary to the concerns that have been expressed about the potentially negative consequences of surrogacy for family functioning, the differences identified between the surrogacy families and the other family types when the children were in their pre-school years indicated more positive parent–child relationships in surrogacy families. However, at age 7, once the children had developed a more sophisticated understanding of the absence of a gestational link to their parents, the surrogacy children showed higher levels of adjustment problems than did the children conceived by gamete donation. This finding parallels that of internationally adopted children at age 7, which has been attributed to their need to struggle with identity issues earlier than domestically adopted children, due to their difference in appearance from their parents. Surrogacy children may similarly face identity issues at an early age; not only are they born to a surrogate mother, which makes them different from other children, but they may also remain in contact with their surrogate mother as they grow up. It is important to point out that the surrogacy children were generally well-adjusted at age 7, with scores within the normal range. Also, the raised levels of psychological problems shown by the surrogacy children disappeared by age 10, which, again, was consistent with the decline in difficulties shown by internationally adopted children by adolescence. By adolescence, the surrogacy families were found to be functioning particularly well. Where differences existed between the surrogacy families and the other family types, these reflected more positive mother–child relationships in the surrogacy families. Despite the expectation that difficulties would arise in the relationship with the surrogate mother, 60% of children were still in contact with their surrogate mother at age 10.

Families with Same-Sex Parents

Lesbian women began to have children through donor insemination in the 1970s. At that time, it was argued that lesbian mothers would be less nurturing than heterosexual mothers and would show higher rates of psychological disorder, and that their children would develop psychological problems as a result. It was also thought that the children of lesbian mothers would show atypical gender development, such that boys would be less masculine in their identity and behavior, and girls less feminine, than boys and girls from heterosexual homes.

There is now a body of research showing that lesbian mothers in general, and lesbian mothers with children born through donor insemination in particular, are just as likely to have good mental health and to have positive relationships with their children as are heterosexual mothers, and that their children are no more likely to show adjustment difficulties or atypical gender-role behavior than are children with heterosexual parents.

The circumstances of gay fathers who have children through surrogacy are somewhat different from those of lesbian mothers who have children using donor insemination in that it is rare for fathers, whether heterosexual or gay, to be primary caregivers. Although

research on fathering has shown that the constructs of fathering and mothering, involving positive engagement, warmth and responsiveness, are largely the same, and that heterosexual fathers influence their children in similar ways to mothers, fathers are generally believed to be less suited to parenting than are mothers. Moreover, gay fathers may be exposed to greater stigmatization regarding their sexual identity than are lesbian mothers. Stigmatization of same-sex-parent families has been associated with emotional and behavioral problems in children.

In a study of parenting in gay father families formed through surrogacy, children in gay-father families were compared to children in lesbian-mother families formed through donor insemination. There were no differences between the gay-father families and the lesbian-mother families in terms of perceived stigma, quality of parenting or parent–child interaction. The children in both family types showed high levels of adjustment with lower levels of children's emotional problems reported by gay fathers. Irrespective of family type, children whose parents perceived greater stigmatization showed higher levels of behavioral problems. The fathers were more likely to maintain a relationship with the surrogate than the egg donor, and most fathers reported a positive relationship with the surrogate.

Single Mothers by Choice

An increasing number of single women are choosing to parent alone and have children through donor insemination. These mothers are often referred to as "single mothers by choice" or "solo mothers." Solo mothers are generally, but not always, well-educated, financially secure women in professional occupations who become mothers in their late 30s or early 40s. Many single mothers by choice report that they would have rather had their children within a traditional family setting, but could not wait any longer because of their increasing age and associated fertility decline; because they wanted to be mothers, they did not actually have a choice.

There is little research on this new family form. However, a comparison between solo mother families and two-parent families, all with donor-conceived children, found no differences in maternal wellbeing or parenting quality apart from lower mother–child conflict in solo mother families. Although the children in solo mother and two-parent families did not differ in psychological adjustment, parenting stress and financial difficulties were associated with children's psychological difficulties in both family types. How best to respond to children's questions about their father was a concern of the single mothers by choice. The mothers reported that their children had begun to ask about their father from the age of about 2–3 years.

Conclusions

The findings of the studies reviewed above show that contrary to the concerns that were raised in the early days of IVF, families created by assisted reproductive technologies – whether through IVF and ICSI, donated gametes and embryos, or surrogacy – are characterized by positive parenting and well-adjusted children. And this remains the case in families formed by assisted reproduction for social rather than medical reasons – families with lesbian mothers, gay fathers, and single mothers by choice.

How can these findings be explained? Parents who have children through assisted reproduction are highly motivated to have children; couples who are less motivated are more likely to have given up along the way. Many have experienced years of infertility and infertility treatment before achieving parenthood, others become parents in the face of significant social disapproval, and still others overcome both hurdles in order to have a child. It seems that those who are successful in surmounting these obstacles become particularly committed parents when their much-wanted children eventually arrive.

Family forms that are currently emerging or are still on the horizon will generate new questions about parenting in assisted reproduction families. Scientific advances in reproductive technologies are leading to new types of parent. In 2017, through developments in mitochondrial DNA transfer, the first child was born with genetic material from three "parents"; a mother, a father, and a woman who donated her mitochondrial DNA. In addition, artificial gametes might soon make it possible for women to produce sperm and for men to produce eggs. Although intended as an infertility treatment, this procedure would allow both parents in same-sex couples to be genetically related to their children.

When Louise Brown was born in 1978, it was unimaginable that, within 40 years, more than 6.5 million babies would be born using IVF; that a woman would be able to give birth to the genetic child of another woman; that, by freezing embryos, parents could give birth to twins years apart; that women would be freezing their eggs until they were ready to become mothers; and that children would be born to gay couples through surrogacy and egg donation. These are just some of the ways in which families have been changed by assisted reproductive technologies. In spite of the concerns that have been raised about the potentially negative consequences for family functioning, the research conducted so far has failed to support the view that creating families through assisted reproduction would have an adverse effect on the psychological wellbeing of children.

Reference

All the material referred to in this chapter can be found in:

Golombok S. 2015. *Modern Families. Parents and Children in New Family Forms.* Cambridge University Press.

Chapter 30

The Commercialization of In-Vitro Fertilization

G. David Adamson and Anthony J. Rutherford

Introduction

Over the past three to four decades, the practice of assisted reproductive technology (ART) has expanded significantly around the globe. Like many other aspects of healthcare, it has been subject, in varying degrees in different areas of the world, to a process many refer to as "commercialization." Merriam Webster dictionary defines commercialization as: (i) management on a business basis for profit, (ii) development of commerce in, (iii) exploitation for profit, or (iv) debasement in quality for more profit. Dr. Fernando Zegers from Chile has said: "In general, commercialization is considered a bad word, especially when used in providing health and happiness . . . All of this is especially tricky when on one hand there is a vulnerable individual suffering from personal and social consequences that result from the incapacity to build a family and on the other hand an educated and powerful giver of happiness." Other terms that have been used to refer to the ever-increasing adoption of business models for the delivery of reproductive care are industrialization, corporatization, commodification, and commoditization. Though each one of these various terminologies may have a specific definition, in the context of in-vitro fertilization (IVF), there is probably a significant overlap in the intended connotation of these words with no mutual exclusivity, encompassing both positive and negative consequences for all parties involved.

In this chapter, a broad perspective will be taken and, rather than presenting just our own perspectives, we will compile and take advantage of the quotes and ideas of 32 respected colleagues in 24 countries around the world who responded to the author's request to comment on "commercialization of IVF." Some responses were short and pithy, others long and very thoughtful. All respondents are listed in the Acknowledgements and some are referenced in the text.

The entire world runs on economics, and profitability is an integral part of any business initiative. Most business enterprises, including those in the healthcare industry, aim to grow and large companies are generally lauded. But do these "business goals" apply to IVF, and should they? Where have we been, where are we and where are we going with "Commercialization of IVF"?

Goals of Healthcare – G. David Adamson

The goal of healthcare depends on the stakeholder being considered. Patients, who should be at the center of healthcare, want access (availability and affordability), effectiveness, and safety; society wants cost-effective care that benefits the health of the general population; physicians and other healthcare professionals would like to be able to provide quality care and be fairly reimbursed for the professional services rendered to patients.

The business objectives of IVF clinics are not that different from other corporations – value creation (through provision of services), differentiation of their product/service (higher cost-effective quality for the patient), and the need for revenue and profit in exchange for the differentiated value. However, the special aspect of medicine is that physicians and healthcare providers have a professional obligation to put the patient's interests above their own; business corporations, on the other hand, have as their first obligation return of investment to owners/shareholders. This is where the confluence of IVF as a medical practice and as a business has the potential for conflict in the different values of medicine and business. In the following sections of this chapter, we will attempt to address the impact of commercialization of healthcare in the IVF sector on all parties involved.

Major Components of Commercialization

Types of Healthcare Systems

Different types of healthcare systems have potentially different levels of commercialization. For example, public systems in which the government pays for, controls, and regulates all medical services have little motivation to commercialize. Likewise, charitable organizations that provide healthcare for social good are not particularly concerned about the profitability of their operations and have little drive to commercialize, but IVF clinics run by charitable organizations are rare. On the other hand, where the private sector is involved in the provision of IVF services, various entities such as companies that own clinics, insurance companies, pharmaceutical companies, laboratory/testing companies, and medical device companies take on financial risks and all have varying degrees of profit motive and employ different strategies to generate that profit. Most countries have varying degrees of mixed models of the above types of systems, with some clinics operating one way and some others. But in countries where there is a preponderance of one model, the influence of the profit motive can be seen.

Dr. Edgardo Rolla shared his perspective from Argentina, stating: "Previously, in December 2010, the Province of Buenos Aires had promulgated the first such law in Argentina. It provided free assisted reproductive techniques to all those living in the province ... most clinics also advertise additional services (not covered by the law) at unregulated fees, such as PGS, PGD, annexin filters for sperm sorting, oocyte cryopreservation for elective and personal reasons (the law covers it only oncological cases), cord blood cell banking, etc. ... If I am allowed to express what I feel, after 30 years in the 'business', it is a 'run for all' commercial competition, with little time left for real quality in some cases." So, Argentina is an example where government regulation had a huge, and most likely unintended, impact on commercialization.

Another example where the nature of the healthcare system has influenced IVF is Japan, where there are some of the biggest clinics in the world. Dr. Osamu Ishihara reports: "Since the first IVF baby was born in 1983, all ART treatments have been done privately at clinics in Japan including national hospitals and university hospitals. There is no legislation regarding ART up to this date and every clinic can theoretically choose their cycle charge as they wish. However, prices still remain very low because of the competition between the clinics, namely around $3,000 US for an IVF cycle and $4,000 US for an ICSI cycle. On the other hand, treatments that require third party are not available in Japan, e.g. donor egg cycles and surrogacy. These require people or organizations to coordinate

care between the clients and foreign clinics; this has the potential for commercialization but has not yet really occurred." Nevertheless, Japan is an example of extremely large clinics where competition has affected the cost of IVF, in this case in a positive way, by keeping the per-cycle cost low and multiple rate low, but not necessarily the per-baby cost.

Organization of Clinics

Although fertility clinics can be organized around a single physician, this practice model has become increasingly difficult to sustain, mainly because of the complexity of IVF services, the need for 24/7 coverage, and increasing regulations in many countries. Nevertheless, this solo practice model offers the single physician almost complete control over the level of profit that the practice attempts to make. Additionally, the physician is directly responsible to the clinic patients who are providing all the revenue. On the other hand, when IVF clinics employ multiple physicians and/or provide services in multiple locations, the pressure to be cost-effective and to maximize profit starts to increase. In these large group practice models, revenue generation becomes less dependent on the individual physician or patient. This distancing increases as group size increases, and even more with larger networks and especially international networks.

Despite the development of many larger centers and organizations, small-scale IVF clinics still exist. Dr. Joel Batzofin commented, "How is it possible for a small, boutique practice to sustain itself in a competitive bustling metropolis when one has to compete with many very large clinics? The only answer is by offering customized services, compassionate care, strategic marketing, and competitive pricing. This is no different than how large companies would attract business – ergo commercialization."

An additional perspective was shared by Dr. Joseph Azoury from Lebanon, "In Arabic countries, IVF commercialization depends mainly on the word of mouth. People rarely go on the internet to find a close IVF clinic. They mainly ask around (neighbors, cousins ...) to decide which Doctor they will visit. Hence the number of patients that visit is directly related to your success rate and to the satisfaction of your patients."

While in many countries a combination of these practice models exists, in many other parts of the world there is very limited access to fertility treatment. Dr. Justin Mboloko Esimo from the Democratic Republic of the Congo reported: "In our country we are not very far with IVF. We are at the beginning of IVF activities. We have only one medical center that provides IVF care. Most patients have to travel to India, South Africa and West African countries for best care. We are doing our best to start another Center." So, there is great variation globally in how the organization of clinics can be affected by commercialization, but even small clinics can be affected.

Profit Motive

Motivation to make a profit is the economic engine of any business and indeed all systems must create sufficient value to someone to merit a financial return commensurate with the cost of staying in business. As Dr. Rudolph Kantum Adageba from Ghana stated: "All IVF centers in Ghana are privately owned, and as private businesses, making profit is one of the motivations of setting up a center."

Difficulties and problems occur when the primary goal of the physician, namely to provide services that are in the patient's best interest, is subjugated to widening the clinic's or physician's profit margin beyond a "reasonable" amount. This can happen in several ways. A major problem occurs when patients are over-treated, i.e. they are recommended to undergo IVF while they could reasonably use less expensive treatments before going on to IVF, or they are treated or continue to be treated with IVF cycles even though the prognosis is very poor. Lord Winston of the United Kingdom was quoted as saying: "It's got worse. It has become more and more private and more and more commercial. IVF is being offered as a blanket treatment when there are a whole variety of other things that you could do that might be more effective." Dr. Robert Norman in Australia concurred: "I think with the commercialization of IVF that's occurring, there's a pressure in every single clinic to use IVF more, and IVF brings in more money for a clinic. This puts pressure on the doctor to use IVF at the expense of simpler interventions."

Furthermore, provided services can be distorted to widen the profit margins; a common example of this approach would be the widespread use of "add-on" services that are either not necessary, or not proven to be of benefit. Interventions such as immunotherapy, herbal medicine, laparoscopy, and hysteroscopy on all patients, may fall into this category. Perhaps an extreme example of this profiteering tactic would be admitting a patient to hospital for a week or more following

embryo transfer to increase pregnancy rates, as one of the surveyed physicians reported. Dr. Gab Kovacs of Australia referred to these add-on services with the old analogy of "snake oil that people take hoping it works without the evidence."

Another example of profit-driven motive is the overuse of technology, demonstrated to be beneficial in certain subgroups of patients, but applied commonly to all patients. Perhaps a prime example of this strategy is the use of intracytoplasmic sperm injection (ICSI) for all ART cycles. Another instance of this is the use of preimplantation genetic testing (PGT) for aneuploidy for all patients. Universal application of such interventions not only incurs unnecessary costs to the patients but may also result in lower cumulative pregnancy rates per initiated cycle.

Other ways to increase profit include providing a valuable service too often, for example ultrasound or estradiol levels, or moving a patient to a more expensive service too early, for example egg donation or PGT.

Norbert Gleicher and colleagues recently reported declines in live birth rates over the last few years in almost all regions of the world. According to Gleicher et al, strongest negative associations were observed with mild stimulation, routine blastocyst-stage embryo culture for patients of all ages, and elective single embryo transfer (eSET). Japan, Australia/New Zealand, and Canada were the regions where these effects were most pronounced. Gleicher and colleagues further concluded that changes introduced to routine IVF practice during the past decade were often made without prior clinical validation of procedures based on economic rather than clinical considerations (i.e., "commoditization" of IVF), often driven by corporate interests assuming control over the provision of clinical IVF services (i.e., "industrialization" of IVF). Australia, the country where industrialization of IVF has so-far made the biggest inroads, with only a handful of corporate entities controlling most of the country's IVF market, represents, likely, the best example how commoditization and industrialization of IVF over the last decade have negatively affected IVF outcomes. These authors also note that Europe and the USA, where commoditization and industrialization quickly follow the Australian model, can expect to see similar consequences on regional live birth rates. In the USA, 2014 live birth rates over the past four years, indeed, have fallen already below 2004 rates.

Another potential source of problems, particularly in jurisdictions where fertility clinics are required by law to publicly publish their success rates, is patient selection biased towards inflating reported success rates. It is possible to refuse services to patients who may be difficult to manage or have a very poor prognosis and who may therefore affect pregnancy rates adversely.

Finally, some clinics could increase profit by opting out of providing costly services, such as patient education, financial counseling, individualized cycle coordination, and psychological support services that are not necessarily essential but certainly are important for patients' overall wellbeing and quality of care. Dr. Steve Ory from the United States said: "Industrialization of IVF has led to the rapid implementation (and more often discarding) of many new techniques often forgoing the classical, previous tradition of development of new technology wherein studies documenting safety and efficacy are completed prior to adoption. This pattern of 'progress' has been most apparent in the US where large expenditures of capital have facilitated the development of new practice models including the appearance of very large ART centers and consolidation of several partner practices under one corporate umbrella. It has also led to the rapid growth of many companies providing essential ART services, supplies and material. This commercialization of IVF has provided a larger population of patients more rapid access to a myriad of new therapies but it has come at a significant cost. The cost is the inevitable conflicts of interest that have arisen between the patients' and broader society's best interests and those of the corporations. There has also been a great amount of resources wasted on ineffective technologies."

Another less-known method by which the profit motive can have a negative impact is in the financial and billing operation of fertility clinics. Manipulative and misleading itemization of multiple essential components of an IVF cycle, and then varying those individual component prices, can be used to maximize total price to the patient and thereby increasing the clinic's profit; for example, the costs associated with freezing and storing embryos can be presented in multiple ways and because of this complexity it may be difficult for the patients to compare pricing from one clinic to another.

Package pricing can be done such that the patient pays just one price for all the services needed. But if the patient then receives less than optimal services to keep the costs of the package services low to the clinic, this increases profit.

In many countries patients finance care, and if the clinic is involved in this it is possible to overcharge the patient for financing or other costs. This issue can be exacerbated in "money-back" or refund guarantee programs where patients might be "cherry-picked" and/or clinics might provide less than optimal care by replacing too many embryos to achieve a pregnancy and not have to pay a refund. Dr. Barry Behr commented, "I think the risk sharing plans when first introduced were one of the turning points in IVF in terms of 'commercializing' it."

Corporatization of Medicine

Corporatization of medicine has been occurring for several decades, at least in the United States (e.g. Kaiser Permanente) and now also in many other countries and regions, e.g. United Kingdom, Australia, India, and the Middle East. Corporatization is intended to bring business principles to medicine. The goal of this for physicians is to improve the quality of care. The goal for reputable companies is to bring cost-effectiveness, such that quality is increased while unit costs go down, so that the patient receives a better financial value while the company can make a better profit than smaller entities. There is no reason that this cannot occur with the corporatization of IVF clinics. However, clearly a potential conflict exists when the primary responsibility of each physician, which is to place the patient's interest above all others, including their own personal interest, must be entwined with the corporate goal of generating a profit for the company. This is where the "rubber hits the road" and physicians and corporations must ensure that their values are coincident, in that the physician recognizes the need for profit for the company, while the corporate structure protects the responsibility of the physician to place the patient first.

Australia may be the most corporatized IVF country. Dr. Michael Chapman explained: "Thus, in Sydney, IVF Australia was formed with four clinics joining together. Venture capital then became involved and with their assistance Virtus Health emerged, with amalgamations with Queensland Fertility Group and Melbourne IVF. Virtus now undertakes over a third of all cycles in Australia. It has clinics internationally in Ireland, Denmark and Singapore. Ultimately Virtus listed on the Stock Exchange in 2013. In parallel Monash IVF, based in Melbourne, linked with Repromed in Adelaide and opened or acquired other clinics around Australia and New Zealand. It listed publicly in 2014."

Corporatization is not necessarily bad. Dr. PC Wong from Singapore stated: "Singapore has eight private and three public hospital IVF clinics. The latest addition was a private clinic started by an Australian publicly-listed IVF group. Prior to this, all the IVF clinics were owned and operated by the hospitals they were located in except for the three private ones which were owned by a physician, an embryologist and a private company. None were owned by companies or corporations. The arrival of the commercialised IVF clinic did not have any adverse impact on the provisions of ART services in Singapore. Perhaps one of the reasons may be that it operated an open system, i.e. any qualified IVF practitioner is welcomed to bring his/her own patients to the clinic for IVF. The IVF practitioners charge their own professional fees, while the IVF clinic charges the laboratory and embryology fees. The encouraging fact is that the cost of IVF in this clinic was not the most expensive in Singapore. How it will be in the future remains to be seen."

Ethical Issues

The four principles of ethical practice are Autonomy – to honor the patients' right to make their own decision; Beneficence – to help the patient advance his/her own good; Nonmaleficence – to do no harm; Justice – to be fair and treat like cases alike. If the individual physician follows these ethical principles and the corporation does not interfere in the provision of services, then the corporation and medicine can co-exist with benefit to all parties involved. However, if the corporation interferes in the practice of medicine, not just in the management of individual patients, but in processes, procedures, budgeting, or control of systems that compromises the physician's capacity to follow these principles, then the practice of medicine and, by direct extension, the patient can potentially be harmed. So, it is essential, but notably not sufficient by itself, to protect physician autonomy regardless of the business environment.

Dr. Michael Chapman explained that in Australia loss of clinical freedom concerned many and, in some early models of practice consolidation, doctors dropped out after their "lock-up" period was over. He stated: "For fertility specialists, the most important aspect of involvement with a corporation is the model to which they are signing up. It must allow clinical freedom, be financially fair to them, and have structures in place to provide confidence that their views are heard. Sympathetic leadership is vital."

It is noteworthy that it is not just the physicians whose ethical boundaries can be challenged

in commercialized IVF. Dr. Duru Shah, the current President of the Indian Society for Reproductive Medicine, stated: "Surrogacy is a good option for a selected few, but the unhealthy combination of profit-driven clinics and financially desperate surrogates, has led to many unethical practices in the unregulated surrogacy industry in India. At one end of the spectrum is the pain of infertility and craving for parenthood, and at the other end is the commercialization of the reproductive capacity of women. If carried out ethically, it is the biggest boon to infertile women who have a problem with their uteri in order to have their own biological children, and a blessing for the surrogates who need those financial resources for better education of their own children. It is hard to tell whether surrogates are exercising their own free will or are being coerced and exploited to fulfill material and financial needs by their husbands and in-laws. Women, as second-class citizens in the third world, are extremely vulnerable to commercialization and exploitation. Undoubtedly, there is also the possibility that surrogacy may be inappropriately used as a convenience for nonmedical reasons, and at times, has been equated to a form of dehumanizing labor and 'organ trafficking'. Surrogacy had become an avenue for medical tourism in India due to its low cost, but as per the latest recommendations from the Government of India, International Surrogacy has been banned." Dr. Shah continued: "Gestational surrogacy should be part of a comprehensive infertility treatment program in accredited centers, with a full back up of lawyers, counselors and ethics committee, and Central Monitoring Agency."

Regulations

Regulations can also affect the commercialization of medicine. For example, the legality or not of payment to gamete donors and gestational carriers (surrogates) has a profound impact on the practice and economics of medicine. While strong arguments are made on both sides of payment issues and reimbursement plans in third-party reproduction, there is no question that these policies affect many patients, both within individual countries and beyond national borders, forcing patients to seek cross-border reproductive care.

Payment policies and practices in this area can be, and are, responsibly undertaken in many countries and by many professionals, but egregious practices also exist in some countries. Whether economics is involved, regulations that limit access to care, for example policies that strictly prohibit third party reproduction, or care for single people, have a profound effect on social justice and discrimination aspects of reproductive rights. Such limiting regulations cause many people to undertake cross-border reproductive care, at great personal financial, time, and emotional cost, and often exposes them to marginal, lower quality care, legal problems, and exploitation.

Dr. Antonio Pellicer from Spain has stated: "Compensation, as well as anonymity, are major drivers of oocyte donation. But Spain has also important rules to protect the donors. For example, they cannot be stimulated more than six times, or OHSS is seriously punished in the Spanish Law. Thus, no one can become a 'professional' of egg commercialization."

And, of course, regulations don't always have their intended effects. Dr Anna Pia Ferraretti from Italy stated: "In Italy, commercialization of IVF has been sometimes paradoxically 'promoted' by legislations that had the aim 'to avoid' some forms of commercialization! The last example is the donation of gametes in Italy." "After 10 years of ban by law (2004–2014), during which period at least 5000 couples per year used to go abroad to receive treatment, gamete donation is now allowed again in Italy. In Europe, the commercialization of gametes is forbidden, but reimbursement for donors is allowed. On the contrary, Italy does not allow any form of reimbursement. To recruit voluntary donors is, therefore, very difficult, mainly for egg donation. But, according to the European Directives, it is possible to import gametes from foreign centers. In this context, several 'banks of eggs' with 'good quality' oocytes are offered to Italian clinics. The result is a 'commercialization' of gametes whereas the intention was to avoid such 'commercialization'!"

Patient Responses to Commercialization

While there are myriad patient responses to commercialization, perhaps nobody stated this better than Ernestine Gwet Bell from Cameroon: "Since 1997 we have two private IVF centers in Douala, the economic City. The first public Center opened in 2016 in Yaoundé, the capital of the country. It was supported by the First Lady of the country. The demand for IVF is very high since tubal obstruction is the most frequent cause of infertility. Social security does not exist and the few private insurance companies? don't support infertility care. Couples are forced to save a lot of money to be

able to undergo an IVF cycle. An IVF cycle including drugs costs $4000. To make it happen couples who do not have means resort to tontines. These are monthly savings contributions that help them save money for one to two years. Patients come from all countries in the sub-region because many of them do not have IVF centers. Other people can sell their belongings such as jewels and cars. Egg donations are quite common; 15% of them are made in the context of 'sharing'. Young women share their oocytes with older ones who, in return, pay for their IVF drugs. We don't have specific companies for the management of IVF. Everything is done in the ART Center."

Another aspect of the patient's perspective came from Dr. Michael Chapman when he said: "Patients are really demanding. Patients want something to happen. If I'm not doing any harm and I may do good, and I don't know whether I'm doing good or not, but if I do no harm, I feel comfortable in prescribing a treatment if the patient thinks that that's going to be of assistance to them."

It is evident that commercialization potentially has major impacts on patients and how they try to access and use IVF services.

Commercialization in the Birthplace of IVF – Anthony J. Rutherford

The first pioneering work by Steptoe and Edwards leading to the birth of Louise Brown, the world's first IVF baby, nearly 40 years ago, began in a National Health Service (NHS) setting, a District General Hospital in Oldham, Lancashire. The two eminent researchers quickly realized the difficulties faced by the confines of the NHS, opening the first commercial IVF clinic in the United Kingdom, at Bourn Hall, in 1980. Prices were expensive, almost half the average yearly wage for one relatively unsuccessful treatment cycle, at the time reflecting the exclusivity of the technology. Another major limitation in the early days of IVF was the need for operating theater facilities for laparoscopy to collect oocytes. As a result, most of the early clinics offering treatment did so in a hospital setting, often associated with an academic department, reflecting the innovative technology as a hot topic for research.

In 1982, the first IVF unit in an NHS setting offering patients IVF treatment opened in St. Mary's Hospital in Manchester, under the direction of Brian Lieberman. One early pioneer of IVF in the UK, Ian Craft, appointed Professor of Obstetrics and Gynaecology at the Royal Free in London, was the first to recognize the commercial potential benefit of opening a private IVF unit in London, initially at Cromwell Hospital, then at Humana Wellington, before opening his own independent unit, The London Gynaecology and Fertility Centre, on Harley Street, in 1990. Professor Lord Winston, an initial sceptic about the value of IVF, opened a clinic at Hammersmith Hospital in 1983. He took the philanthropist approach, and used income generated by treating private patients and an extensive private surgical practice to promote IVF treatment, offering "free" IVF before NHS funding existed. In the mid-1980s major academic centers, working with clinicians with a fertility background, developed dedicated IVF clinics throughout the UK.

The advent of transvaginal ultrasound, initially introduced in the UK in 1986, allowing oocytes to be collected under conscious sedation as a day-case procedure, and the use of GnRH analogs to program cycles simplifying the IVF procedure, opened the door for IVF clinics to be developed outside of hospital facilities. Multiple IVF units opened in the center of private medicine in London, Harley Street. The subsequent development of large IVF conglomerates across the UK was originally organized by clinicians and scientists with business acumen, but during the past decade venture capitalists have entered the IVF market in the UK. In addition, more recently, large overseas IVF consortia have also moved into the UK market. There has been an eagerness to purchase IVF units, and, on behalf of NHS hospitals with large deficits, a keenness to sell. As a result, the IVF map in the UK has seen a radical overhaul in the last five years. The main drive to develop commercial organizations in the UK was patient demand. Initially, the NHS provision of IVF remained extremely limited, as it was regarded by many in the echelons of the NHS as a relatively unsuccessful research technique. The Human Fertilisation and Embryology Act 1990 established the Human Fertilisation and Embryology Authority (HFEA) in 1991 to regulate IVF in the UK, and to promote good practice. At the same time, a national infertility awareness campaign (NIAC), started by professionals, patient organizations, and funded through the pharmaceutical companies, to promote NHS IVF. Unfortunately, despite these endeavors, in terms of state funding, the UK fares relatively poorly compared to the rest of Europe. Great store was placed on the National Institute for Health and Care Excellence (NICE) guidelines, first published in 2004, which recommended three full cycles of IVF

on the NHS. However, this has never been achieved nationally, with less than 50% of Clinical Care Groups (CCGs) funding the whole recommendation, and most funding just one cycle with wide exclusion criteria. Private treatment flourished, with approximately 60% of all IVF cycles performed in the UK funded privately, accessed by young couples not normally accustomed to private medicine. Interestingly, in Scotland, where NHS funding is generous, complying with the NICE guidelines and lacking some of the restrictive criteria used to ration access to treatment, such as children in previous relationships, the private sector fails to thrive.

"New technologies, such as intracytoplasmic sperm injection (ICSI 1992), broadening the appeal of IVF, allowing an ever-greater proportion of infertile couples to benefit from treatment, at a premium price. During this same decade, new medications were developed, highly purified urinary gonadotrophins, recombinant gonadotrophins, and GnRH antagonists, which allowed subcutaneous injection instead of deep intramuscular injection and simplified the treatment process. While these advances in medication did not bring about a substantial improvement in clinical outcomes, with no significant increase in live birth rates, there was inevitably an increased cost. In the monitoring of the IVF cycle itself, there are wide variations in practice, some advocating multiple endocrine assays, increasing the invasiveness and cost of the procedure without any real evidence of benefit. There have also been substantial improvements in IVF technology, in our understanding and recognition that embryos grow best in a low oxygen culture, and more complex culture media."

"Of course, most IVF cycles will not result in a live birth (HFEA), and there is an inevitable quest to try and find an explanation. NICE developed an evidence-based guideline initially, published in 2004 and updated in 2013, summarizing which interventions were of proven benefit. However, many fringe interventions with limited evidence are widely practiced, including a variety of adjunct therapies and modified diets to improve response, and immunomodulation using a variety of techniques to improve implantation. Another controversial topic is the use of pre-implantation genetic screening (PGS). Embryo biopsy and PGS at the early cleavage stage is clearly unsuccessful. However, there is growing evidence that by using more advanced technology with Next Generation Sequencing (NGS), and blastocyst biopsy, knowledge of the embryo karyotype will improve live birth rates. In many of these adjunct treatments, where clinical trials are available, there are conflicting reports of value, which are difficult for a doctor to interpret, let alone the patient. These 'add-ons' quickly inflate the base price of an IVF treatment cycle, often more than two- or three-fold. In 2007, the widespread use of these non-evidence based adjuncts prompted Professor Lord Robert Winston to raise concerns about the commercialization and exploitation of women stating "Information used to populate websites can be highly misleading, with wildly inaccurate claims of success in relatively selected small patient populations."

Advantages and Disadvantages of Commercialization

Commercialization of IVF, no matter how assessed, has occurred since Louise Brown was born in 1978. Some aspects of commercialization have been advantageous: scale can bring resources that enable first quality facilities and personnel, enable physicians to focus on clinical medicine and research, increase standardization and quality control, enable more sophisticated assessment and improvement of systems, and help improve care for patients.

At the same time, commercialization can lead to a focus on profit over the best interests of any given patient or even groups of patients. "Cherry picking" patients to improve outcomes and financial results, encouraging unproven "add-on" services, providing unnecessary services or not providing necessary services, opaque bundled or unbundled pricing, inadequate investment in necessary facility, personnel and operations resources, and other manipulations to raise real or apparent profit can result in profoundly unethical behaviors by physicians and/or corporations.

Dr. Bill Ledger of Australia has stated: "Australia has an almost completely commercialized ART sector, very different from the University led initiatives of a generation ago. This has brought benefits including speedy referral and treatment and competitive success rates, but has sometimes led to money driving medicine. We see this in the practice of some clinics billing large amounts for fertility preservation for cancer patients and in the exclusion of the less well off from ART due to the cost of treatment. Uniquely, Australian Medicare provides substantial (but partial) reimbursement for almost every IVF cycle, with no cap on cycle number or female age. This leads to occasional abuses by a minority of clinicians, with continuation of (State funded) treatment beyond what is medically realistic.

However, the flip side of this generosity is that our SET and singleton term birthrate is amongst the highest in the world as patients are not pressurized by large personal expenditure to maximize their chances of pregnancy in one hit."

Dr. James Olobo-Lalobo from Uganda stated: "There is no country in the world providing unlimited, and nearly–free IVF treatment between the adult reproductive age of 18–45 years. That means there is no automatic public or charity based healthcare system, with policies and resource capacity to achieve the right enshrined in Article 16 of the Universal Declaration of Human Rights that states that: "men and women of full age . . . have the right to found a family." Therefore, there's a significant and definable role for commercialism, in the provision of IVF, in particular, in regard to access and availability of treatment.

Dr. Heinz Strohmer from Austria commented, "Industrialization needs simplification and standardization leading to a decreasing need of human input. Since the fascinating scientific breakthrough of the first successful IVF delivery, ART shows a definite trend regarding industrialization. The method is established, benefits by standardization, process control and there is an increasing demand. I expect two factors to speed up this tendency further: 1) More and more centers are owned by institutional investors or IVF chains and they definitely are interested to support this trend. 2) The recent slogan 'industry 4.0' will be adapted analogously as 'IVF 4.0' as all machines in an IVF center, US machines, incubators etc. will be linked and will contribute to big data. This allows a central software to determine the main parameters of the treatment (stimulation dosage, selection of embryos for transfer, chances of an individual couple, performance of staff, etc.) without any human input. I expect this to happen within the next 5 years and it will lead to a worldwide trend that I call the 'McIVF' concept."

Conclusion

Despite the obvious challenges that commercialization has brought to IVF, the reality is that the clear majority of patients in most countries get good to excellent care. Success rates have risen dramatically since IVF was introduced, and issues of safety with multiple births are being mitigated in almost every country. There are probably close to 10 million babies born from IVF globally. Almost all are healthy, almost as healthy as the general population. Tens of millions of family

247

members have benefited from IVF babies, and society has benefited from their productivity. Undoubtedly, some people have paid too much to unscrupulous and greedy doctors and/or corporations; but they almost all believe that their babies were worth it.

The authors believe that IVF has become commercialized, much as other services have become more commercialized when there is an absence of societal responsibility for that service. Since the United Nations charter states that every person has the right to found a family, every person should have the right to reproductive care consistent with the level of health care in their country. The major problem with IVF now is not commercialization, but lack of access to care because of lack of clinics or, more commonly, lack of affordability because of limited government or insurance coverage. More government and insurance coverage would not only increase access but also reduce, but not eliminate, the influence of commercialization on IVF, and therefore would be of major benefit to patients.

Commercialization of all aspects of global business is occurring at a rapid pace, and in many areas of healthcare. It is not surprising that IVF, a sector of healthcare that has had limited societal support in most countries, has fostered an entrepreneurial environment. This has undoubtedly harmed some patients financially and otherwise. However, it has also resulted in rapid expansion of the number of IVF clinics and their size, dramatic scientific advances, outstanding clinical care in many clinics and a competition to increase quality. The value of a child is so high that many who can afford it overlook the price. Unfortunately, the price is preventing most people needing IVF from ever receiving the service.

It is the responsibility of all of us as physicians and as healthcare professionals to practice evidence-based medicine so that our patients' best interests always come first. However, we can also strive to utilize the benefits of commercialization while avoiding the intrusion of its negative aspects into patient care. This is an ongoing challenge, but one I believe our professionals can successfully manage if we always remember and practice that the patient comes first.

Acknowledgments

The following have given invaluable help with the preparation of this Chapter, some of whom have been quoted within the text above.

Argentina: Edgardo Rolla

Australia: Michael Chapman, Bill Ledger, Rob Norman

Austria: Heinz Strohmer

Brazil: Carlos Petta

Camaroon: Ernestine Gwet Bell

Chile: Fernando Zegers-Hochschild

China: Jie Qiao

Democratic Republic Congo: Justin Mboloko Esimo

Egypt: Moustafa Eissa

Germany: Markus Kupka

Ghana: Rudolph Kantum Adageba

India: Sabahat Rasool, Duru Shah

Israel: Ziona Haklai

Italy: Anna Pia Ferraretti

Japan: Osamu Ishihara

Lebanon: Joseph Azoury

Russia: Vladislav Korsak

Singapore: PC Wong

South Africa: Silke Dyer

Spain: Antonio Pellicer

Tunisia: Kharouf Mahmoud

Uganda: James Olobo-Lalobo

United Kingdom: Ian Cooke, Tony Rutherford

USA: Joel Batzofin, Barry Behr, Max Ezzati, Norbert Gleicher, Steve Ory, Mark Surrey

Index

Abate, Vincenzo, 104
abortion, 143, 158
  spontaneous, 185, 186
accessibility, treatment, 158, 162–165, 174
accreditation program, 144–145
Acosta, Dr. Anibal, 66, 67, 70
add-on services, 242, 247
adoption, 234, 236, 238
Africa, 158–170
  ART registration, 161–162
  IVF, accessible and affordable, 162–165,
    245
  IVF, history of, 159
  IVF, lack of expertise, 166
  IVF, unmet need for, 160
  lack of consumables, 166
  major challenges and hurdles, 166
age
  and aneuploidy, 185
  ethical issues, 149
  fertility and, 78
  social freezing and, 138
Agrawal, Rina, 148–151
Ahrén, Professor Kurt, 111
Alberda, Bert, 15, 130
Ali, J., 193
Alpha society, 33, 200
amenorrhea, 133
American Society for Reproductive
    Medicine (ASRM), 71–72, 78
amniocentesis, 53, 80
ANARA (African Network and Registry for
    Assisted Reproductive Technology),
    161
Andrews, Dr. Mason C., 66
aneuploidy testing, 79, 185, 187
animal studies, 38. See also mouse embryos;
    rabbit studies
  1950s and 1960s advances, 4
  embryo biopsy, 180
  from human IVF, 8–19
  Heape experiments, 1
  ovarian tissue cryopreservation, 198
  Pincus experiments, 2
Argentina, 229, 241
arrayCGH, 187–188
ART cycles. See IVF cycles
artificial insemination with donor sperm
    (AID), 84
Ascaris megalocephala, 10
Asch, Dr. Ricardo, 76, 81
Asherman, Joseph, 132
assisted hatching, 78, 136
Asztély, Dr. Mats, 116

Austin, Bunny, 43
Austin, C.R., 3
Australia, 46–65
  1980 onwards, 54–60
  commercialization, 242, 243, 244, 247
  early success with IVF, 48–49
  first human embryos, 47–48
  IVF births, 52–54, 59, 60
  IVF workshop, world's first, 60
  legislation, 183, 224–228
  Melbourne, 46–63
  New South Wales, 63–64
  Queensland, 64
  South Australia, 64–65
  West Australia, 64
Austria, 87–100
  first IVF outpatient clinic, 93–96
  first IVF trials, 87
  IVF program grows, 88, 89–91
  IVF road to success, 89–91
  Jovanovic family. See Jovanovic family
  preliminary studies at 2nd VUWH, 87
Avery, Dr. Sue, 33
azoospermia, 77, 84, 85, 86, 178
  DAZ gene, 210
azoospermia factor (AZF) gene, deletion, 77

Baby Joseph, 178
Baby M, 80
back to nature principle, 12
bacterial artificial chromosomes
    (BAC), 187
Balfour Studentship, 1
Balfour, Professor Francis, 1
Balmaceda, Dr. Jose, 81
Bartoov, Benjamin, 137
Bavister, Barry, 4, 14
Ben-Rafael, Zion, 132–138
Berlusconi, Silvio, 106
Biggers, John D., 1–6, 12, 13, 78
birth-associated tissues, stem cells from,
    219–220
Blakemore, Jennifer, 21–26
blastocentesis, 109
blastocysts
  biopsy, 185, 246
  cryopreservation, 154, 193
  culture, 79, 215–216
  embryonic stem cells from, 216–217
  hatching, 195
blastomere biopsy, 19, 79
BlueGnome, 187, 188
BMOC2 medium, 13
Bomsell, Ondine, 102

bone marrow stem cell transplantation,
    216, 221
Bongso, Ariff, 214–222
Borini, Andrea, 195, 196
Bourn Hall clinic, 8, 15, 16, 28–35
  commercialization issues, 245
  cryopreservation prohibition, 18
  first IVF international meeting, 32, 90,
    114–115
  numbers of births, 32
  research papers from, 36
  site of, 31, 35
Bourn-Hallam Group of IVF Clinics, 33
Boveri, Theodor, 10–11
Boveri–Sutton chromosome theory, 10
Braude, Peter, 42
Brave New World (Huxley), 11
Brinsden, Peter, 28–35
Brinster method, 14
Brinster, Ralph, 13, 14
British Medical Association (BMA), 43
Brown, Leslie, 15, 30
Brown, Louise
  birth of, 15, 30, 52
  birth of, media on, 30, 31, 41
  birth of, public backlash, 5–6
  fortieth birthday, 35
  twenty fifth party, 35
Brown, Professor James, 50
Brüel and Kjaer (company), 117
Brussels, 84–86
Bull, Graham, 43
Bunge, Raymond, 11
Burt, Elizabeth, 148–151
Buster, John, 76, 182

Canada, 229
Cannon, Graham, 43
capacitation, 3, 13
Carr, Elizabeth, 31, 67, 75
Carter, President Jimmy, 5
Catholic Church, 30, 61, 72, 80, 104
  Latin America, 141, 143–144
cell theory, 9
centrifugation-migration technique, 177
centriole, 10
centrosome, 10
Certificate of Need, 6
CFTR gene mutation, 77
CGH. See comparative genomic
    hybridization (CGH)
Chalmers, Theo, 38
Chambers, Joanna, 42
Chambers, Robert, 9

Chang, M.C., 3, 11, 12, 22, 25
Chang's medium, 216
Chapman, Dr. Michael, 243, 244, 245
Chen, Zi-Jiang, 152–156
Chile, 141–147
China, 152–156
  development of IVF, 152
  IVF techniques, 153–156
  surrogacy, 156
choline, 196
chromosomes, 10
  abnormalities, 154, 180–190
  aneuploidy, 185
  bacterial artificial, 187
  diploid and haploid, 10
  model of inheritance, 10
  sex chromosomes, 10, 184, 188
Cittadini, Ettore, 104
Clayton, Stanley, 40
cleavage stage embryos, cryopreservation,
  192–193
Clinical Care Groups (CCGs), 246
clinical embryologists, first, 17
clomiphene, 47, 50, 51, 90, 92
clomiphene citrate (CC), 203
Cobo, Ana, 197
co-culture systems, 193, 215, 216
Coddington, Charles C., 66–73
Cohen, Jacques, 8–19, 79, 136, 193
Cohen, Jean, 102, 103
colchicine, 184
collaboration
  Bob Edwards and Patrick Steptoe, 14
  regional, in Latin America, 141–147
  regional, in Scandinavia, 116–119
Comisión Nacional de Reproducción
  Humana Asistida (CNRHA), 121
commercialization, 63, 172–176, 240–248.
  See also funding
  advantages and disadvantages, 247
  birthplace of IVF, 245–247
  definition, 240
  ethics, 244
  goals of healthcare, 240
  patient responses to, 245
  profit motive, 242–243
  regulations, 244–245
  surrogacy, 227
  types of healthcare system, 240–241
comparative genomic hybridization
  (CGH), 182
  arrayCGH, 187–188
  metaphase, 186–187
compensation, donors, 121, 245. See also
  reimbursement
Conant, James, 23
congenital bilateral absence of vas deferens
  (CBAVD), 77
Conn, Clare, 188
Connell, Matthew, 75–82
Contraceptive Research and Development
  (CONRAD) Program, 68
controlled ovarian hyperstimulation
  (COH), 67, 75
controlled ovarian stimulation (COS),
  75–76, 133, 206

Controversies in Obstetrics Gynaecology
  and Infertility (COGI) Congress, 132
corporatization of medicine, 243–244
Costa Rica, 143
costs. See compensation; funding;
  reimbursement
Cox, Lloyd, 64
Craft, Professor Ian, 32, 42, 54, 245
Creutzfeld-Jakob disease (CJD), 202
criminal offence, 227
CRISPR, 155, 190
Croxatto, Horacio, 11
cryopreservation, 15, 18–19, 192–200
  blastocysts, 154, 193
  China, 153–154
  embryo, 18, 31, 62, 153, 154
  human embryo, 192–194, 215
  human ovarian tissue, 198–200
  oocytes, 78, 153, 154
  oocytes, human, 194–198
  social freezing, 77, 137–138, 198
cryotop, 197
cryptozoospermia, 85
Culture Club, 78
culture media, 12–14
  in IVF tests, 4
  KSOM, 78
culture systems, 12–14
  blastocyst, 79, 215–216
  co-culture, 193, 215, 216
cystic fibrosis, 77, 174, 186, 188
cytoplasm, donor oocyte, 79
cytotoxic therapies, 192, 194, 197, 198

DAZ (deleted in azoospermia) gene, 210
de Kretser, David, 60, 177–179
deafness, 154
DeCherney, Alan H., 81, 75–82
Delhanty, Dr. Joy, 184, 188
Del-Zio, Doris, 80
developing countries. See also Africa; India;
  Latin America
  fertility rates, 165
  infertility and, 158, 165
  Special Task Force on infertility, 159, 166
Devroey, Paul, 84
diabetes, 219
  gestational, 220
diathermy, 39
Dickey-Wicker Amendment, 81
Diczfalusy Egon, 111
Diedrich, Klaus, 129–130
Dignitas Personae, 80
Dill, Sandra, 228–231
dimethyl sulfoxide (DMSO), 15, 192, 194,
  198
DNA
  mitochondrial, 155, 239
  recombinant, 76, 205
donor anonymity, 234
donor disclosure, 234–237, 237
donor embryos, 156, 234, 236
donor gametes, 155–156
  ban on, 108
  families, 234–237
  legislation, 224, 225, 226

donor insemination, 61, 155
  AID, 84
  early 20th century, 11
  lawsuit, 81
donor oocytes, 76, 98, 155, 197
  cytoplasm, 79
  pregnancies, 61–62
  Spain, 121–122
Donor Sibling Registry, 235, 236
donors
  compensation, 121, 245
  reimbursement, 108, 245
Dor, Dr. Jehoshua, 134
Driscoll, Geoffrey, 63
Dunstan, Gordon, 5

East Virginia Medical School (EVMS), 16,
  66, 68, 69
ectogenesis, 11–12
Edgar, David, 192–200
Edwards, Sir Robert, 4–5, 5, 12, 26, 28–35,
  132
  awards and honors, 32
  blastomere biopsy, 19
  early years, 29
  first successful human IVF, 14
  forecasting future directions of IVF, 34
  France, speaking in, 102
  hostility to work, BMA and, 43
  hostility to work, early inklings, 37–38
  hostility to work, MRC and, 41–42
  hostility to work, Nature 1969 paper, 38
  hostility to work, Parliament and, 42
  hostility to work, referees' reports, 38–41
  Howard Jones and, 66
  Nobel Prize, 8
  ovarian stimulation protocol, 202
  psychological/social aspects of IVF, 232
  Spain and, 120
  Steptoe collaboration, 14
  supporters of work, 43
  Zegers-Hochschild, Influence on, 141
Elder, Dr. Kay, 33
embryo biopsy, 14, 62, 180–182, 190
embryo cryopreservation, 18, 31, 62,
  153, 154
  human, 192–194, 215
embryo donation, 156
  families, 234, 236
embryo transfer (ET)
  first attempts, 1
  frozen vs fresh, 154
  multiple, 134, 177, 192
  single, 34, 79, 85
embryo vitrification, 193
embryonic stem cells
  blastocyst culture, 215–216
  first, 34
  from blastocysts, 216–217
  human. See human embryonic stem cells
  (hESCs)
embryotrophic factors, 215
endometrial scratching, 137
Ennals, David, 41
Enzmann, E.V., 2
Estes operation, 1

Estes, W.L., 1
estradiol, 75
ethics, 40, 41, 232, 244
    approval sought, 84
    donor egg pregnancy, 61–62
    donor insemination, 81
    four principles of practice, 244
    France, 103
    India, 149
    Nuffield Council on Bioethics, 235
Ethics Advisory Board, 81
ethylene glycol, 197
European Convention on Human Rights,
    228
European Society of Human Reproduction
    and Embryology (ESHRE), 109, 120
    award from, 186
    Bonn meeting, 129
    Special Task Force on infertility, 159, 166
European Study of Assisted Reproduction
    Families, 233, 235
Evans, Martin, 8
experimental embryology
    hundred years of, 10–11
    Nobel prizes for, 8
eye diseases, 218

Fabbri, Raffaella, 196
fallopian tubes
    blockage, 1, 92
    environment, 50, 215
    gamete intra-fallopian transfer, 76
    microsurgery, 211
families, 232–239
    gamete donation, 234–237
    IVF and ICSI, 232–234
    lesbian, 237, 238
    same-sex parents, 227, 238
    single-mother, 237, 238
    surrogacy, 237–238
Fanconi's anemia, 189
Fasolino, Antonio, 105
Fauser, Bart, 125–131
federal regulations, 81–82
Fehilly-Willadsen, Carole, 8
Feichtinger, Dr. Wilfried, 87–100
feminists, 61, 183
Ferraretti, Anna Pia, 104–109
Fertility Clinic Success Rate and
    Certification Act, 81
Fertility Society of Australia (FSA), 64
fertility tourism, 106, 121, 149, 151, 244
fibrin sealant glue, 136
Ficoll, 178
First World Congress on IVF, 97
Fishel, Simon, 8, 14
fluorescent in situ hybridization (FISH), 79,
    182, 188
    multi-probe, 185
    single cell, 183–186
fluorochromes, 184, 185, 186
Follicle Programme, 89
follicles. See ovarian follicles
follicle-stimulating hormone (FSH), 16, 76,
    111, 177
    characteristics, 202

dosages, 134
    recombinant-hFSH, 205
follitropin alfa, 205
Ford Foundation, 56, 87
Fowler, Bob, 208
Fowler, Norman, 42
France, 102–103
frozen embryo pregnancies, 62, 154
Frydman, René F., 102–103
funding
    Africa, 158, 162–165, 245
    government, lack of, 8, 16
    India, 148, 149
    lack of, 30, 38, 41, 42
    Latin America, 144
    misappropriation, 81
    Russia, 174

gamete donation. See donor gametes
gamete intra-fallopian transfer (GIFT), 29,
    76, 154
gamete intrauterine transfer (GIUT), 154
Garcia, Dr. Jairo, 66
Gardner, David, 79, 193
Gardner, Richard, 19, 37
gay father families, 238
gender inequality, 148
gene editing, 154–155
Germany, 129–130
Gianaroli, Luca, 104–109, 185
Gibbons, William, 70
GIERAF (Groupe Inter Africain d'Etude,
    de Recherche et d'Application sur la
    Fertilité), 162
Gleicher, Norbert, 17, 242
glucose, 13
glycerol, 18, 193, 198
Godfrey, Malcolm, 43
Golombok, Susan, 232–239
gonadotrophin releasing hormone
    (GnRH), 32
    agonists, 16, 204
    antagonists, 205, 206
gonadotrophins, 202, See also follicle-
    stimulating hormone (FSH);
    luteinizing hormone (LH)
    hCG. See human chorionic gonadotropin
        (hCG)
    hMG, 75, 76, 132, 134
    HPG, 50, 51
    introduction of, 132–134
    stimulation, 67, 70
    superovulation from, 13
    urinary, 205
Gook, Debra, 192–200
Gorbachev, M., 173
Gosden, Roger, 198
Goswamy, Rajat, 31
Gothenburg, 111–113
    Bourn Hall meeting, 114–115
    time-lapse photography, 113
    ultrasound, 115
Gould, Donald, 42
government
    restrictive legislation for IVF, 229–230
    view on infertility, 228

government funding, lack of, 8, 16
government opposition
    Edwards and Steptoe, 42
    Indian, 148
    Italy, 106
    PGD, 183
Gowans, James, 41, 42
grafting, ovarian tissue, 199
Gray, Sir John, 41
Greece, 125–131
Griffin, Darren, 184, 188
Gruzdev, V.S., 172
Gurdon, Jon, 8

Haan, Nick, 187
hemophilia, 184
Haldane, J.B.S., 11
Hamberger, Lars, 17, 97, 111–119
Hammarberg, Karin, 112
Hammersmith Hospital, 183, 246
Hammond, John, 12
Handyside, Alan, 180, 182, 184, 188, 189
haploblocks, 189
Harris, Muriel, 43
Hartman, Carl, 3
Harvard, Dr. John, 43
hCG. See human chorionic gonadotropin
    (hCG)
health insurance, 138, 174
Heape, Walter, 1–2, 11
heart failure, 219
hemagluttination assay, 204
hematopoietic diseases, 216, 220, 221
hematopoietic stem cells (HSCs), 219
Hennessey, John, 64
Hertwig, Oscar, 10
hESCs. See human embryonic stem cells
    (hESCs)
heterotopic grafting, 200
Hillensjö, Torbjörn, 111–119
hiPSCs. See human induced pluripotent
    stem cells (hiPSCs)
HIV, 163, 165
HLA testing, 189
hMG. See human menopausal gonadotropin
    (hMG)
Hoagland, Dr. Hudson, 23
Hochfellner, Christa, 94
Hodgen, Gary D., 68, 69
Holm, Dr. Hans Henrik, 115, 116
hormonal contraception, 26
hostility. See government opposition;
    media backlash; professional
    hostility; public backlash; religious
    opposition
Howarth, Sheila, 38, 41
Howles, Colin M., 202–206
Hughes, Mark, 188
human chorionic gonadotropin (hCG), 16,
    47, 48, 50
    protocol, 203
human embryo
    cryopreservation, 192–194, 215
    development, 214
human embryo research, 42
    moratorium on, 16

251

human embryonic stem cells (hESCs), 216
   beneficial uses of, 219
   characterization and differentiation, 217
   clinical grade, 217
   clinical trials using, 218
   hurdles in using, 217–218
Human Fertilisation and Embryology Act
   1990, 5, 246
Human Fertilisation and Embryology
   Authority (HFEA), 82, 230, 246
Human Genome Project, 187
human induced pluripotent stem cells
   (hiPSCs), 218, 221
   beneficial uses of, 219
   clinical trials using, 218
human IVF. *See also* in-vitro fertilization
   (IVF)
   1960s and 1970s work on, 14–16
   1980s and 1990s work on, 16–19
   controversiality of, 183
   first successful demonstration, 14
   from animal IVF, 8–19
human menopausal gonadotropin (hMG),
   75, 76, 132, 202
   dosages, 134
   protocol, 203
human oocyte cryopreservation, 194–198
human ovarian tissue cryopreservation,
   198–200
human pituitary gonadotrophin (HPG),
   50, 51
human recombinant leukemia inhibitory
   factor (hLIF), 216
Humana Wellington Hospital, 32
Hunter, Dr. John, 11
Huxley, Aldous, 11
hypo-gonadotrophic hypogonadism, 177
hypoxanthine phosphoribosyl-transferase
   enzyme (HPRT), 180
hysterosalpingogram (HSG), 92, 163

ICSI. *See* intracytoplasmic sperm injection
   (ICSI)
identity issues, 238
idiopathic infertility, 60
immuno-rejection, 217
incubators, earliest, 9
India, 148–151
   current legislation, 150
   National Registry, 149–150
   reproductive medicine bills, 150–151
   reproductive medicine in, 148–149
   subfertility in, 148
   surrogacy, 244
infant of the diabetic mother (IDM), 220
infections, screening for, 163
infertility
   Africa, 158, 168, 245
   China, 152
   consumers as partners, 230
   diagnosis and treatment, 11
   India, 148
   isolating experience, 228
   limited resources argument, 165
   low priority in investing, 39
   low priority in solving, 40

male factor. *See* male factor infertility
   medical condition, 228–229
   microsurgery, 208–213
   neglected problem, 158, 165
   one-stop clinic for diagnosis, 163
   overpopulation argument, 165
   real costs of, 230–231
   Steptoe and Edwards committment to
      help, 34
   stigma, 148, 149, 158
   treatment in Israel, 132
Infertility Medical Procedures Act 1984, 62,
   224, 225
Infertility Treatment Authority (ITA), 226
informed consent, 150
inner cell mass (ICM), 214, 216
Institute of Medicine (IOM), 82
Instituto Valenciano de Infertilidad (IVI),
   120, 122, 123
International Consumer Support for
   Infertility (iCSi), 229
International Fertility Congress,
   Berlin, 113
intracytoplasmic morphologically selected
   sperm injection (IMSI), 137
intracytoplasmic sperm injection (ICSI), 14,
   18, 77, 78, 84–86, 178, 179, 210
   China, 153
   commercialization, 246
   families, 233
   Israel, 135
   overuse of, 242
Investigational New Drug (IND) review
   process, 218
in-vitro fertilization (IVF), 214–215
   alternatives to traditional techniques, 76
   American roots of, 21–26
   birthplace of, 245–247
   commercialization, 63
   early instruments and equipment, 9
   families, 232–234
   First World Congress, 97
   historical outline, 1–6
   professional hostility to, 37–43
   psychological aspects, 232
   sixth World Congress, 136
   unmet need for, 160
in-vitro maturation (IVM), 153
in-vivo fertilization, 214
Ishihara, Dr. Osamu, 241
Israel, 132–138
   first IVF clinic, 134–135
   IVF cycles *per capita*, 138
   legislation, 136
   OHSS, 135
   social egg freezing, 137–138
Italy, 104–109
   commercialization, 245
   current and future issues, 108–109
   late 1980s and 1990s, 105–106
   legislation, 104, 106–108, 195, 229
   pioneers, 104–105
   year 2000 onwards, 106–108
IVF births
   Australia, 52–54, 59, 60
   Baby Joseph, 178

Baby M, 80
Bourn Hall clinic, 32
chronology in different countries, 54
Elizabeth Carr, 67, 75
France, 103
Greece, 126, 129
ICSI treatment, 85
India, 148, 149
Italy, 104
Latin America, 146
Louise Brown. *See* Brown, Louise
numbers, 238
numbers worldwide, 8, 247
Scandinavia, 119
IVF clinics. *See also* Bourn Hall clinic
   Africa, 160, 161
   Bologna, Italy, 105
   business objectives, 240
   China, 153
   corporatization, 243–244
   early ones worldwide, 16
   India, 149
   Israel, 134–135
   numbers worldwide, 19
   organization of, 242
   profit motive, 242–243
   Russia, 173, 174
   types of, 240–241
   UK, 246
   USA, 6, 75
   world's first, 8, 16
   world's first outpatient, 93–97
IVF cycles
   Africa, 160, 162
   Africa, access to, 161
   Bourn Hall clinic, 31
   China, 152
   monitoring, 115
   per capita in Israel, 138
   reimbursement, 160, 247
   Russia, 174

Jacobson, Dr. Cecil, 80
Janisch, Herbert, 88, 89, 90, 92
Jansen, Rob, 63
Janson, Per Olaf, 111
Japan, 241
Jeffcoate, Norman, 38, 39, 40
Johnson, Martin, 14, 37–43
Johnston, Dr. Ian, 46, 52
Jones catheter, 66
Jones Institute, 6, 26, 67–69, 71
Jones, Georgeanna, 6, 16, 26, 66–73
   profile of, 72
Jones, Howard, 4, 6, 16, 26, 54, 66–73
   vision and legacy, 72–73
Jovanovic family, 87
   25th celebrations, 100
   IVF treatment, 92
   pregnancy and birth, 92–93

karyomapping, 189–190
karyotyping, 182
   metaphase CGH, 186–187
Keefe, David, 21–26
Keen, Dr. Jeffrey, 76

keloids, 220
Kemeter, Peter, 87, 89, 93–96, 100
Kennedy, Senator Edward, 81
Kirkman family, 62
Klinefelter's syndrome, 77
Kola, Ismail, 182
Korsak, Vladislav, 172–176
Kovacs, Gabor, 46–65, 177, 242
Krasovskaya, O.V., 172
Krebs, Professor D., 129
Kruger, Thinus, 70
KSOM media, 78
Kuang, Professor Yanping, 153
Kumar, Dr. Anand, 149

Lancet, letter in, 15, 30
laparoscopy, 4, 16
    Australia, 46
    drawbacks to, 76
    ethics of, 40
    introduction, 15
    opposition to, 39
    Steptoe's work in, 28, 29
laparotomy, 48
Lassalle, B., 192
Latin America, 141–147
    regional collaboration, 144–146
Latin American Registry (RLA), 144, 145,
    161
Laurentian Hormone Research
    Conferences, 23
Law 40, 107–108, 109, 229
Lawson, R.A.S., 47, 48
Ledger, Dr. Bill, 247
Leeton, John, 46, 47, 49, 51, 62, 102
legal actions
    Baby M, 80
    Costa Rica, 143
    Del-Zio v. Vande-Weile, 80
    Edward's for defamation, 43
    Jacobson v. United States, 80
legislation
    Australia, 183, 224–228
    commercialization, 244–245
    effect on infertile couples, 228–231
    Germany, 129
    Greece, 127
    India, 150–151
    information and its disclosure, 226–227
    Israel, 136
    Italy, 104, 106–108, 195, 229
    Spain, 120, 121
    surrogacy, 227
    USA, 16
    USA, federal regulations, 81–82
Leibo, Stanley, 9, 192
lesbian families, 245, 246
Lesch-Nyhan syndrome, 180
leukemia, 189
life expectancy, 166
limited resources argument, 165
Lithuania, 109
London Gynaecology and Fertility Centre,
    246
Lopata, Alex, 31, 46–65, 89
Lunenfeld, Bruno, 132

luteinizing hormone (LH), 16, 76, 114, 177,
    202
    surge, 202–206

M16 medium, 13
Macdonald, Alastair, 30
Macnamee, Dr. Mike, 33
Maddox, John, 38
Magli, Maria Cristina, 104–109, 185
Male Factor Group, Monash, 177
male factor infertility, 15, 17, 18, 77, 177–179
    Africa, 163
    Australia, 60
    ICSI, 85, 210
    microsurgery, 208–213
male infertility program, 67, 70–71
malignant disease, 78, 192, 194, 195
Malta, 109
Malter, Henry, 18
mammalian reproductive cycles, 2
Marle, Gerard van, 9
Mashiach, Shlomo, 134
Mason, Dr. Bridget, 33
Massouras, Dr. Harris, 126, 127
Mathews, Dr. Thomas, 33
Matthews, Colin, 64
Mazur, Peter, 9, 192
McBain, John, 50, 52
McLaren, Anne, 13, 41, 180
media, 231
    Austrian, 93
    birth of Louise Brown, 30, 31, 41
    Edward's research, 43
    India, 148
    professional antagonism towards, 39
media backlash
    birth of Louise Brown, 5
    Chile, 143
    Italy, 107
    IVF treatment, 1, 19
    Nature 1969 article, 38
    Pincus experiments, 2
media, culture. See culture media
medical insurance, 247
Medical Research Council (MRC)
    change of policy, 41
    changing stance, 41
    experimental subjects/procedures, 40
    human embryo research, 42
    lack of support, 16, 38
    taking a stand, 41–42
medical tourism, 106, 122, 149, 151, 244
Medical, Ethical and Social Aspects of
    Assisted Reproduction (WHO), 159
Medicare, 247
medication, 16, 76
meiotic spindle, 194, 195
Meirov, D., 137
Mendel's laws, 10
Menezo, Yves, 193
Menkin, Miriam, 3, 12, 24
menotrophin, 202
mesenchymal stem cells (MSCs), 219
metaphase CGH, 186–187
methotrexate, 98
micro-drop method, 14

microepididydimal sperm aspiration
    (MESA), 77
microepididymal sperm aspiration
    (MESA), 210
microinjection, sperm, 178
micromanipulation, 9, 14, 16, 17, 18, 84, 180
micropipettes, 180
microsurgery, 208–213
microtools, 197
Mills, Ivor, 43
MINC incubator, 10
mineral oil, 14
miscarriage, spontaneous, 155, 185
mitochondrial DNA, 155, 239
mitochondrial replacement, 155–156
mitochondrial transfer, 82
Mohr, Linda, 62
Monash clinic, 46, 63, 64, 177, 243
Monk, Marilyn, 180
monogenic disease, 154, 180–190
Morris, R.T., 1
Mortimer David, 10
motile sperm organelle morphology
    examination (MSOME), 137
mouse embryos
    cryopreservation, 192
    culturing, 4, 13, 180, 182, 183
Muasher, Dr. Suheil, 67, 70
Muggleton-Harris, Audrey, 180
Mukerji, Dr. Subhas, 148, 149
multiple annealing and looping-based
    amplification cycles (MALBAC), 155
multiple embryo transfers, 134, 177, 192
multiple pregnancies, 73, 130, 134, 177, 192
multiple sclerosis, 80
multi-probe FISH, 185
Munné, Santiago, 106, 185
muscular dystrophy, 184

Naftolin, Frederick, 21–26
National Cooperative Program on Non-
    Human In Vitro Fertilization and
    Preimplantation Development, 12
national infertility awareness campaign
    (NIAC), 246
National Institute for Health and Care
    Evidence (NICE) guidelines, 246
National Institute of Health (NIH)
    backlash on IVF, 5
National Research Act 1974, 81
Nature, 1969 paper, 38
Netherlands, 9, 130–131
neural progenitor cells, 217
New England Journal of Medicine,
    editorial, 2, 11
New Zealand, 229, 235
next generation sequencing (NGS), 187,
    190, 246
NHS provision of IVF, 245, 246
Nikitin, A., 172–176
Nilsson, Lars, 111, 115
Nilsson, Lennart, 113, 114
Nobel prizes, 8, 10, 33, 120, 132
Norfolk Clinic. See Jones Institute
Norfolk system, 14
Nuffield Council on Bioethics, 235

Oehninger, Sergio C., 66–73
Oktay, Kutluk, 200
Oldham General Hospital, 43, 245
oligospermia, 77
oligo-terato-astenospermia (OTA), 135
Ombelet Willem, 158–170
oncofertility, 77
Oncofertility Consortium, 77
one-stop clinics, infertility diagnosis, 163
oocyte donation. *See also* donor oocytes
    pregnancy, 61–62
oocyte recovery with tubal insemination
    (ORTI), 29
oocytes
    cryopreservation, 78, 153, 154
    cytoplasm, 79
    fertilization *in vitro*, 4, 22, 41
    human oocyte cryopreservation, 194–198
    maturation, 5
    pick-up, 115, 116, 135
    recovery and fertilization rates, 47, 51
    recovery and yield, 50
    recovery, laparoscopic, 4
    recovery, mistimed, 203
    retrieval, 76
orchidometer, 178
orthotopic grafting, 199
ovarian follicles
    atresia, 204
    monitoring, 50
    recruitment, 16, 211
ovarian hyperstimulation syndrome
    (OHSS), 122, 133, 134, 206
    controlled, 67, 75
    Israel, 135
ovarian stimulation, 50, 51, 69, 98,
    202–206
    China, 153
    controlled, 75–76, 133, 206
    improving, 50
    protocols in Africa, 164
ovarian tissue
    cryopreservation, 198–200
    transplantation, 137
ovary transplant, 211
overpopulation argument, 165
overseas surrogacy, 227
over-treatment, 242
ovulation induction (OI), 133
ovulation, timing of, 16

package pricing, 243, 247
Papiernick, Professor Emile, 102
paraffin oil, 14
parthenogenesis, 22
partial zona dissection, 84, 136
payment. *See* compensation;
    reimbursement
Pellicer, Antonio, 120–123
pelvic infections, 158, 163
Pennings, Guido, 235
Pepperell, Professor Roger, 54
Pergonal clinic, 133
Perrutz, Max, 40
Petri dish, 14, 97
Petrov, G.N., 172

PGD. *See* preimplantation genetic diagnosis
    (PGD)
PGS. *See* preimplantation genetic screening
    (PGS)
Pincus, Gregory, 2, 3, 12, 19, 22–24
Poland, 109
polar body biopsy, 185
Polge, Chris, 11
polycystic ovary syndrome, 148, 153, 154
polymerase chain reaction (PCR), 19, 182,
    188, 189
polyspermy, block to, 17
poor ovarian response (POR), 153
poor responders, 75, 137
Pope Benedict XVI, 143
population-control, worldwide priority, 39
Porcu, Eleonora, 107
Powell, Enoch, 42
Pratt, Hester, 42
prednisolone, 98
pregnancies
    donor egg, 61–62
    multiple, 73, 130, 134, 177, 192
pregnanediol, 48
preimplantation genetic diagnosis (PGD),
    19, 85, 107–108, 180–190
    China, 154–155
    early techniques, 182–183
    public controversy, 183
    single gene, 188–189
preimplantation genetic screening (PGS),
    79, 106, 185
    overuse of, 242
pre-pronuclear transfer (PPNT), 155
professional hostility
    PGD work, 183
    to Steptoe and Edwards, 37–43
profit motive, 242–243
Progress campaign group, 42
PROH-sucrose method, 192, 194, 196
psychological effects
    donor disclosure, 235, 237
    ICSI, 234
    IVF, 232
public backlash, 81
    birth of Louise Brown, 5–6
    Italy, 107, 109
    IVF treatment, 1, 15
    PGD treatment, 183
    Pincus experiments, 2
Purdy, Jean, 8, 28–35, 37
pyruvate, 4, 13

Qin, Yingying, 152–156
quality control, 17
Queen Victoria Medical Centre (QVMC),
    46, 47, 51

Rabau, Ervin, 132
rabbit studies, 22, 180
    first, 1, 2
Racowsky, Catherine, 1–6
Ragni, Guido, 104
Rawlings, Dr. Richard, 144
Rechitsky, Svetlana, 189
reciprocal translocations, 188

recombinant DNA, 76, 205
recombinant human insulin, 205
recombinant-hFSH, 205
red-green fluorescence ratio, 186, 187
Reed, Candice, 31, 53, 58, 224
Reed, Linda and John, 53
referees' reports, 38–41
regulations. *See* legislation
reimbursement, 230
    donors, 108, 245
    IVF cycles, 160, 247
    policies, 244
religious opposition, 30, 61, 73, 80
    Australia, 224
    Italy, 104, 107, 109
    Latin America, 141, 143–144
religious support, Israel, 135
reproduction, 21
    control of, 21
    lectures on, 37
reproductive cycles
    first work on, 1
    mammalian, 2
reproductive endocrinology and infertility
    (REI), 66
retinal macular degeneration, 218
Right to Life organization, 183
Rijkmans-Verhamme, Camilla, 15
Rios, Mario and Elsa, 62
Robertson, Robert, 6
Robertsonian translocations, 188
Rock, Professor John, 2–3, 3, 4, 11, 12, 22,
    24–25
Rolla, Dr. Edgardo, 241
Rosenwaks, Dr. Zev, 67, 79
Royal Women's Hospital (RWH), 46, 52
Rudak, Dr. Edwina, 134
Russia, 172–176
    commercialization of IVF, 172–176
Russian Association of Human
    Reproduction (RAHR), 174
Rutherford, Tony, 245–247

salt solutions, 4, 12
same-sex parents, 227, 238
Sarris, Dr. Spyros, 126
Saunders, Doug, 63
saviour sibling PGD, 189
Scandinavia, 111–119. *See also* Gothenburg
    collaboration within, 116–119
Schenk, M., 10
Schoolcraft, William, 79
Schrurs, Bridget, 184
second polar body transfer (PB2T), 155
Second Vienna University Women's
    Hospital (2nd VUWH), 87,
    93–96, 97
sepsis, pregnancy-related, 158
Sermon, Karen, 187, 189
sex chromosomes, 10, 184, 188
sex selection, 79, 150, 184, 188
sexually transmitted diseases (STDs), 148,
    158, 163, 165
Sgargi, Serena, 104–109
Shah, Dr. Duru, 244
Shanghai protocol, 153

Sherman, Jerome, 11
Shettles, Landrum, 4, 25, 80
Short, Roger, 38, 40, 41
sickle cell anemia, 79
Silber, Sherman, 77, 208–213
Simons, Roger, 18
simplex optimization, 12
Singapore, 243
single cell fluorescent in situ hybridization (FISH), 183–186
single embryo transfer, 34, 79, 86
single gene PGD, 188–189
single nucleotide polymorphisms (SNPs), 187
single-mother families, 237, 238
Sjögren, Anita, 112
slow freezing
    cleavage stage embryos, 192–193
    human oocytes, 196
Smith, John Lawrence, 9
smoking, 137
social freezing, 78, 137–138, 198
Society for Assisted Reproductive Technologies (SART), 72, 78, 81
somatic cell nuclear transfer (SCNT), 218
Soupart, Pierre, 113
Southwick, Graeme, 178
Spain, 120–123
Special Task Force on infertility in developing countries, 159, 166
Speirs, Andrew, 53
sperm
    cryopreservation, 153
    donation. See donor insemination
    ICSI. See intracytoplasmic sperm injection (ICSI)
    microinjection, 178
    preparation, 13, 50
    production rate, 177
    subzonal injection, 62, 84–85, 178
    transfer, 11
sperm banks
    China, 153, 155
    world's first, 11
spermatogenic stem cells (SSCs), 211
spinal cord injury, 219
spontaneous abortion, 185, 186
spontaneous miscarriage, 155, 185
St Mary's Hospital, Manchester, 245
stakeholders, 240
Standing Review and Advisory Committee on Infertility (SRACI), 183, 224, 225
Stargardt's disease, 218
stem cells
    birth-associated tissues, 219–220
    embryonic. See embryonic stem cells
    spermatogenic, 211
    transplants, 216, 221
    umbilical cord Wharton's jelly, 219, 220–222
Stephen, Sir Ninian, 228
Stephens, Douglas, 208
Steptoe, Patrick, 4, 5, 8, 18, 28–35
    awards and honors, 32
    early years, 28
    Edwards collaboration, 14

hostility to work, BMA and, 43
hostility to work, early inklings, 37–38
hostility to work, MRC and, 41–42
hostility to work, Nature 1969 paper, 38
hostility to work, Parliament and, 42
hostility to work, referees' reports, 38–41
lack of cooperation with Australia, 51
ovarian stimulation protocol, 202
role in British Fertility Society, 32
supporters of work, 43
Stern, Elizabeth and William, 80
stigma
    infertility, 148, 149, 158
    same-sex parents, 238
Stock-Myer, Sharyn, 189
Stokes, Julian, 59
Stone, Dr. Sergio, 81
Strohmer, Dr. Heinz, 247
stromal cells, 219
subzonal sperm injection (SUZI), 62, 84–85, 178
success rates, annual improvements in, 8
sucrose, 192, 193, 194
    concentration, 196, 197
Sundström, Per, 114
superovulation, 13
surrogacy, 62–63, 77, 80, 227
    China, 156
    ethics, 244
    families, 237–238
    India, 150
    Israel, 135
    overseas, 227
Sutton, Walter, 10
Suzuki, Nao, 199
Svetlov, Professor P.G., 172
Sweeney, Dr. William, 80
swim-up technique, 50, 177
Szalay, Stefan, 88, 89, 90, 97

Tarkowski, Andrzej, 180
Tarlatzis, Basil C., 125–131
Tasca, Dr. Richard, 78
Taylor, Dr. Patrick, 33
Taylor, Ian, 208
Taymor, Melvin, 5
Temple-Smith, Peter, 178
teratomas, 218
Testart, Jacques, 102, 103
testicular biopsy, 179
testicular size, 178
testicular sperm extraction (TESE), 77, 210
testicular transplants, 208
thalassemia, 189
Thibault, Charles, 12, 13, 102
threshold theory, 133
Time to Tell campaign, 227
time-lapse microscopy, 17
time-lapse photography, 113
Toner, James, 70
total reproductive potential, 70
translocation testing, 188
transplants
    bone marrow stem cell, 216, 221
    ovarian tissue, 137

ovary, 211
testis, 208
transport IVF program, 131
transvaginal ultrasound-guided oocyte retrieval (TVOR), 117, 135
Treff, Nathan, 187
trehalose, 196
Trounson, Alan, 15, 51, 52, 56, 90, 178, 180
    frozen embryo pregnancies, 62
    open attitude, 183
    subzonal sperm injection, 62
tubal environment, 50–51, 215
tubal microsurgery, 211
tumorigenesis, risk of, 217, 218
Turner Syndrome, 149, 188
TWE lab method, 164
Tygerberg criteria, 70

UK Longitudinal Study of Assisted Reproduction Families, 234, 235, 237
ultrasound, 16, 52, 98
    Gothenburg team, 115
    oocyte pick-up, 116
    TVOR, 117, 135
    vaginal, 116
    vaginal retrieval, 76
umbilical cord Wharton's jelly, 219, 220–222
United States
    commercialization, 243
    federal regulations, 81–82
    first IVF clinic, 6
    IVF post-Joneses, 75–82
    IVF, roots of, 21–26
    Jacobson v. United States lawsuit, 80
    Joneses and Jones Institute, 66–73
    legislation bans, 16
Universal Declaration of Human Rights, 228, 247
urinary gonadotrophins, 205
uterine abnormalities, 164
Utian, W.H., 77

Van Blerkom, Jonathan, 164
van der Ven, Professor K., 129
Van Steirteghem, André, 84–86, 178
Vande Wiele, Dr. Raymond, 80
varicocoelectomy, 211
vasectomy reversal, 208, 209
Vatican, 30, 72, 80, 143
Veeck, Lucinda, 66
Verlinsky, Yuri, 173, 174, 185, 189
Victorian Assisted Reproductive Treatment Authority (VARTA), 226, 227
Victorian IVF Committee, 61, 224, 228
    information and its disclosure, 226–227
    regulatory experience, 225–226
Victorian Law Reform Commission (VLRC), 226
Virtus Health, 63, 243
vitrification, 19, 78, 154, 206. See also cryopreservation
    embryos, 193
    unfertilized oocytes, 196–198
von Baer, Karl Ernst, 172
Voullaire, Lucille, 186

255

Walking Egg Project, 164, 166–168
Waller, Louis, 224–228
Wang, Jianfeng, 152–156
Warnock Committee report, 5, 42
Warnock, Dame Mary, 5
Watson, James, 30, 40
Waxman, Henry, 81
Wei, Daimin, 152–156
Weinberger, Casper, 81
Wells, Dagan, 186
whalebone bougie, 1
Wharton's jelly stem cells, 219, 220–222
Whitehead, Mrs, 80
Whitten, Wesley, 13
Whittingham, David, 3, 4, 9, 192
Wide, Leif, 111
Wikland, Matts, 17, 111, 111–119

Williamson, Professor Bob, 186
Wilton, Leeanda, 62, 180–190
Winston, Lord Robert, 39, 125, 183, 194, 242, 246, 247
Wiquist, Nils, 111, 113
Wiscott-Aldrich syndrome, 189
Wood, Gillian, 56
Wood, Professor Carl, 31, 46, 47, 51, 52, 54, 56
    frozen embryo pregnancies, 62
Woodruff, Dr. Theresa, 77
Worcester Foundation for Experimental Biology, 23
World Congresses
    first, 97
    sixth, 136
wound healing, 220

Yale University program, 125
Yamanaka, Shinya, 8
Yanagimachi, Ryuzo, 25
Yovich, Dr. John, 33, 64, 126, 127

Zaccheddu, Eleanora, 104
Zegers-Hochschild, Fernando, 141–147, 240
Zeilmaker, Gerard, 9, 14, 15, 130
Zhang, Professor Lizhu, 152, 154, 155, 156
Zika virus, 220
zona drilling, 17, 84
zona hardening, 194, 195
Zondek, Bernard, 132

Printed in the United States
By Bookmasters